Pharmacology for Dental Students

Second Edition

F.S.K. Barar

M. Sc. (Med), M.D. (Pharmacology)
Former Senior Professor and Head
Department of Pharmacology
SMS Medical College
Jaipur
Former Associate Director (Pharmacy)
Lachoo Memorial College of Science and Technology
Jodhpur

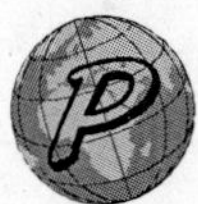

PEEPEE

PUBLISHERS AND DISTRIBUTORS (P) LTD.

Pharmacology for Dental Students

Published by
Pawaninder P. Vij and Anupam Vij
Peepee Publishers and Distributors (P) Ltd.
Head Office: 160, Shakti Vihar, Pitam Pura
Delhi-110 034 (India)

Correspondence Address:
7/31, First Floor, Ansari Road, Daryaganj
New Delhi-110 002 (India)

Ph: 65195868, 23246245, 9811156083

e-mail: peepee160@yahoo.co.in

e-mail: peepee160@rediffmail.com

e-mail: peepee160@gmail.com

www.peepeepub.com

First Edition: 2009
Second Edition: 2014

ISBN: 978-81-8445-157-3

Dedicated to
My Wife, My Children
and
My Students

Preface to the Second Edition

It is not the marble halls which make for intellectual grandeur – it is the spirit and brain of the worker.

— *Sir Alexander Fleming*

The text-material has been reviewed. In dental practice commonly employed procedures are *prosthetic, periodontal, endodontic, restorative,* and *surgical* in nature. During or postoperatively certain medical emergencies can occur, and have to be managed urgently. *Appendix-III* provides working guidelines for managing such situations. Moreover, drugs which the dentist uses in everyday practice include the local anaesthetics, analgesics, antibiotics, antifungals, antivirals, and anxiolytics. *Appendix-IV* provides essential information and dosage schedules for such commonly used drugs. In addition, the dentist must take into account the drug history of the patient before prescribing any drug to avoid untoward drug interactions.

Last but not the least, I am thankful to Mr. Pawaninder P. Vij, Director, Peepee Publishers & Distributors (P) Ltd., New Delhi and his team for their efficient cooperation towards the printing and publication of this work.

F.S.K. Barar
Jodhpur
February, 2014

Preface to the First Edition

"You cannot hope to build a better world without improving the individuals. To that end each of us must work for his own improvement, and at the same time share a general responsibility for all humanity, our particular duty being to aid those to whom we think we can be most useful".

— *Marie Curie (1867-1934)*

Dentistry is that branch of medicine and surgery which deals with the diagnosis, prevention, and treatment of diseases of the mouth, the teeth, the maxilla, and the face. In addition to general dentistry, there are many dental specialities, including Dental Public Health; Endodontics; Oral and Maxillofacial Pathology, Radiology and Surgery; Orthodontics; Dentofacial Orthopaedics; Dental Anaesthesiology; Periodontics; Paediatric Dentistry; Geriatric Dentistry; and Prosthodontics. For the safe and effective practice of dentistry basic knowledge about the actions, uses, adverse reactions, and interactions of drugs used in man is essential. Here comes in the role of pharmacology for which a fairly comprehensive syllabus has been chalked out for the graduate and postgraduate courses in the subject, which is covered in this book.

The text has 15 Chapters, 2 Appendices, and an Index for rapid consultation and revision. Basics about general pharmacology and systemic pharmacology have been covered in the book. Special topics in Dental Pharmacology are covered in Sub-Chapter 1.10, and include Dentifrices; Tooth Bleaching Agents; Demulcents and Astringents; Dental Protectives and Dressings; Obtundents; Mummifying Agents; Root Canal Fillings; Dental Caries; and Emergencies in Dental Practice. Subject matter has been collected from standard drug compendia and the following websites: www.nim.nih..qov/medicine/print/dru qinfo; www.netdoctor.co.uk/medicines; www.rxlist/cgi/qeneric; www.healthresource.com/library; and www.medclik.com.

Last, but not the least, I have to record my profound thanks to Mr. Pawaninder P. Vij, Director, Peepee Publishers and Distributors (P) Ltd., New Delhi-110002 and his team for their prompt and efficient cooperation towards the printing and publication of this work.

F.S.K. Barar
Jodhpur
May, 2009

Contents

Abbreviations

ACh	Acetylcholine	IM	Intramuscular
AChE	Acetylcholinesterase	IV	Intravenous
ACTH	Adrenocorticotrophic hormone, Corticotrophin	l	Litre
ADH	Antidiuretic hormone	LH	Luteinizing hormone
ADP	Adenosine diphosphate	log	Logarithm
AIDS	Acquired Immunodeficiency Syndrome	LSD	Lysergic acid diethylamide
ANS	Autonomic nervous system	M	Molar
ATP	Adenosine triphosphate	MAO	Monoamine oxidase
BP	Blood pressure	MAOI	Monoamine oxidase inhibitor
c-AMP	Cyclic adenosine 3', 5' monophosphate	mcg	Microgram
ChE	Cholinesterase	mg	Milligram
CNS	Central nervous system	MIC	Minimal inhibitory concentration
CoA	Coenzyme A	min	Minute
COMT	Catechol-O-Methyltransferase	mol	Mole (gram molecular weight)
CSF	Cerebrospinal fluid	mRNA	Messenger ribonucleic acid
CTZ	Chemoreceptor trigger zone	NA	Noradrenaline
CVP	Central venous pressure	NADP	Nicotinamide adenine dinucleotide phosphate
DNA	Deoxyribonucleuic acid	NADPH	Nicotinamide adenine dinucleotide phosphate (reduced)
DOPA	Dihydroxyphenylalanine	ng	Nanogram
ECF	Extracellular fluid	PABA	Para-aminobenzoic acid
ECG	Electrocardiogram	PG	Prostaglandin
ECT	Electroconvulsive therapy	pH	Negative log of hydrogen ion concentration
EEG	Electroencephalogram	P450	Cytochrome with maximum absorption at wavelength 450 nm
FSH	Follicle stimulating hormone	RNA	Ribonucleic acid
g	Gram	SC	Subcutaneous
GABA	Gamma-aminobutyric acid	SRS-A	Slow reacting substance of anaphylaxis
GFR	Glomerular filtration rate	t½	Half-life
GH	Growth hormone	THC	Tetrahydrocannabinol
G-6-PD	Glucose-6-phosphate dehydrogenase	tRNA	Transfer RNA
HCG	Human chorionic gonadotrophin	TSH	Thyroid stimulating hormone, Thyrotrophin
HMG	Human menopausal gonadotrophin	v/v	Volume per unit volume
5-HT	5-Hydroxytryptamine	WHO	World Health Organization
HVA	Homovanillic acid	w/v	Weight per unit volume
Hz	Hertz (1 Hertz is 1 cycle per second)	w/w	Weight per unit weight
Ig	Immunoglobulin		

General Pharmacology

1

1.1 SCOPE OF PHARMACOLOGY

DEFINITIONS

Pharmacology is the science of drugs. It deals with sources of drugs; their absorption, distribution, metabolism and excretion; their mechanism of action; and their toxicity. It has the following subdivisions:

Pharmacognosy is the study of the sources of drugs derived from plants and animals, and of the physical and chemical properties of such substances.

Pharmacy is the study of the preparation, compounding, and dispensing of medicines.

Pharmacokinetics is the study of the fate of drugs in body, right from the time they (drugs) enter the body until they, or their by-products, are eliminated from the body. This includes absorption, distribution, metabolism and excretion of drugs.

Pharmacodynamics is the experimental study of actions of drugs on the living organism, including their mechanism of action.

Pharmacotherapeutics is the treatment of disease by means of drugs.

Therapeutics is the practical branch of medicine dealing with the science and art of the treatment of disease.

Chemotherapy deals with the use of drugs capable of inhibiting or destroying invading bacteria, viruses, parasites or cancer cells; while having minimal effect on healthy living tissues.

Toxicology is the science of poisons–their source, chemical composition, actions, tests for detection, and antidotes. It forms a major part of forensic medicine.

Pharmacogenetics deals with the study of genetically determined variations in drug response.

Clinical pharmacology deals with the pharmacologic effects of drugs in man.

DRUG INFORMATION SOURCES

The Pharmacopoeias

The term **pharmacopoeia** is derived from the Greek words *pharmakon*, meaning "drug" and *poiein* meaning "make". The pharmacopoeias contain monographs on drugs and ancillary substances. A pharmacopoeia is periodically revised. The **National Formulary** is a smaller and much more handy book containing formulations of therapeutic value. Drugs included in the current edition of a pharmacopoeia are designated as *official*.

The **International Pharmacopoeia** is published by the World Health Organization (WHO). This pharmacopoeia is meant for use and adoption all over the world.

India

1. **Pharmacopoeia of India** (The Indian Pharmacopoeia), Two Volumes, Government of India, Ministry of Health & Family Welfare,

New Delhi.
2. **National Formulary of India**, Government of India, Ministry of Health, New Delhi.

Great Britain

1. **British Pharmacopoeia**, Two Volumes, Her Majesty's Stationary Office (HMSO), London.
2. **The (British) Pharmaceutical Codex** (BPC), The Pharmaceutical Press, London.
3. **British National formulary** (BNF), Joint publication of the British Medical Association and the Pharmaceutical Society of Great Britain, London.
4. **The Extra Pharmacopoeia** (Martindale) The Pharmaceutical Press, London.
5. **Dental Practitioner's Formulary**, Joint publication of the British Dental Association, the British Medical Association, and The Pharmaceutical Society of Great Britain.

USA

1. **The United States Pharmacopeia** (USP) and **The National Formulary** (NF), United States Pharmacopeial Convention Inc., Rockville, MD, USA (In one cover).
2. **Physicians Desk Reference** (PDR) published by Medical Economics Inc. Oradell, N.J., USA (published every year).
3. **AMA Drug Evaluations**, prepared by the AMA Division of Drugs with the American Society for Clinical Pharmacology and Therapeutics, WB Saunders Co., Philadelphia, USA.

Some hospitals maintain their own special formularies and handbooks for the drugs and formulations frequently prescribed in their institutions.

1.2 SOURCES AND NOMENCLATURE OF DRUGS

The term 'drug' is derived from the French word 'drogue' meaning a dry herb. It is defined as a substance used for the *diagnosis, prevention treatment* or *palliation* (relief from symptoms) of disease. A *fifth* category of drug usage is for prevention of pregnancy, i.e., contraception. *Sixthly*, drugs may also be used for maintenance of optimal health.

SOURCES OF DRUGS

Drugs are derived from *four* main sources:

i. **Plant drugs:** The roots, leaves and barks of plants were used to treat disease earlier. Later, the active principles were extracted and used in modern medicine. Plant products like *quinine, morphine, ephedrine* and *digoxin* continue to be important drugs.
ii. **Animal drugs:** Animal products used for the treatment of disease are *insulin*, extracted from pork and beef pancreas used for diabetes mellitus; *thyroid powder* for hypothyroidism; and *heparin* as an anticoagulant.
iii. **Mineral drugs:** Minerals as simple elements or their salts provide useful drugs, like *ferrous sulphate* for anaemia, *magnesium trisilicate* for hyperacidity and peptic ulcer.
iv. **Synthetic drugs:** Majority of drugs in use today are prepared synthetically, e.g., *sulphon amides, thiazide diuretics, oral antidiabetics, synthetic corticosteroids, sympathomimetics* and other autonomic agents.

Recombinant DNA technology: This innovative technology is now being used for production of *human insulin* by introducing coded DNA into harmless strains of *Escherichia coli*.

DRUG NOMENCLATURE

Drugs may be divided into *two* main groups: (i) *non-prescription drugs*, which are sold "over the counter" (OTC) as they are judged to be safe for use without medical supervision; and (ii) *prescription drugs*, which are considered to be unsafe for use except under medical supervision, and are dispensed only on a physician's prescription.

Every drug has *three* names: (i) the *chemical* name; (ii) the *approved* name (non-proprietary); and (iii) the *trade* (proprietary, brand, registered) name. The chemical name gives the chemical constitution of the drug. Chemical names are generally too complex to be widely used.

1.3 DOSAGE FORMS AND ROUTES OF DRUG ADMINISTRATION

A *dosage form* of a drug is a product suited for administration to the patient by various routes.

VEHICLES

Vehicles or solvents are used to dissolve or suspend drugs. **Waters** are solutions of volatile oils or other aromatic substances in distilled water, e.g., Peppermint, Cinnamon and Anise waters. **Syrups** are solutions of flavouring or medicinal substances in an almost saturated solution of sugar (sucrose) in water. *Simple syrup is a saturated solution of sugar in water*, which is used to make other syrups. **Elixirs** are sweetened, pleasantly flavoured hydroalcoholic solutions of medicinal substances.

COLOURING AGENTS

Colouring agents are harmless substances used for lending colour to drugs to make them more acceptable to patients. *Amaranth* solution colours red; *Caramel* (burnt sugar) colours brown; *Cochineal* colours bright red.

SWEETENING AGENTS

Solid sweetening agents usually employed are: (i) **Sucrose** or cane sugar for syrups and elixirs; and (ii) **Aspartame** which is 200 times sweeter than sugar. Lately there has been a controversy about its safety as a sugar substitute. *Low-calorie artificial sweeteners*, not metabolized in the body, used in diabetic patients are: (i) **Sucralose** made from sugar, (ii) **D-tagatose** with a similar structure to fructose; and (iii) **Ace-sulfame K** which has been lately approved by the US FDA.

AQUEOUS SOLUTIONS

Aqueous solutions contain one or more drugs dissolved in water. They are of *two* categories: (i) **Solutions for oral use**, e.g., Strong iodine solution and (ii) **Solutions for injection**, which are sterile liquids or suspensions, packaged in suitable containers to maintain sterility, and are intended for parenteral use. The aqueous vehicles mostly used for preparing injections are: *Water for Injection and Sodium Chloride Injection.* Injections are available in sealed glass ampules or vials. **Ampules** are sealed glass containers and contain one dose of the drug, e.g., eostigmine (Prostigmin) Injection, Nalorphine hydrochloride (Nalline) Injection etc. **Vials** are glass containers with hermetically (airtight) sealed rubber stoppers, and contain multiple doses of the drug, e.g., Insulin injection; Isophane Insulin suspension etc.

AQUEOUS SUSPENSIONS

Aqueous suspensions contain one or more chemical substances dispersed in water by means of harmless suspending agents. They are preparations of finely divided, undissolved drugs dispersed in liquids. Suspensions for oral use are as under:

Emulsions are suspensions of fats or oils in water with the aid of an emulsifying agent (gum acacia). *Examples*: Cod Liver Oil Emulsion, Castor Oil Emulsion.

Gels are colloidal aqueous suspensions of hydrated inorganic substances. *Example*: Aluminum Hydroxide Gel.

Mixtures are preparations where the drug or drugs are in solution or suspension meant for oral administration.

ALCOHOLIC SOLUTIONS

Spirits or **Essences** are concentrated alcoholic solutions of volatile substances. *Examples*: Peppermint Spirit, Lemon Spirit, Compound Orange Spirit, Aromatic Ammonia Spirit.

EXTRACTIVE PREPARATIONS

Extractive preparations are made from vegetable drugs and contain the active principles in a hydroalcoholic solvent.

Tinctures are alcoholic or hydroalcoholic preparations of vegetable drugs. *Examples*: Belladonna Tincture, Digitals Tincture and Tincture Iodine.

Fluid extracts are alcoholic or hydroalcoholic extracts of vegetable drugs which are highly concentrated. *Example*: Aromatic Cascara Sagrada Fluid Extract.

Extracts are concentrated, solid or semisolid preparations made by percolation and evaporation of the percolate. *Example*: Belladonna Extract.

Solid Dosage Forms

Powders are medicinal substances in a dried and finely divided form. They may be *simple* (one active ingredient) or *compound* (more than one active ingredient). Powders are used internally or externally. Effervescent powders like Seidlitz powder when dissolved in water liberate carbon dioxide.

Capsules are small containers usually made of gelatin and may be hard or soft. Sizes of capsules range from 5 (small) to 000 (big). They dissolve readily in the stomach. Capsules may be coated with substances that resist the action of gastric juice, and do not disintegrate in the stomach. On reaching the intestines they dissolve in alkaline juices and release the drug. They are called *enteric coated capsules*.

Spansules are delayed action capsules prepared by variably coating the drug particles with material that permits gradual release of the drug in the gut.

Tablets are solid dosage forms, containing granulated or powdered drugs that are compressed or moulded into round or discoid shapes. Some tablets are *scored* (marked with an indented line across the surface) so that they may be easily divided if smaller doses are required.

Compressed tablets contain solid drugs subjected to great mechanical pressure and pressed into tablets. *Examples*: Aspirin tablets, Erythromycin tablets.

Moulded tablets are prepared by mixing the moistened powdered drug with sugar, milk sugar or some other inert diluent. The resulting plastic mass is then moulded into discoid forms and dried. They may be used for oral, sublingual or buccal administration (sublingual or buccal tablets). *Examples*: Ergotamine tartrate tablets. Nitroglycerin tablets.

Hypodermic tablets are compressed or moulded tablets that dissolve completely in water, making a solution suitable for injection. These tablets are dissolved in water for injection just before administration. *Examples*: Atropine Sulphate Hypodermic tablets, Morphine Sulphate Hypodermic tablets.

Pellets are sterile spheres formed by compression of certain steroid hormones. They are suitably implanted subcutaneously, and form a depot from which the hormone is slowly released. *Examples*: Desoxycorticosterone Acetate Pellets, Testosterone Pellets.

Pills are powdered drugs mixed with adhesive substances like honey or glucose. This adhesive mass is moulded into globular, oval or flattened bodies convenient for swallowing.

Troches or **lozenges** are flat, round or rectangular preparations that are kept in the mouth till they dissolve liberating the drug or drugs they contain. They are used to treat local conditions in the mouth and throat.

DOSAGE FORMS FOR EXTERNAL ADMINISTRATION

Liniments are liquid suspensions or dispersions, applied to the skin by rubbing. They contain one or more active ingredient in a liniment base of a fixed oil, soap or alcohol. They relieve pain and swelling by counter-irritation and improvement in circulation. *Example*: Camphor Liniment

Lotions are liquid preparations applied to the skin without rubbing. Their base is usually aqueous. Lotions can be protective, emollient, cooling, cleansing, astringent or antipruritic depending on their content. *Example*: Calamine Lotion.

Ointments are semisolid greasy substances intended for local application to the skin or mucous membranes. The usual ointment has a petroleum base. Ointments serve as soothing agents, astringents and antiseptics. *Examples*: Zinc Oxide Ointment, Sulphur Ointment, Bacitracin Ointment.

Ophthalmic ointments are sterile medicated ointments for use in the eye. *Examples*: Chloramphenicol Ophthalmic Ointment, Oxytetracycline Ophthalmic Ointment.

Pastes are ointment-like preparations of one or more medicaments and some adhesive material. They are applied to oozing surfaces and afford greater protection, and more absorptive action than ointments. *Example*: Zinc Oxide Paste.

Suppositories are mixtures of drugs with a firm base that can be moulded in shapes suitable for insertion into a body cavity or orifice. They melt at body temperature, releasing the drug to come in contact with the mucous membrane to produce a local or systemic effect. *Rectal suppositories* are conical or bullet shaped; *vaginal suppositories* are conical or spherical; and *urethral suppositories* are pencil shaped. Suppositories should be stored in a refrigerator.

Plasters are solid adhesive preparations, applied to the skin to protect, support, soothe and lessen pain. *Examples*: Zinc Oxide Plaster, Mustard Plaster.

Transdermal system is a unique and new drug delivery method applied through the skin. It provides for a prolonged and uniform release of a drug like *scopolamine* or *nitroglycerin*. The adhesive matrix contains a mineral oil and polyisobutylene.

Ophthalmic solutions (collyria) are sterile usually isotonic, buffered solutions for instillation in the eye. *Example*: Silver Nitrate Ophthalmic Solution.

Sprays are solutions of one or more drugs in oil or water, administered by atomizers. Air forced through the atomizer by squeezing the rubber bulb carries with it a coarse liquid spray containing the drug into the nose or throat. *Example*: Tyrothricin Spray.

Inhalants are drugs which because of their high vapour pressure can be carried into the nasal passages with the inhaled air. They are available in portable inhalers. *Example:* Propylhexedrine Inhalant.

Inhalations (Aerosols) are stable suspensions of extremely small liquid or solid particles (0.5 to 5 microns) in a medium such as air or oxygen. They are produced and administered by nebulizers. The nebulized mist reaches the bronchi or even the alveoli.

ROUTES OF DRUG ADMINISTRATION

The major routes are *oral, parenteral* and *topical.*

Oral Route

The oral route of administration is the safest, most economical, and the most convenient way of giving medicines. The dosage forms for oral route include *tablets, capsules, powders, mixtures, emulsions* and *gels*. Drugs in solution are more quickly absorbed than solids. If a rapid effect is desired, the substance should be diluted and given with water before meals. If the drug is likely to cause gastrointestinal irritation, it is given with or immediately after meals.

On oral administration, drug action has a slower onset and more prolonged but less potent effect than when drugs are given parenterally.

Drugs may also be given through tubes placed in the gastrointestinal tract, like the nasogastric or gastrostomy tubes.

Disadvantages of oral administration of certain drugs are: (i) an objectionable odour or taste; (ii) damage or discolouration of teeth; (iii) irritation of the gastric mucosa, causing nausea and vomiting; (iv) aspiration into the lungs in seriously ill or uncooperative patients; and (v) they may be destroyed by digestive enzymes.

Sublingual: Some drugs like *isoprenaline* and *nitroglycerin* may be given sublingually by placing them under the patient's tongue, where they are retained until dissolved and absorbed, or the desired effect is produced. The thin epithelium and the rich capillary network under the tongue permit rapid absorption and drug action, in addition the drug is saved from hepatic inactivation and destruction by digestive enzymes, as it reaches the general circulation without passing through the liver.

Rectal administration can be used advantageously when the stomach is non-retentive due to vomiting; when the drug has an objectionable taste or odour; or when it can be destroyed by digestive enzymes.

Parenteral Routes

The term parenteral route refers to any route other than gastrointestinal (enteral), but is commonly used to indicate *subcutaneous, intramuscular,* and *intravenous* injections. These routes may be selected when a rapid effect is desired.

Aseptic technique must be employed when the drug is given parenterally. A cotton pledget soaked in a germicidal solution (or rectified spirit) is applied at the site of injection in a circular motion, moving from the centre outwards. Poor technique may cause infection.

Drugs for injection: Parenteral drugs must be packaged, prepared and administered in a manner which maintains sterility. Multiple dose vials can be reused if sterility is maintained. Medication of once broken ampules must be discarded, as it no longer remains sterile.

SYRINGES AND NEEDLES

Drugs in solution are administered parenterally by means of a **syringe-needle unit**, or an **intravenous infusion set**. The common syringe is made of glass, and **consists of a plunger** and a **barrel.**

Syringes are available in various sizes – 1, 2, 5, 10, 20 and 50 ml. There are specialized insulin and tuberculin syringes. An insulin syringe may be marked so that there are 40 calibrations per 1 ml, or 80 calibration per 1 ml. The U 40 syringes are usually marked in *red,* while the U 80 syringes are marked in *green.* The *tuberculin* syringe has a capacity of 1 ml and calibrated in 0.01 ml markings. Now *sterile disposable syringes* and *needles* are available.

Needles precisely called *hypodermic needles* are made of high quality stainless steel which is strong flexible and rust resistant. The needle size is designated by two numbers, the gauge and the shaft length. The gauge numbers run from 27 (finest) to 13 (thickest). The shaft is measured from the junction of the hub to the tip of the point. The tip of the needle is bevelled to different grades (regular, short or very short bevel). Choice of the needle gauge and length depends on the route of administration; the viscosity of the solution; and the size of the patient. Usually a 25-gauge, 5/8 inch needle is used for *subcutaneous* injections and a 22 or 20 gauge, 1.5 inch needle is used for *intramuscular* or *intravenous* injections. For 'drawing up' of a dose from an ampule, the ampule is clean broken at the constricted portion by applying lateral pressure following gentle filing by a *serrated* metal file. For 'drawing up' of a dose from a rubber stoppered vial, a hypodermic needle is inserted into the vial, and some air is injected first to facilitate withdrawal of the liquid medication. Then the vial is inverted to withdraw the desired amount of the material.

Jet injection syringe (hypospray) is a devise for administration of a drug parenterally without a needle. It resembles a flash light. It forces a fine jet of the medicament of almost microscopic size, under high pressure through the skin into the tissues. The procedure is almost painless, and the efficacy equals that of *subcutaneous* injection. It is mostly employed in mass immunization programmes.

The various types of injections for parenteral administration of drugs are: *intradermal, subcutaneous* (SC), *intramuscular* (IM), *intravenous* (IV) *intramedullary, Intra-arterial, Intrathecal, epidural, intracardiac, intra-articular* and *intraperitoneal.*

Intradermal (intracutaneous) injection: The drug is injected into the outer layers of the skin. The amount of drug given is small and absorption is slow. The medial surface of the forearm is the site frequently used. This injection is best made with a fine (26 gauge), short needle and a tuberculin syringe. Local anaesthetics are first injected intradermally, and then further deeper injections are made through the superficially anaesthetized tissues. Also used for *sensitization testing* in patients.

Subcutaneous (hypodermic) injection (SC): The injection is made into the loose subcutaneous tissue under the skin. Common sites for SC injections are the outer surface of the upper arm, abdomen, and front of the thigh. This route is used to inject a small amount of the drug (2 ml or lesser). The piston of the syringe should be withdrawn slightly before injecting the drug to make sure that a blood vessel has not been entered. The angle of insertion should be 45 to 60 degrees. Drugs like *adrenaline, morphine* and *insulin* are usually administered subcutaneously.

Hypodermoclysis is a form of SC injection that permits the slow administration of large amounts (500 to 1000 ml in adults) of fluid such as isotonic saline or glucose solution. A large bore needle is inserted into the loose subcutaneous tissue over the anterior aspect of the thigh, or elsewhere, and the fluid is slowly infused. Occasionally the spread of such locally injected fluid is facilitated by adding the enzyme *hyaluronidase* to the solution, which temporarily decreases the viscosity of the ground substance in connective tissues. Hypodermoclysis is particularly useful in infants and young children to treat dehydration.

Intramuscular injection (IM): The injection is given with a longer and heavier needle that penetrates the subcutaneous tissues, and the drug is deposited deep between the layers of the muscle mass. This route is suitable for administration of solutions or suspensions. Absorption from the site is more rapid than from subcutaneous injection sites. Small volumes (upto 3 ml) are injected in the *deltoid muscle.* Small or large volumes (upto 10 ml) are injected into the *gluteal mass* underlying the upper and outer quadrant of the left or right buttock. The *vastus muscle* underlying the lateral surface of the thigh is an alternate area. Needles from 1 to 3 inches in length (gauge 19 to 22) are used for IM injections. A precaution is that after the needle is inserted (at almost a 90 degree angle) the plunger should be slightly withdrawn to make sure that the needle is not in a blood vessel. Care is required to avoid injury to nerves. The needle is held perpendicular to the skin, and the inserting movement should be quick and smooth to prevent undue discomfort to the patient.

The IM route is used for administering long-acting *esters of sex hormones, corticosteroids,* or poorly soluble salts like *benzathine penicillin G* or *procaine penicillin G.*

Intravenous injection (IV): When an immediate drug effect is desired, or when for any reason the drug cannot be injected into other tissues, or when absorption may be inhibited by poor circulation, it may be introduced directly into a vein as an *injection* or *infusion.* The *cubital vein* at the bend of the elbow is selected, although any other suitable vein, or even the *superior longitudinal sinus* in children may be selected. This technique requires skill and asepsis. The IV injection is of great value in emergencies.

A vein that is distended with blood is much easier to enter than a collapsed vein. If an arm vein has been chosen, a tourniquet is applied tightly around the middle of the upper arm to distend the vein, the air is expelled from the syringe, and the needle (20 or 22 gauge) is introduced quickly and forcefully pointing upwards towards the heart. A few drops of blood aspirated into the syringe indicate that the needle is in the vein; the tourniquet is then removed; and the solution is injected slowly and steadily.

An **infusion** is the intravenous administration of larger amounts of fluid, varying from 1 to 2 litres. The solution flows by gravity from a graduated glass bottle or plastic bag through a drip set (a system of sterile tubes consisting of a drip chamber and tubing inserted above into a bottle/bag of infusion fluid and below through a connecting tip into the needle or catheter placed in the vein). Such a set up provides for a continuous slow administration of fluid into the body at a uniform rate. Ordinarily 3 to 4 hours are required for every 1000 ml of fluid. For children the rate is slower.

Insoluble drugs, oily substances or drugs in suspension, or markedly acid or alkaline salts incompatible with blood should never be administered by the IV route.

Intramedullary injection: This route is also designated as *bone marrow injection* and the material is injected into the bone marrow of the *sternum* or *tibia*. Rapidity of drug effect is comparable with IV injection. This route is used when the veins are not available, specially in children, and a special needle is used. Whole blood, normal saline or glucose may be administered by this route.

Some injection routes are used to achieve high local concentrations of certain drugs. The following are some examples:

Intra-arterial injection: In this highly specialized procedure the needle is placed in an artery, through which an arterial blood sample may be withdrawn for *blood gas studies* or a radio opaque substance may be injected to make arteries of the part visible on an X-ray film (arteriography). Certain cytotoxic drugs may be perfused through the artery for treating specific areas, specially in cases of malignancy involving the limbs (regional perfusion).

Intrathecal (intraspinal) injection: By this method a drug is injected into the subarachnoid space. These injections are made by inserting the needle through the vertebral interspinous spaces into the spinal fluid, usually by lumbar puncture.

Epidural injection: By this method the drug is deposited through a vertebral interspace between the dura of the spinal cord and the periosteal lining of the spinal canal (also known as peridural or extradural injection). It is used to produce epidural nerve block by depositing the local anaesthetic solution in the space where the spinal nerves emerge from the dural membrane and enter the intervertebral foramina.

Intracardiac injection: In some emergencies like sudden cardiac arrest of an otherwise normal heart (as happens during anaesthesia, electrocution or drowning) injections of adrenaline directly into the heart may restart the heart beat. The injection is given by a long needle in the left fourth intercostal space close to the sternum.

Intra-articular injection: The drug (usually a glucocorticoid) is injected into the joint without much danger of systemic steroid toxicity. Strict asepsis must be maintained.

Intraperitoneal injection: A needle or trocar is inserted into the peritoneal space and a special fluid is cyclically circulated through the space for removal of toxins or drugs in cases of acute poisoning, and in renal failure.

INHALATION

Two classes of substances may be administered by inhalation–**volatile** and **non-volatile.** Volatile substances like *gaseous anaesthetics; vapours of liquid anaesthetics; gases* like oxygen and carbon dioxide; and drugs like *amyl nitrite* produce rapid effects when inhaled. Non-volatile substances have to be broken down into small particles and inhaled as aerosols. **Aerosols** are liquid or solid particles, so small that they remain suspended in air for a long time instead of setting down rapidly due to gravity. The particle size influences the rate of absorption through the alveoli, i.e., smaller the particle size, greater amounts reach the alveoli and are absorbed. Common aerosol producing devices are: *vaporizers, humidifiers, atomizers, nebulizers, inhalers* and *spinhalers*. Bronchodilators like adrenaline, isoprenaline and salbutamol may be administered by inhalation for prompt action.

DERMAL APPLICATION

The dosage forms applied topically (locally) to the skin are *powders, lotions, liniments, ointments, creams, pastes* and *jellies*. These preparations are used mostly for their local antiseptic, antipruritic, analgesic, emollient and healing effects.

Absorption of drugs through the skin is proportional to their lipid solubility, as the **epidermis** acts like a lipid membrane barrier. The **dermis** is freely permeable to many fluids. Absorption through the skin may be enhanced by: (i) suspending the drug in an oily vehicle (ointment), and rubbing it into the skin, known as **inunction**; and (ii) **iontophoresis** (Greek *phorein* = to carry) in which the absorption rate of lipid insoluble ions is enhanced by the passage of a galvanic current through a solution of the drug applied to the skin in contact with an electrode. The other electrode is placed elsewhere on the body.

MUCOSAL APPLICATION

Local application is often used in the nose, throat, rectum, or vagina to produce systemic effects, because of the good absorption through the highly vascularized mucosa of these areas. Dosage forms include **lozenges, sublingual tablets, buccal tablets, suppositories, otic solutions, aerosols, nasal solutions,** and **ophthalmic solutions. Demulcents,** i.e., substances which protect and soothe the mucous membranes from irritation are also applied locally.

Thus, there are **enteral** and **parenteral** routes of drug administration. The enteral method includes **sublingual, oral and rectal routes**. The parenteral method includes **injections**, **inhalation**, and **application to the skin** and **mucous membrane.**

1.4 FACTORS INFLUENCING DOSAGE AND DRUG ACTION

A **dose** (Greek, *dosis*) is the amount of the medicament to be administered to the patient, as directed by the physician. It is expressed in terms of **weight** (g, mg, mcg), **volume** (ml) or **in standard units.** The official doses mentioned in the pharmacopoeias are oral doses for adults, unless mentioned otherwise. The change in the activity of the cell or tissue produced by the drug is called the **response.** Both, the dose and the response are closely related, termed as the **dose-response relationship.**

Many patient factors affect drug action qualitatively and quantitatively.

AGE AND BODY WEIGHT

Many formulae are available to calculate the dose.

1. **Young's rule:** This is used for children from 2 to 12 years of age.

$$\text{Child's dose} = \frac{\text{Age in years} \times \text{Adult dose}}{\text{Age} + 12}$$

Example: To calculate the dose of paracetamol (official adult dose 500 mg orally) for a 3 years old child substitute:

$$\text{Child's dose} = \frac{3 \times 500}{3 + 12} = 100 \text{ mg}$$

2. **Body surface area rule:** A more accurate method for calculating the dose for children or adults is to determine the **body surface area** (BSA). **Nomograms** are available for determining the BSA of infants, children and adults from the patient's weight and height. On obtaining the BSA use the following formula:

$$\text{Child's dose} = \frac{\text{BSA in } M^2 \text{ of child} \times \text{Adult dose}}{1.7}$$

M^2 = Square metres of BSA

1.7 = Average BSA in an adult

(Same formula is applied for adult dosages)

Example: To calculate the dose for a child weighing 50 pounds (height 47 inches), and the adult dose of the drug is 60 mg, determine the BSA from the nomogram (BSA from nomograms is 0.86 M^2). Then substitute:

$$\text{Child's dose} = \frac{0.86 \times 60}{1.7} = \frac{51.6}{1.7} = 30 \text{ mg}$$

The above formulae provide a *first approximation* only, which has to be further adjusted for the individual patient.

SEX FACTORS

Women require smaller doses of drugs, probably due to their lesser body weight. Drugs must be used with special care during pregnancy as they may have a **teratogenic** (embryopathic) effect on the foetus.

TIME AND PLACE FACTORS

Presence of food in the stomach and intestines delays absorption of drugs, whereas when the stomach is empty, the absorption of the drug is faster. Administration of a drug with food may be taken advantage of to reduce its irritant action on the gut.

The time of the day affects drug action. Daylight is a stimulant and enhances the effect of **stimulant drugs**, while the action of **hypnotics** is diminished.

PHYSIOLOGICAL FACTORS

Hormones like **ACTH** and **cortisol** exhibit a cyclic 24 hour rhythm (diurnal or circadian rhythm). This knowledge is applied to administer glucocorticoids only when the glandular cells are least sensitive to damage, i.e., as a **single early morning dose** or as **alternate day therapy** for chronic diseases.

PATHOLOGICAL FACTORS

Diseases of the liver and kidney interfere with the **detoxification** and **excretion** of drugs, and usual doses can accumulate to toxic levels in the body. In patients with impaired renal function, drugs like **streptomycin**, **gentamicin** and **kanamycin** may accumulate to toxic levels causing serious eighth cranial nerve damage.

PHARMACOGENETIC FACTORS

Genetic factors sometimes account for differences in the response of patients receiving similar doses of the same drug. For example some people are **rapid inactivators** of **isoniazid,** while others are **slow inactivators**. The latter are more likely to suffer the ill effects of isoniazid like polyneuritis. This ability to inactivate isoniazid by acetylation is genetically determined.

Idiosyncrasy is an old term, and stood for an extraordinary and peculiar response to a drug which was different from its pharmacologic response. Lately, with the development of pharmacogenetics, most idiosyncratic reactions to drugs are now being attributed to genetically determined defects in certain enzyme systems.

IMMUNOLOGIC FACTORS (DRUG ALLERGY)

The first (primary) exposure of the patient to the drug stimulates the immunologic mechanisms to produce antibodies. Later when the patient receives the same drug again, a reaction may occur which manifests in different ways, ranging from a breathing difficulty to skin, joint and blood disorders. Such manifestations are due to **drug allergy** or **hypersensitivity.** History of allergy to a certain drug is an *absolute contraindication* for the use of that drug.

PSYCHOLOGICAL AND ENVIRONMENTAL FACTORS

Some patients even respond to administration of a pharmacologically inert material, or **placebo** (*Latin*, I shall please). Placebos are inactive dosage forms, usually tablets or capsules containing sucrose or lactose. A placebo produces a variety of positive responses in about 30 to 35 percent of patients classified as **"placebo responders".**

Environmental factors influence effects of drugs of abuse like **alcohol**, **Cannabis** and **LSD**, i.e., it depends on the *set* and *setting*.

TOLERANCE

Tolerance is said to develop if the effect of a drug diminishes when it is given repeatedly, so that larger doses are required to produce the same effect.

Congenital tolerance: Certain species of animals like rabbits are tolerant to large doses of *atropine*.

Acquired tolerance: This form of tolerance is produced by drugs like cocaine, heroin, morphine, alcohol, nicotine, barbiturates, amphetamine and nitrites.

Tachyphylaxis (acute tolerance): It is an acute development of tolerance to the rapid and repeated administration of a drug. *Ephedrine* on repeated intravenous doses at short intervals elicits smaller and smaller hypertensive responses on the blood pressure in an anaesthetized animal (dog).

Cross-tolerance: This is a type of acquired tolerance developed as a result of repeated use of a drug, and which is manifested also towards other drugs closely related chemically, or related in their pharmacological actions.

CUMULATION

Cumulation occurs when the rate of removal or inactivation of a drug is slower than the rate of administration. Such a phenomenon can lead to dangerous overdose or toxicity. *Digitoxin* is a cumulative drug.

PHARMACOKINETIC FACTORS

Half-life (t½): With most drugs the rate of elimination is proportional to the amount in the body, i.e., the amount of drug eliminated is *not* constant, but is a *constant fraction* of the total amount in the body at any one time. The time a drug takes to reach an effective concentration, or steady-state level depends upon its rate of elimination from the body. *This is expressed in terms of the drug's biological half-life or, i.e., the time it takes for the amount of drug in the body to decrease to one-half of the peak previously attained.* **Penicillin G** has a short half-life (< ½ hour). **Digoxin** has a long half-life (about 1 week).

Loading and maintenance doses: In emergencies it is often necessary to raise the drug concentration rapidly to an effective level. For this, the drug is given initially in doses that exceed their elimination rate from the body. Such a **loading dose** is usually administered within a short period of time in several small doses. On attainment of a **steady-state level,** the dose is reduced which is intended to make up for the portion of the drug metabolized or eliminated from the body each day. This is the **maintenance dose.** For *example*, the initial digitalizing (loading) dose of digoxin is 1.0 to 1.5 mg orally, and the daily maintenance dose is 0.25 to 0.75 mg orally.

COMBINATION OF DRUGS

When one drug is given together with a second drug, the effects produced by the first drug may either be **increased** or **decreased** by the administration of the second drug. The terms usually employed to describe the combined effects of drugs are **addition**, **potentiation** and **antagonism.**

Addition or summation: The combined effect of the two drugs is equal to the algebric sum of their independent effects (2 + 2 = 4). Strictly speaking when the two drugs act by the same mechanism (receptors), the combined effect is an additive effect, e.g., **aspirin** and **paracetamol** exemplify **addition.** In contrast, when the two act by different mechanism (receptors) producing the same response, the combined effect is **summation,** e.g., aspirin and codeine produce analgesia by summation.

Potentiation or synergism: The combined effect of the two drugs is greater than the algebric sum of the independent effects of each drug (2 + 2 = 5).

Potentiation describes combined drug action by two drugs, only one of which produces a particular effect, while the other is inactive in that respect, e.g., *physostigmine* potentiates *acetylcholine* action by saving acetylcholine from destruction.

Synergism is seen when two drugs produce the same type of effect, but by acting at different sites and by different mechanisms, e.g., combination of **hydrochlorothiazide** with **methyldopa** in the treatment of essential hypertension. Slightly varying definitions of these terms are found in different texts.

Antagonism: The combined effect of the two drugs is lesser than the algebric sum of the individual effects of each drug (2 + 2 = 1). The opposing action of certain drugs has been utilized in **toxicology** in the treatment of poisoning as **antidotes.** In short, an **agonist** is an agent which is capable of producing a response by stimulating a **receptor**, like **acetylcholine** and **noradrenaline.** The **antagonist** is a drug which prevents the action of an agonist, and may be used as an **antidote** to reduce or abolish the effect of an overdose of the agonist. There are *four* mechanisms by which one drug may oppose the action of another.

Pharmacologic antagonism is **competitive** when the antagonist combines reversibly with the same receptor sites as the agonist, and can be displaced from these sites by an excess of the agonist, e.g., *diphenhydramine and histamine; atropine* and *acetylcholine*. Pharmacologic antagonism is **non-competitive** when the antagonist combines irreversibly with same receptor sites as the agonist, but it can not be displaced from these sites by an excess of the agonist, e.g., *phenoxybenzamine* and *noradrenaline*.

Physiologic antagonism is observed when two agonists, acting at different sites, counterbalance each other by producing opposite effects on the same physiologic function, e.g., **acetylcholine** induced contraction of the isolated intestine or uterus is antagonized by **adrenaline.**

Biochemical antagonism is observed when one drug indirectly decreases the amount of the second drug that would otherwise be available to its site of action in the absence of the first drug (antagonist). This type of antagonism is the **opposite of synergism**, e.g., *phenobarbitone* induces the hepatic microsomal enzyme activity and increases the rate of metabolism of drugs like *phenytoin, warfarin, dicumarol, griseofulvin* and *digitoxin*, whereby their effect is indirectly decreased by phenobarbitone.

Chemical antagonism is simply the reaction between an agonist and an antagonist to form an inactive product. The agonist is inactivated in direct proportion to the extent of chemical interaction with the antagonist, e.g., neutralization of excess gastric hydrochloric acid by antacids like **aluminium hydroxide** or **sodium bicarbonate.**

1.5 ABSORPTION, DISTRIBUTION, METABOLISM AND EXCRETION OF DRUGS (PHARMACOKINETICS)

In order to achieve its effect, a drug must first be **administered** in a suitable dosage form at an appropriate site. It must then be **absorbed** from the site of administration, and **distributed** in the body to reach its site of action. After its action the drug must be **metabolized** and the **metabolites excreted** from the body.

Absorption and distribution comprise the **disposition** of a drug, i.e., its placement in the body. Metabolism and excretion comprise the **fate** of a drug.

Simply speaking, **absorption** is the entry of the drug molecules into the blood via the mucous membranes of the alimentary or respiratory tracts, or from the site of injection. **Distribution** is the movement of the drug molecules between the water, lipid and protein constituents of the body. **Metabolism** or **biotransformation** is the process of alteration in the structure of the drug molecule in the body, specially the liver, and **excretion** is the removal of the original drug molecule or its metabolites from the body.

The above mentioned four processes are studied quantitatively in the mathematical science of **pharmacokinetics.**

DRUGS AND CELL MEMBRANES

The processes of absorption, distribution, biotransformation and excretion require the **passage of the drug across cell membranes**. These membranes consist of a bimolecular layer of lipid molecules, coated with a protein layer on each surface **(Fig. 1.1)**. The cell membrane also has small 'pores' and active transport systems.

The chemical structure of a drug determines whether a drug will be more *fat-soluble* or *water-soluble*.

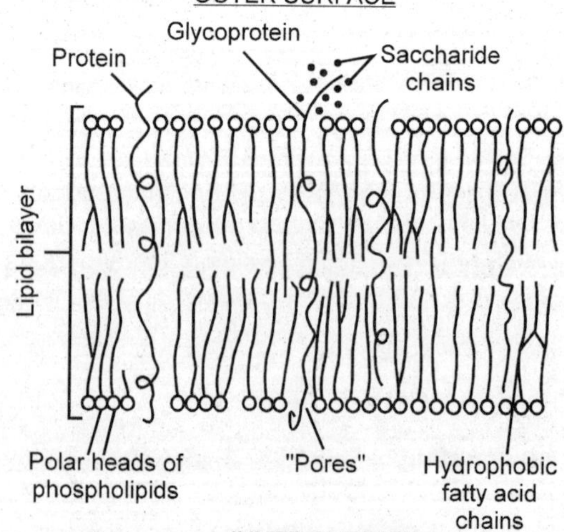

Fig. 1.1: Major features of a lipid bilayer cell membrane.

Drugs may cross body membranes by the following mechanisms:

1. **Passive transfer**
   Simple diffusion
   Filtration
2. **Specialized transport**
   Active transport
   Facilitated diffusion
   Pinocytosis

Passive Transfer

Simple diffusion requires no energy and depends on the difference in concentration of the drug on either side of the membrane. Both fat-soluble and water-soluble molecules of small size may cross the membrane by simple diffusion. The term **filtration** is used when a porous membrane exists which allows the flow of substances of a certain size only, with the larger molecular sizes being blocked. The glomerular membrane of the kidney is an example of a filtering membrane.

Most drugs are weak organic acids or bases and at the physiological pH of body fluids (7.35 to 7.45), drug molecules exist as a mixture of the **non-ionized** or uncharged molecular form, and the **ionized** or charged form. **Cell membranes are more permeable to the non-ionized form** of a drug than to an ionized form.

Specialized Transport

Active transport of a drug refers to a situation when the drug is moved against a concentration gradient, by the use of energy. **Facilitated diffusion** is a form of transport in which the drug attaches to a special 'carrier' which facilitates the diffusion of the drug across the membrane, and then releases the drug. **Pinocytosis** describes the ability of cells to surround and engulf small droplets. This process is of importance in the uptake of large molecules.

DRUG ABSORPTION

Most drugs are given **orally** and they must pass through the gut wall to enter the blood stream. There are five main factors which determine its fate in the body: (i) **molecular weight;** (ii) **chemical stability;** (iii) **lipid solubility;** (iv) **degree of ionization;** and (v) **pharmaceutical formulation of the drug**.

Molecular weight: Substances with a high molecular weight are not usually absorbed intact except in minute quantities. **Insulin** undergoes enzymatic breakdown in the gut, and is not effectively absorbed.

Chemical stability: Unstable drugs are inactivated in the gastrointestinal tract. **Benzylpenicillin** is unstable in an acid medium, and cannot produce satisfactory results on oral administration. In contrast, **phenoxymethylpenicillin** is more stable in an acid medium than benzylpenicillin, and oral doses are effective.

Lipid solubility: As cell membranes are lipid in nature, the degree and rate of penetration of the drug through them is dependent on the lipid solubility of the drug.

Degree of ionization: Under physiological conditions some substances like **ethanol** (ethyl alcohol) are un-ionized, while others like **acetylcholine** are highly ionized. The absorption of unionized molecules is favoured because they are more lipid-soluble than the ionized form.

Pharmaceutical formulation: Various formulations of a drug can greatly influence the amount and rate at which it is absorbed, e.g., effervescent aspirin (0.6 g orally) produced more than double the plasma level produced by an equivalent dose of ordinary aspirin (both measured after 30 minutes).

Absorption via Gastrointestinal Tract

For most drugs, the **proximal small intestine** is the major site of absorption. **Acidic drugs** such as aspirin and barbiturates can be absorbed from the stomach. **Basic drugs** including antipsychotics, anticholinergics, narcotics and sympathomimetics are absorbed only in the intestine. Their absorption is delayed if taken with food.

First-pass metabolism refers to the biotransformation of drugs during absorption through the intestine, and their transport through the **liver**

in the portal circulation. It can significantly reduce the percentage of an oral dose that reaches systemic circulation. Drugs like **propranolol** are extensively metabolized as they pass through the liver—the '*first-pass effect*'. **Sublingual** administration may be an alternative to the oral route, e.g., **isoprenaline** and **nitroglycerin.** Nitrates such as **nitroglycerin** and **isosorbide dinitrate** are more effective when given sublingually.

On **oral** administration *three* processes precede absorption: (i) **Disintegration** of the solid dosage form (tablet or capsule) into granules. The **disintegration rate** (in terms of time) is dependent on the dosage form. **Compressed tablets** take some time to break up in the stomach, which delays absorption. Disintegration is deliberately delayed in **enteric coated tablets**, by a special acid-resistant coating material which is soluble only at a high pH in the intestine; (ii) **Deaggregation** of the granules forms fine particles;and (iii) **Dissolution** of the active material from fine particles into a solution. On these three processes **(Fig. 1.2)** depends the ultimate absorption and *bioavailability* of the drug.

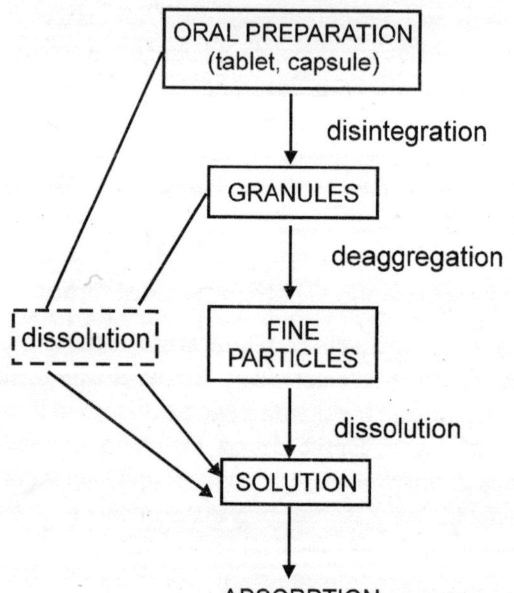

Fig. 1.2: Diagrammatic representation of the fate of oral preparations in the gut (see text).

Other factors which govern drug absorption from the gut are: (i) **Surface area of absorption;** (ii) **Gastric emptying speed;** (iii) **Splanchnic blood flow;** (iv) **Contents of the gut**; (v) **Certain disease states;** and (vi) **pH within the gut**.

Absorption via Parenteral Sites

The factors which influence the rate of absorption from intramuscular (IM), and subcutaneous (SC) injection sites are: (i) **Drug concentration**; (ii) **Solubility of the drug;** and (iii) **Local blood flow.**

The dosage **formulation** can also affect absorption from parenteral sites, e.g., drugs in aqueous **solutions** are usually absorbed more rapidly than drugs in **suspension,** e.g., benzathine penicillin with procaine penicillin G.

Absorption of drugs from IM sites is more rapid than from SC sites because of the higher vascularity of the muscle compared to subcutaneous tissue. Decreased peripheral blood flow in conditions of 'shock' significantly reduces the rate of absorption of injected drugs.

Absorption via Lungs (Inhalation)

Drugs presented in the correct form to the trachea and lungs are absorbed by **simple diffusion.** The correct form is a **vapour**, an **aqueous solution,** or a **suspension** of particles small enough to be evenly distributed over the mucous membrane. *Examples* include volatile anaesthetics and disodium cromoglycate.

Absorption via Topical Sites

Absorption of most drugs through the intact skin is poor, as the keratinized epidermis behaves like a barrier. Absorption through the skin is proportional to the lipid solubility of the drug, and the surface area to which the drug is applied. It can be enhanced by dissolving the drug in an oily base, and vigorous massaging of the area.

Lately, drugs intended for systemic action are being formulated in a way that topical application is utilized as the route of administration. For example, the **nitroglycerin transdermal system patch**

(Chap. 1.3). This drug impregnated patch is applied to the skin of upper torso in patients of angina pectoris.

BIOAVAILABILITY

Bioavailability of a drug is the percentage of a dose that reaches the systemic circulation after administration via a stated route. The application of this concept to the comparison of various formulations of the same drug is referred to as **bioequivalence.**

The bioavailability of any drug after IV administration is 100 percent, and is assumed to be close to this value when given IM or SC.

BIOEQUIVALENCE

Bioequivalence is said to exist when the bioavailability of a drug from different formulations is the same. Bioinequivalence of formulations of the same drug has been used by the pharmaceutical industry as a rational argument in favour of prescribing drugs by their **brand names,** rather than their **generic names.**

PRODRUGS

To improve bioavailability, the drug molecule is modified to form a better absorbed compound, which liberates the active drug after absorption. Such modified drugs are known as **prodrugs**. For example: *dipivalyladrenaline* is a prodrug of *adrenaline.* As dipivalyladrenaline is better absorbed, less drug is required and side effects are minimized.

DRUG DISTRIBUTION

Drug distribution describes the process which transports a drug to its site of action, to other storage sites in the body, and to organs of metabolism and excretion. The movement of drug molecules in these areas determines its **effectiveness, duration of action,** mode of **metabolism** and rate of **excretion. Lipid-soluble** drugs tend to distribute more widely in the body compared to **lipid-insoluble** drugs. **Initial distribution** of a drug is primarily dependent on the **cardiac output,** and the **local blood flow.** Subsequently, other factors come into play that govern the **final distribution pattern** of a drug:

1. Physicochemical characteristics.
2. Route of drug administration.
3. Binding to plasma proteins.
4. Regional blood flow.
5. Availability of active transport systems.
6. Special compartments and barriers.

Physiochemical characteristics: Drugs reach the extracellular space by **passive diffusion** through junctions or 'pores' between the endothelial cells, except in the brain which has tight junctions between these cells. Only lipid-soluble drugs cross cell membranes effectively.

Route of administration: Drugs given intravenously are preferentially distributed in organs with a high regional blood flow. In contrast drugs which are well absorbed from the gut are extracted and concentrated in the liver during their "first pass", e.g., **propranolol** and **tricyclic antidepressants.**

Binding to proteins: Drugs bind either to plasma proteins, usually albumin or to proteins of cells (nucleoproteins). Drugs bound to plasma protein are in equilibrium with free drug in the plasma water, but only the **free drug** exerts a pharmacological effect. Plasma protein binding of a drug slows the disappearance of the drug from the plasma, limits its access to its site of action, and prolongs the time the drug remains in the body by slowing its renal filtration.

Regional blood flow: The brain, endocrine glands, the heart, kidneys, liver and the lung are well perfused. Muscle and skin are moderately perfused, whereas adipose tissue (fat) is poorly perfused, and the bones and teeth receive the least blood supply. Tissues with a good regional flow equilibrate rapidly with the drug present in the blood. Drug distribution is altered when tissue perfusion is reduced like in **heart failure, cardiogenic shock** or **hypothyroidism.**

Availability of active transport systems: Some drugs are concentrated in certain tissues as a result of uptake by selective transport systems, e.g., the **adrenergic neurone blocker** (guanethidine) into the adrenergic nerve terminal; and **iodine** is actively concentrated into the thyroid cells.

SPECIAL COMPARTMENTS AND BARRIERS

The plasma space: Drugs leave the plasma by diffusing across the capillary membrane which has the characteristics of a lipid membrane. All drugs other than proteins can readily diffuse into the extracellular space.

Blood-brain barrier: Anatomically there is a dual barrier in the CNS–the blood-brain barrier and the blood-CSF (cerebrospinal fluid) barrier. Some drugs enter the CNS with relative ease, while others do not enter at all.

Thus, a highly lipid-soluble barbiturate like **thiopentone** readily enters the CNS, whereas, drugs which are highly ionized, like most **penicillins** and **gentamicin**, penetrate very slowly.

Placental barrier: The passage of most drugs from the maternal to foetal circulation occurs quite easily. The placental membrane is **lipid in nature,** and readily allows the transfer of non-ionized, lipid soluble drugs by **simple diffusion** down a concentration gradient. Thus, most drugs that are well absorbed orally can easily enter the foetal circulation, e.g., **chlorpromazine, gaseous anaesthetics, sulphonamides, barbiturates, morphine, pethidine, heroin** and **alcohol.**

Eye: The conjunctiva, sclera, iris and the ciliary muscle receive moderate blood supply (cornea and lens are avascular). Lipid-soluble drugs can penetrate and reach these structures and the aqueous humour from the conjunctival sac, e.g., **prednisolone sodium phosphate, atropine, chloramphenicol and cocaine.**

DRUG METABOLISM (BIOTRANSFORMATION)

Termination of drug effect, also termed as **drug elimination,** involves two processes: (i) *metabolism*, mainly in the liver and kidneys; and (ii) *excretion of the unchanged drug* and/or its metabolites by the kidneys, gut, lungs, sweat glands, breasts and salivary glands.

Drug metabolism occurs predominantly in the liver by way of **hepatic microsomal enzyme systems.** Lipid-soluble drugs easily gain access to these metabolizing enzymes in liver cells.

Biotransformation generally results in the conversion of a drug to a metabolite that is less active, less lipid-soluble and hence easily excreted. Some drugs are administered in the form of an inactive **prodrug,** which is then converted to an active metabolite in the body.

The activity of **hepatic microsomal enzymes** can be altered by a number of factors. Enzymatic function is reduced in the presence of **liver diseases** or **impaired circulation.** Drugs like monoamine oxidase inhibitors (MAOIs), and organophosphorus insecticides also adversely affect the liver microsomal enzyme system. Decreased enzymatic activity results in slowed metabolism of drugs, leading to **cumulation** and **toxicity.**

Microsomal enzyme function can also be increased by a number of drugs and is termed as **enzyme induction**. Prolonged administration of **barbiturates, phenytoin, carbamazepine, ethanol,** and a number of other drugs accelerate metabolism of drugs by the hepatic microsomal system. This effect is responsible for the development of **tolerance** to those drugs.

In the liver biotransformation of drugs usually occurs in two phases: (i) **Phase I reactions;** and (ii) **Phase II reactions.**

Phase I reactions: These **preconjugation** reactions produce a chemical change in the drug molecule. Such reactions include **oxidation**; **reduction;** and **hydrolysis.** The majority of phase I metabolites are generated by a common hydroxylating enzyme system known as cytochrome $P_{450.}$

Phase II reactions: These **conjugation** or **synthetic** reactions involve the coupling of the drug or its metabolites formed in phase I to another chemical group (e.g., sulphate, acetate), or substrate (carbohydrate, amino acid). The end products formed are more water-soluble and can be eliminated in bile or urine.

DRUG EXCRETION

Drugs can be excreted in their unchanged form or as metabolites by several routes including the *kidneys, lungs* and *intestines*, and to a lesser extent by the *sweat, salivary* and *mammary glands*.

Renal Excretion

Three major processes are involved in the excretion of drugs by the kidneys: (i) **Glomerular filtration;** (ii) **Tubular secretion;** and (iii) **Tubular reabsorption**. The first two processes remove drugs from the plasma, whereas the third process retains drugs in the body by returning them to the plasma. The **net excretion** of a drug therefore, depends on the sum total of the three processes.

Biliary Excretion

Excretion in the bile is a relatively minor route of elimination of unmetabolized drugs, but it is a **major** route of elimination of drug metabolites, particularly water-soluble conjugates like glucuronides.

Pulmonary Excretion

This route of excretion is important primarily for **gaseous** and **volatile liquid general anaesthetics,** which can be excreted from the blood stream across the alveolar membrane into the expired air.

Excretion of drugs in **sweat, saliva, milk** and **gastric juice** is mainly by passive diffusion of the non-ionized form. Some drugs are transferred to the suckling infant in breast milk in significant amounts. Hence, drug use by a breast feeding mother should be restricted to the minimum.

PHARMACOKINETICS

Phamacokinetics is the study of drug absorption, distribution, metabolism and excretion. These factors interact to produce a definite pattern for the time course of **absorption**, **distribution** and **excretion** of each drug and its metabolites. Strictly speaking phamacokinetics is the science which uses mathematical models to describe and quantify processes which determine the time course of drug action. It is a complex science.

Drug plasma concentration: An assumption is made that the time course of drug concentration at its site of action is determined by its plasma concentration.

Volume of distribution (Vd): This is the apparent volume into which the drug is distributed on intravenous administration. Vd can be calculated by the following equation:

$$\text{Vd (in litres)} = \frac{\text{Amount of drug in the body (dose in mg)}}{\text{Concentration of drug in plasma (mg/l)}}$$

The Vd can be used to calculate the clearance of the drug.

Clearance is analogous to renal clearance, i.e., the total volume of plasma from which the drug has been removed per unit time. It can be calculated from the equation:

$$\text{Clearance (clp)} = \frac{\text{Vd} \times 0.693}{\text{half-life } (t½)}$$

The whole body clearance of a drug is the volume of plasma 'cleared' of the drug per minute, regardless of the means by which it is cleared or removed from the plasma. Thus, Clp = Clm (metabolic clearance) + clr (renal excretion).

Half-life (t½): It is the time taken for the concentration of a drug in the plasma to fall by half its original value. The **plasma half-life** is the most used measure, and is closely related to the concentration of the drug at the site of action. It is comparatively easily measured. Further, plasma t½ determines the time taken to achieve a *steady-state* or an equilibrium with any constant dose rate. In practice a useful estimate of time required to reach a steady-state is obtained by the equation:

Time to 95% steady-state = 4.3 x t½

As a working rule it is followed that it will take five half-lives to reach a steady-state on regular dosing.

Drug dosage: Ideally, in drug treatment, a **steady-state plasma concentration** is required within a known safe and effective therapeutic range. This steady-state will be achieved when the rate of drug entering the systemic circulation (dosage rate) equals the rate of elimination.

THERAPEUTIC DRUG MONITORING (TDM)

There is at times marked variability between patients in their pharmacokinetic parameters, and in drug responsiveness. This renders the concept of a generally accepted 'therapeutic dose' rather inaccurate. Alternatively monitor and maintain drug plasma concentrations at a level which is necessary to produce a therapeutic effect. Such a procedure is designated as **therapeutic drug monitoring (TDM).** Some commonly monitored drugs are **carbamazepine, digoxin, lithium, phenytoin, sodium valproate** and **theophylline.**

Basic knowledge about drug disposition and pharmacokinetics is essential for safe drug therapy.

1.6 MECHANISMS OF DRUG ACTION (PHARMACODYNAMICS)

Pharmacodynamics is concerned with the **actions, interactions** and the **mechanism (mode) of action** of drugs. Drugs can be divided into *two* major groups: those acting on **pharmacological receptors** situated on or within the cells, and those in which the **receptors are not involved.**

Drugs which **act via receptors:** (i) act at low concentrations; (ii) react with specific receptors; (iii) show structure-activity relationships; and (iv) can be antagonized by specific antagonists. *Examples* are **acetylcholine, adrenaline, noradrenaline** and **histamine.**

In contrast drugs which **do not act via receptors:** (i) act at higher concentrations; (ii) do not react with specific receptors; (iii) tend not to show structure-activity relationship; and (iv) do not have specific antagonists. *Examples* are general anaesthetics like **diethyl ether** and **halothane; diuretics** like the **thiazides;** and **detergents** which non-specifically destroy cell membranes.

BASIS OF DRUG ACTION

Drugs do not create new functions. They can only modify inherent functions of the tissues or the cells concerned. Considering these processes briefly: **stimulation** is an increase in rate of the functional activity of a cell or tissue, e.g., **caffeine** and **amphetamine** stimulate the CNS; **depression** denotes a reduction in such activity, e.g., **barbiturates, alcohol** and **trimethadione** depress CNS; **replacement** is done for conditions associated with the underproduction of a natural substance, e.g., **insulin** for diabetes mellitus; and **irritation** signifies the effect of drugs inducing a change in function, e.g., **liniments** to relieve muscular pain. **Bacteriostatic** (inhibition of bacterial growth and multiplication), and **bactericidal** (death of bacteria) activity is induced by complex mechanisms by **antibiotics** and other **chemotherapeutic drugs,** e.g., **penicillin** and **tetracyclines.**

There are *five* patterns of action:

1. Drug -receptor interactions.
2. Drugs acting on enzymes.
3. Non-receptor mechanisms:
   i. Antimetabolites.
   ii. Chelation.
   iii. Drugs affecting the permeability of membranes.
   iv. Drugs acting by their physical or chemical action.
   v. Drugs acting as antiseptics.
4. Drugs acting through antibodies.
5. Placebo effects.

DRUG-RECEPTOR INTERACTIONS

Receptor Theory of Drug Action

The structure of the **drug** is related to the correlative structure of the **receptor**, and as just one key can fit in one lock, so also one drug is specific for one receptor type. This specificity is based on the **chemical structure** of the drug, which is termed as the **structure-activity relationship** (SAR) of the drug **(Fig. 1.3).**

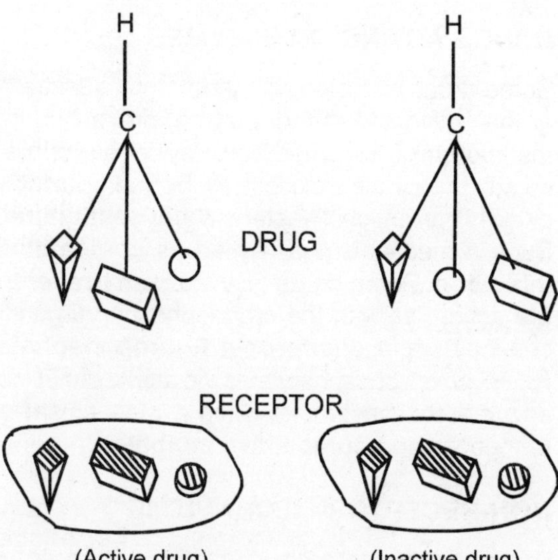

Fig. 1.3: The receptor concept

Terminology: A pharmacological **receptor** is a macromolecule with **special** sites to which **specific substances,** i.e., drugs bind. Drug-receptor binding triggers a sequence of events resulting in a **response** of the tissue or organ, e.g., **acetylcholine** induces contraction of intestinal smooth muscle.

An **agonist** is a drug (or hormone, or neurotransmitter) which combines with its **specific receptor**, activates it and initiates a response, e.g., **acetylcholine** and **noradrenaline** activate cholinoceptors and adrenoceptors respectively.

An **antagonist** is a drug which binds to the receptors, but does not activate it. It prevents the action of the agonist by rendering the receptors unavailable for interaction with the agonist, e.g., **atropine** antagonizes acetylcholine, and **phentolamine** antagonizes noradrenaline. A **pure antagonist** has no action of its own.

A **partial agonist** binds to the receptor , but activates it weakly and prevents the action of a full agonist. In fact, it is a drug that acts on a receptor with an **intrinsic activity** or **efficacy** of less than 1 (See later). Practically, an activity of 1 means the ability of a drug to elicit a maximal response.

A **mixed agonist-antagonist** is a drug that acts simultaneously on a mixed group of receptors with an **agonist action** on one set, and with an **antagonist action** on another set. *Examples* are found among the **opioids.**

Thus at any receptor *four* types of drugs may act (agonists, antagonists, partial agonists, mixed agonist-antagonists) by attachment to receptor site.

The **pharmacological receptors** are named according to either (a) the principal endogenous agonist that activates them (**adrenoceptors, cholinoceptors, glucocorticoid receptors** etc.), or (b) the first exogenous agonist found to activate them (**opioid receptors, benzodiazepine receptors**).

LOCATION OF DRUG RECEPTORS

The sites where drug receptors are found are as under:

1. **On or within cell membranes:** These are of two types: (i) those that act on membrane permeability with a very fast response time, or (ii) those that act on intracellular second messenger with a slower response time.
2. **Inside the cells:** The **cytoplasmic glucocorticoid receptors** alter DNA transcription with a slow response time, such as produced by **corticosteroids.**

AFFINITY AND INTRINSIC ACTIVITY

The term **affinity** describes the ability of a drug to form and maintain a complex with a receptor site. The term **intrinsic activity** describes the ability of a drug to evoke a pharmacologic response on combining with a receptor. Thus agonists possess both affinity and intrinsic activity, whereas antagonists display only affinity. In contrast, a **partial agonist** possesses less intrinsic activity than a full agonist, but may have equal affinity.

INTENSITY OF DRUG RESPONSE

Simply speaking, an **agonist** is a drug capable of interacting with a receptor to produce a response. When an **antagonist** attaches itself to the receptor, no response is produced and in the presence of an antagonist, the normally elicited response by the agonist is diminished or totally blocked. In most instances a specific chemical structure is required for a drug to act as an agonist or an antagonist **(Fig. 1.4).**

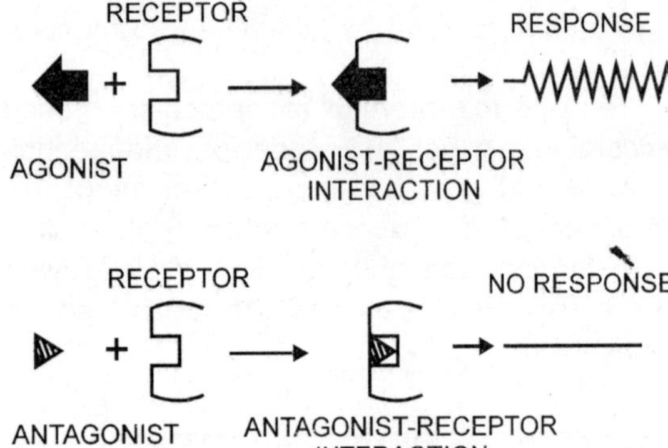

Fig. 1.4: *Drug-receptor interactions. The agonist neatly fits and interacts with the receptor site to produce a pharmacologic response. Whereas, the antagonist only partially fits the receptor site, hence it is unable to produce a response itself, and prevents the agonist from combining with the receptor.*

Currently *three* theories attempt to explain the nature of *drug-receptor* interactions: (i) the **receptor occupation theory;** (ii) the **rate theory;** and (iii) theories involving **drug-induced protein changes** at receptor site.

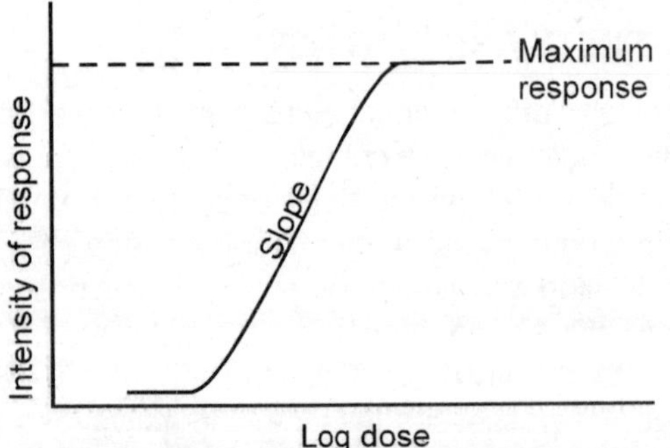

Fig. 1.5: *A typical log dose-response curve for a drug.*

A typical curve illustrating the intensity of a drug effect with increasing dosage (conventionally plotted as log dose) is shown in (**Fig.1.5**).

DRUGS ACTING ON ENZYMES

Some drugs compete with the normal substrate at the active site of the enzyme, preventing its metabolism. This competition may be **reversible,** as with the xanthine oxidase inhibitor **allopurinol,** or with the anticholinesterase **physostigmine.** Such a mechanism is termed as **competitive inhibition.** Some drugs may exert an **irreversible** action, as with the organophosphorus anticholinesterase **diisopropyl fluorophosphate** (DFP), which phosphorylates the active site of the enzyme cholinesterase. Such a mechanism is termed as **non-competitive inhibition.**

NON-RECEPTOR MECHANISMS

Some drugs do not act by combining with receptor sites. For example, **gastric antacids** act by neutralizing the hydrochloric acid secreted by partial cells in the stomach. **Osmotic diuretics,** like mannitol remove excess of fluid from the body by increasing the osmolarity of plasma and the glomerular filtrate resulting in diuresis. **Volatile general anaesthetics** produce anaesthesia without directly involving receptors. **Metal chelating agents**, like EDTA are employed in the treatment of poisoning by heavy metals. The **vaccines** produce their effects by stimulating the defence mechanisms in the body and induce production of antibodies, while **antisera** contain antibodies which neutralize toxins in the body.

PLACEBO EFFECTS

A **placebo** (means, I shall please) is an inactive substance given to satisfy the patient's demand for medicine. Inert medicines (placebos) can lead to improvement in more than one-third of all patients (about 35 percent). This is termed as a placebo response. Sometimes doctors use the placebo response to reinforce the effects of treatment.

THERAPEUTIC INDEX

An "ideal" drug should cure all patients in a dose that kills none. The therapeutic index gives a measure of the safety margin of a drug, although it does not take into account the possible occurrence of an abnormal response, like an allergic or hypersensitivity reaction.

REPEATED DOSAGE

When a drug is administered repeatedly the absorbed fraction of each dose is added to the amount remaining in the plasma at the particular time. Thus the **maximum** and **minimum** plasma levels slowly rise until the rate of elimination **equals** the rate of administration. At this point, assuming that the drug is being given in fixed dosage at constant time intervals, **a steady-state plasma range** is attained, and the concentration of the drug in the plasma reaches a **plateau.** The plateau concentration of a drug is dependent on the **dose,** the **frequency** of administration, and the **elimination half-life** (t½). Once the desired steady-state plasma concentration has been attained changes in dosage or frequency of administration must be avoided.

To ensure therapeutic plasma levels the following measures have to be adopted:

1. Maintain a consistent dosage and frequency pattern for drugs.
2. Plasma levels of drugs are reliable only if the blood is drawn at the correct time interval after dose administration.
3. Loading doses of drugs may be given to facilitate rapid attainment of therapeutic plasma levels.

The above mentioned *three* factors have important nursing implications for effective drug therapy.

COMBINED EFFECTS OF DRUGS

The combined effects of drugs are discussed in **Chap. 1.4** as they influence dosage. Sometimes the presence of the second drug alters the response to the first drug in a *positive* or a *negative* manner. **Adverse drug interactions** are detailed in **Chap. 1.7.**

1.7 ADVERSE DRUG REACTIONS AND TREATMENT OF POISONING

When a drug is administered to a patient, essentially two types of reactions can occur, **desired** effects, and the **undesired** effects. The undesired drug effects are divided into those that are **innocuous**, and those that are harmful to the patient. The latter group is commonly referred to as **adverse drug reactions**.

DEFINITION

An **adverse drug reaction (ADR)** is any response to a drug which is injurious and unintended, and which occurs at doses used in man for prophylaxis, diagnosis, or therapy of disease.

Strictly speaking, ADRs exclude therapeutic failures and consequences of administration of the wrong drug, to the wrong patient, in a wrong dosage, at the wrong time, or for the wrong disease. Any single 'wrong' may result in unwanted effects or cause a reaction.

CLASSIFICATION OF ADRs

1. *Pharmacologic ADRs:*
   i. Extension of therapeutic effect.
   ii. Non-therapeutic adverse effects.
2. *Non-pharmacologic ADRs:*
   i. Hypersensitivity (drug allergy).
   ii. Idiosyncrasy (pharmacogenetics).
   iii. Photosensitivity.
3. *Disease-related ADRs.*
4. *Multiple drug reactions.*
5. *Miscellaneous ADRs:*
   i. Carcinogenicity.
   ii. Teratogenicity (dysmorphogenesis).
   iii. Drug dependence.
   iv. Overdosage.

Pharmacologic ADRs

Extension of therapeutic effects: Overdosage with a drug usually elicits an excessive reaction to the primary effect of the drug, e.g., **tranquillizers** used as daytime sedatives in excessive doses will produce drowsiness and hypnosis.

Non-therapeutic adverse effects: Some adverse effects caused by drug administration are the result of one or more secondary effects produced by a drug, e.g., **antihistamines** cause profound drowsiness; **anticholinergics** produce dry month, blurring of vision, and some degree of urinary retention and constipation; and **diuretics** produce hypokalaemia.

Non-pharmacologic ADRs

Such reactions are **not** predictable on the basis of the pharmacologic profile of the drug, and occur in a small proportion of patients.

Hypersensitivity (Drug Allergy)

Allergic reactions are usually **not** dose-related and independent of the pharmacologic properties of the drug. Macromolecules (proteins, peptides) can act as **complete antigens**, but most drugs are small molecules and do not stimulate antibody production. They combine with other carrier macromolecules and function as **haptens** or **partial antigens** resulting in production of antibodies to the drug molecule. Subsequent exposure to the same drug elicits an antigen-antibody reaction that produces symptoms like itching, oedema, congestion and wheezing. Allergic drug reactions are either **immediate** (anaphylaxis, urticaria) or **delayed** (serum sickness).

Immediate hypersensitivity develops within minutes of drug exposure. Upon re-exposure the antigen combines with the antibodies on the target tissue, and certain natural substances like histamine, 5-hydroxtryptamine, slow-reacting substance (SRS-A), bradykinin and prostaglandins are liberated. These substances produce characteristic signs of the allergic reaction like bronchoconstriction and vasodilation. Immediate immune reactions like **anaphylactic shock, asthma, rhinitis** and **angioneurotic oedema** occur within a few minutes of re-exposure, e.g., penicillin allergy. Quick recognition and treatment are essential to avoid serious consequences.

Delayed hypersensitivity reactions develop slowly following drug challenge. The clinical picture of delayed hypersensitivity includes a **diffuse rash, fever, angioedema, swollen lymph nodes** and **stiff joints.**

Idiosyncrasy (Pharmacogenetics)

Strictly speaking, indiosyncrasy refers to a peculiarity of bodily function that causes an individual to react in an abnormal manner to a drug. These reactions are not caused by formation of an antigen-antibody complex, but result from a **genetically determined defect** in the patient's ability to handle a particular drug. Idiosyncrasy today is a term of the past.

A specialized field of a study termed **pharmacogenetics** deals with those altered drug responses that are under hereditary control, e.g., in glucose-6 phosphate dehydrogenase (G-6 PD) deficiency a usual dose of **primaquine** may cause **haemolytic anaemia;** in individuals who lack normal plasma cholinesterase activity **suxamethonium** may cause **prolonged apnoea;** slow acetylators are more likely to develop polyneuritis with **isoniazid.**

Photosensitivity

A unique type of skin hypersensitivity reaction following use of many drugs is observed on exposure to sunlight, and is termed **photosensitization.** *Examples* of photosensitizing drugs include antimalarials, carbamazepine, chlordiazepoxide, contraceptives, frusemide, griseofulvin, haloperidol, phenothiazines, phenytoin, sulphonyureas, tetracyclines and thiazide diuretics.

Disease-Related ADRs

Hepatic disease: Since the liver plays a major role in metabolism of many drugs, impaired liver function may result in abnormally high plasma levels of drugs for a long period of time.

Renal disease: In renal disease doses of drugs excreted by the kidneys need to be reduced to avoid accumulation and toxicity, e.g., most *amino-*

glycoside antibiotics are excreted by glomerular filtration in an unchanged form. Thus, they are potentially toxic even in normal doses in patients with impaired renal function.

Emotional disorders: Mentally unstable patients should not be allowed to monitor their own drug therapy. Often they do not follow proper dosage schedules, and this can lead to over dosage with drugs.

Other disease states: Existence of certain diseases increases the likelihood of an ADR to a particular drug. Patients with **bronchial asthma** must avoid nonselective beta-blockers (nadolol, propranolol), since their bronchospastic action can worsen ventilatory function. Patients with a healed **duodenal ulcer** are likely to suffer from increased bleeding if given non-steroidal anti-inflammatory agents like *indomethacin* or *naproxen*.

Multiple Drug Reactions

The presence of a second drug may modify the actions of a simultaneously administered drug. This domain of **drug interactions** would be covered in **Chapter 1.8.**

Miscellaneous ADRs

Some drugs generally recognized as being potentially carcinogenic are: *androgens, antineoplastic agents, busulphan, carbon tetrachloride, clofibrate, corticosteroids, cyclamates, griseofulvin, metronidazole, oestrogens,* and *tobacco smoke*.

Teratogenicity (Dysmorphogenesis)

The term 'teratogenic' means monster-producing (*teratos* = monstor), and similarly 'dysmorphogenic' means causing a derangement in form. Administration of certain drugs to pregnant women, specially during the **first trimester** of pregnancy, has resulted in foetal deformities. Such drugs are said to be **teratogenic**. In the early 1960s the teratogenic effects of **thalidomide** came to be known.

Drugs with known teratogenic effects include antiepileptics (phenytoin, phenobarbitone); antithyroid drugs (carbimazole); antineoplastics (methotrexate, cyclophosphamide, busulphan, chlorambucil); sex hormones (androgens, progestogens); corticosteroids; sulphonylureas; and ethyl alcohol.

In general, no drug should be used during the **first trimester** of pregnancy, unless very necessary.

Drug Dependence

The use of drugs particularly those acting on the central nervous system for 'non-medical' or 'recreational' purposes is becoming increasingly common specially among the youth. **Drug dependence** varies in intensity from **habituation** to **psychologic dependence**, to **true physical dependence (Chapter 2.10).**

Overdosage

With overdosage ill effects occur in direct relation to the total amount of drug present in the body. The term **toxicity** is used for these undesired and detrimental effects of a drug.

ACUTE POISONING

A poison is a substance which when consumed endangers life due to derangement of certain vital physiological functions. The study of the poisonous effects of drugs, and other chemical substances is known as **toxicology.**

Diagnosis: Some drug poisonings produce characteristic physical signs. However, a large number of patients are brought to the hospital in a comatosed state. If facilities exist, the **Poison Control Centre** or the hospital emergency department must be promptly informed.

General Principles of Management of Poisoning

1. **Identify the poison.**
2. **Ensure and maintain a clear airway.**
3. **Ensure adequate ventilation.**
4. **Suppress convulsions:** If convulsions provoked by the poison are not controlled by

adequate ventilation, **diazepam 10 mg IV** should be administered in adults.

5. **Fluid and electrolyte therapy:** For this **isotonic saline** (0.9% w/v), or **isotonic glucose** (5% w/v), or **plasma** may be used. The **urine volume** and **fluid balance** should be recorded.
6. **Decontamination:** The stomach should be emptied by **gastric lavage** in a conscious patient. Vomiting may be induced by apomorphine or syrup of ipecac (15-20 ml orally). **Gastric lavage** and **induction of vomiting are contraindicated** if the patient is drowsy or unconscious. Induction of vomiting is also contraindicated if a caustic alkali or corrosive mineral acid has been ingested. **Activated charcoal** 10-30 g suspended in 100 to 400 ml of water may be introduced in the stomach to bind the unabsorbed drug. **Universal antidote** (or burnt toast) 2 parts; magnesium oxide (milk of magnesia) 1 part; and tannic acid (or strong tea) 1 part mixed together may be administered orally.
7. **Specific antidotes:** These antagonists may be administered with advantage. They are listed in (**Table 1.1**).

Table 1.1: *Some antidotes used against drug overdosage (poisoning)*

Drug in overdose	*Antidote*	*Mechanism*
Narcotic analgesics (morphine,	Nalorphine	Partial agonist
pethidine, pentazocine)	Naloxone	Antagonist
Irons salts	Desferrioxamine	Chelation
Lead salts	Penicillamine	Chelation
Mercury salts	Dimercaprol	Chelation
Paracetamol	Acetylcysteine	Reduction of oxidized glutathione
Anti-cholinesterases (physostigmine, neostigmine)	Atropine	ACh antagonist
Organophosphorus anticholinesterases	Pralidoxime	Cholinesterase reactivation

8. **Non-specific pharmacological antidotes** like **anticonvulsants** in convulsant; and **analeptics** in narcotic poisoning may be employed.
9. **Promote elimination of the drug:** Forced diuresis (fluid load and diuretic) reduces the transit time through the nephron, and lessens reabsorption of drugs.
10. **Haemodialysis or peritoneal dialysis:** These specialized techniques are more effective than diuresis. Haemodialysis is 5 to 10 times more effective than peritoneal dialysis, but peritoneal dialysis is a much easier technique, whereas haemodialysis can only be done in bigger hospitals or special centres.
11. **General supportive and nursing measures** have to be simultaneously instituted.

1.8 DRUG INTERACTIONS

When two drugs are administered in close sequence to each other, they may interact either to **enhance** or **diminish** the intended effect, or they may produce an unintended and potentially harmful reaction.

DEFINITIONS

The term **drug interaction** is defined as an alteration in the **duration** or **magnitude** (or both) of the pharmacological effect of one drug produced by another drug. When more than one drug is administered simultaneously the combined effect may be **antagonistic** or **synergistic.** The incidence of drug interactions has increased mainly due to *three* factors: (i) **drug explosion;** (ii) **availability of potent drugs;** and (iii) **irrational poly-**

pharmacy, i.e., indiscriminate prescribing of combined preparations by the clinician.

The term **polypharmacy** covers the practice of multiple drug therapy in the management of disease. Judicious use of drug combinations (rational polypharmacy) can be of considerable benefit in treating disease like tuberculosis, hypertension, coronary artery disease, and diabetes mellitus.

Some over 1600 potential drug interactions have been described in man. It is impossible to remember them, but ready information is available in pocket books, manuals on drug interactions, drug interaction discs, or from hospital *drug information centres.*

CLASSIFICATION AND MECHANISMS OF DRUG INTERACTIONS

Drug interactions may occur **outside the body** (*in vitro*), or **inside the body** (*in vivo*):

- **I. Outside the body**
  1. Physical.
  2. Chemical.
- **II. Inside the body**
  1. Pharmacokinetic interactions.
  2. Pharmacodynamic interactions.

Outside the Body

These interactions may occur during formulation and mixing of drugs. They may either be:

1. **Physical interactions:** The physical state of either drug is altered when the chemicals are mixed, e.g., **amphotericin** precipitates if mixed with normal saline instead of 5 percent dextrose.
2. **Chemical interactions:** The components of a drug mixture interact to form chemically altered products, e.g., methicillin and kanamycin; aminophylline and chlorpromazine; dopamine and sodium bicarbonate; furosemide and ascorbic acid.

General guidelines to avoid such interactions occurring *in vitro:* (i) Do not add drugs to blood or amino acid solutions; (ii) In the absence of special knowledge, a drug should only be added to simple solutions (normal saline, dextrose, dextro-saline); (iii) Interactions may occur without any visible changes in the solution; (iv) Drugs should be mixed with the infusion fluid immediately before use; (v) Single drug additions to simple solutions are likely to be safe; and (vi) Drug firm package inserts should be consulted.

Inside the Body

Most of the drug interactions occurring inside the body can be categorized as either **pharmacokinetic** or **pharmacodynamic** interactions.

Pharmacokinetic Interactions

Interactions During Gastrointestinal Absorption

Decreased gut motility by agents like **atropine** increases the total absorption of drugs. The **purgatives** decrease drug absorption by speeding the passage of material through the intestine.

Antacids that contain calcium, magnesium or aluminium interfere with the absorption of **tetracycline** which forms chelates with these metals.

Interactions During Distribution

Plasma Protein Binding

The portion of the drug which is being transported in the **bound** form is pharmacologically inactive, and only the **free** molecules that diffuse into the tissues exert their effect. The presence of a second drug with a **higher affinity** for protein, competes with the first drug, producing serious toxicity. **Tolbutamide** can be displaced by **dicoumarol** resulting in severe hypoglycaemia. Certain drugs which have a higher binding affinity to plasma proteins displace agents with lower binding affinities **(Table 1.2).**

Interactions During Biotransformation

Table 1.2: *Displacement of drugs from plasma protein binding sites*

Drug displaced (lower binding affinity)	*Displacing agent (higher binding affinity)*
Acetaminophen	Clofibrate, phenytoin, salicylates
Methotrexate	Salicylates, sulphonamides
Sulphonamides	Warfarin, salicylates, tolbutamide
Warfarin	Clofibrate, salicylates, phenytoin, sulphinpyrazone

Enzyme induction: Liver microsomal enzymes involved in drug metabolism can be stimulated by drugs including *barbiturates, hydantoins, griseofulvin, chlorinated hydrocarbon insecticides,* and many others. This is termed as enzyme induction and results in a reduced therapeutic response to those drugs that are metabolized by microsomal enzymes **(Table 1.3)**.

Table 1.3: *Drugs that induce the metabolism of other drugs*

Inducer	*Drugs affected*
Alcohol	Tolbutamide
Haloperidol	Warfarin
Phenobarbital	Adriamycin, barbiturates, bishydroxycoumarin, cortisol, cyclophosphamide, digitoxin, griseofulvin, phenytoin, progesterone, testosterone, thyroxine, warfarin
Phenytoin	Steroid hormones
DDT	Steroid hormones

Enzyme inhibition: Compounds that interfere with the activity of inactivating enzymes can potentiate the action of other drugs.

A therapeutically useful interaction based on enzyme inhibition is the combination of **carbidopa** with **levodopa.** Carbidopa competitively inhibits the enzyme dopa decarboxylase peripherally (outside the brain). Thus, peripheral dopa decarboxylase inhibition permits a greater fraction of the dose of levodopa to enter the brain, leading to increased formation of dopamine, and relieve symptoms of parkinsonism.

Interactions During Excretion

Interactions occurring during excretion of drugs may involve any of the renal excretory processes, i.e., glomerular filtration, tubular reabsorption or active tubular secretion.

Pharmacodynamic Interactions

Interaction at adrenergic nerve terminals: They are of *two* major types: (i) those between monamine oxidase inhibitors (MAOIs) and food stuffs/drugs; and (ii) those between tricyclic antidepressants and catecholamines/hypotensive drugs.

The MAOIs inhibit intraneuronal MAO, and the sensitivity to infused or injected indirectly acting sympathomimetics (amphetamines) is increased. Any foodstuff or beverage which contains *tyramine* may cause the release of accumulated noradrenaline from the adrenergic nerve terminals causing a *hypertensive crisis.* The substances which can interact with MAOIs are: **foodstuffs** - cheese, yoghourt, yeast extract, liver, broad beans; **beverages** - sherry, beer, and **drugs** - levodopa, tricyclic antidepressants.

Interactions in the CNS: The aminoglycoside antibiotics (streptomycin, kanamycin, gentamicin), and the potent loop diuretic frusemide when used concurrently may cause severe ototoxicity.

Interactions in the bronchial tree: Bronchial relaxation depends upon the formation of cyclic 3'5' AMP (c-AMP). The formation of this 'second messenger' is increased when adenylcyclase is stimulated by catecholamines. Alternatively, the breakdown of c-AMP can be inhibited by aminophylline. Thus, the combination of the two may be useful in the treatment of bronchial asthma.

Receptor blockade: The development of drugs that selectively block receptors particularly those of the automonic nervous system, has led to several important interactions, e.g., alpha-adrenoceptor blockade with *phenoxybenzamine* prevents the action of noradrenaline and other alpha-sympathomimetics; beta-blockade with *propranolol* reduces or abolishes the cardiac stimulating activity of adrenaline and isoprenaline.

Interactions in the heart: Interactions at this site mainly involve the beta-adrenoceptor blockers and cardiac-glycosides. The beta-blockers can produce a profound bradycardia, and delay auriculoventricular conduction. The cardiotoxicity of **cardiac glycosides** increases to 3-fold by hypokalaemia induced by diuretics.

ADVERSE DRUG INTERACTIONS

The number of potential drug interactions is large. Caution must be exercised whenever drugs are prescribed concurrently with *digitalis glycosides, anticonvulsants, oral anticoagulants, oral hypoglycaemics, cytotoxic agents, hypotensives* and *MAOIs* **(Table 1.4)**.

Table 1.4: *Some clinically observed adverse drug interactions*

Major symptoms	*Interacting drugs*
Hypertensive crisis	MAOI + Tyramine (cheese)
	MAOI + methamphetamine
Haemorrhagic episodes	Warfarin + sulphinpyrazone
Hypoglycaemic reaction	Tolbutamide + sulfisoxazole
Cardiac arrhythmias	Digitalis + chlorothiazide
Respiratory paralysis	Neomycin + succinylcholine
	Neomycin + ether

Here mention must also be made about *fixed dose combination products* available in the market. Majority of fixed-dose combinations have certain *disadvantages*: (i) the dosage of individual ingredients cannot be adjusted to suit a particular patient; (ii) there is a likelihood of some ingredients being administered unnecessarily to the patient; and (iii) the higher cost of the product is to be borne by the patient.

There are, however certain *advantages* of fixed dose combinations like: (i) the synergistic effect of aspirin with codeine for analgesia; and (ii) improved compliance by the patient.

1.9 DISCOVERY AND DEVELOPMENT OF NEW DRUGS

In ancient times, most drugs were derived from naturally occurring substances of plant origin, e.g., **opium** from poppy, **quinine** from cinchona, and **digitalis** from foxglove. Presently the majority of new drugs are **synthetic** in nature.

DRUG DISCOVERY

The starting point for the discovery of a new drug is mainly by the following **five** procedures:

i. **Random screening:** New chemical entities are subjected to a battery of screening tests designed to determine different types of biological activity.
ii. **Molecular manipulation:** Chemical analogues of existing drugs are synthesized and tested for their biological activity.
iii. **Molecular designing:** This is the most rational form of drug research and development. It aims at designing of substances to fulfil a specific biological task, e.g., **dopamine** for cardiogenic shock; **levodopa** for parkinsonism; **allopurinol** for gout.
iv. **Metabolites of drugs:** Sometimes active metabolites of drugs are found to possess therapeutic advantages over the parent compound, e.g., **paracetamol** is a metabolite of phenacetin and is effective as an analgesic, but does not cause renal damage.
v. **Serendipity:** It means 'happy observation by chance' and has led to the introduction of many useful remedies in the past, e.g., **penicillin** as an antibacterial agent;

lignocaine and **phenytoin** as antiarrhythmics; **amphetamines** to control hyperkinetic behaviour in children.

DRUG DEVELOPMENT

Chemical synthetic activity is mostly carried out by the **synthetic chemist.** The structure-activity relationships (SAR) are determined. After synthesis the structure of the new compound and its purity is determined, and confirmed by the **analytical chemist**. The study of a promising compound can be divided into *two* stages: (i) **preclinical pharmacology** (animal studies); and (ii) **clinical pharmacology** (human studies).

These preclinical data are scrupulously screened and analysed by the **Drug Control Authority** of the country, and if considered safe, permission for human trials is granted. The drug is then subjected to a **clinical trial** under the guidance and supervision of a **clinical pharmacologist**, and a specialist **clinician.**

To *summarize*, the following steps are involved in the development of a new drug:

1. Preliminary synthesis and physico-chemical analysis.
2. Preliminary biological evaluation.
3. Secondary and specific biological evaluation.
4. Range finding toxicological studies.
5. Target organ toxicological studies.
6. Acute and subacute toxicological studies.
7. Metabolic studies.
8. Synthesis and quality control of bulk material.
9. **Phase I clinical evaluation** (human toxicity and metabolic studies).
10. Final formulation, and final physico-chemical analysis.
11. **Phase II clinical evaluation** (Broad efficacy and tolerance studies in a large population of patients; chronic toxicological studies).
12. **Phase III clinical evaluation** (Broad efficacy and tolerance studies in a large population of patients; chronic toxicological studies).
13. **Phase IV clinical evaluation** (Surveillance during general clinical use).

Steps 1, 8 and 10 involve **medicinal chemistry** and **pharmaceutics.** Steps 2 to 7 are covered by **preclinical pharmacological evaluation** of the drug in animals. Step 9, 11 and 12 are in the domain of **clinical pharmacological evaluation** of the drug in humans. Step 13 is an ongoing process of surveillance to ensure safe use of the drug. If all these steps are satisfactorily passed by the drug, it is granted **registration as a new drug** for use in man.

Preclinical Evaluation (Animal Studies)

The candidate drug is subjected to extensive pharmacological testing *in vivo* in animals and on *in vitro* preparations. In addition, its pharmacokinetics is studied in animals.

The *three* major areas of preclinical evaluation are:

1. Acute, subacute and chronic toxicity studies (toxicity profile).
2. Therapeutic index (safety and efficacy evaluation).
3. Absorption, distribution and elimination studies (pharmacokinetics).

Therapeutic Index

Therapeutic index refers to the relative **margin of safety** of a drug. The **median lethal dose** (LD_{50}) for the drug, which is lethal to 50 percent of the test population of animals is determined. Then the dose which is effective in 50 percent of the test population, termed as the **median effective dose** (ED_{50}) is estimated. The ratio of the LD_{50} to the ED_{50} is the therapeutic index (TI).

$$\text{Therapeutic index (TI)} = \frac{LD_{50}}{LD_{50}}$$

The TI indicates how close the effective dose is to the lethal dose for 50 percent of the test population.

Absorption, Distribution and Elimination (Pharmacokinetics)

All promising new compounds are subjected to pharmacokinetic studies in several species of animals, usually rats, dogs and sometimes monkeys. These studies establish the relative **bioavailability** of the compound on oral or parenteral administration.

CLINICAL EVALUATION (HUMAN STUDIES)

Preclinical data obtained from animal studies provide a **general pharmacological**, **toxicological,** and **pharmacokinetic profile** of the new drug. The New Drug Application, must be submitted to the **Drug Control Authority** for scrutiny, and sanction obtained before clinical evaluation studies are initiated.

In U.K. the introduction of new drugs is regulated by the **Committee on Safety of Medicines** (CSM); and in the USA by the **Food and Drug Administrations** (FDA). In India the **Drug Controller, Government of India**, based in New Delhi is responsible for the organization of this system.

Clinical Pharmacology

In short, clinical pharmacology deals with the effect of drugs on the body, and the effect of the body on drugs in man, i.e., the **pharmacodynamic** and **pharmacokinetic** studies in man. It has **three** distinct parts: (i) **Confirmatory pharmacology** in which studies are carried out in healthy volunteers; (ii) **Human biotransformation** studies about the absorption, distribution and elimination of the drug carried out in volunteers; and (iii) **Clinical trials.**

CLINICAL TRIALS

Some salient guidelines are:

i. **Ethics and patient selection:** The Declaration of Helsinki of the World Medical Association (1964) codified recommendations for guidance of doctors in clinical research. **Informed consent** must be obtained in writing from subjects (patients or volunteers), or their guardians if the patient is incapable of giving consent.
ii. **Response measurements:** The end points should be clearly defined.
iii. **Experimental design:** The design of the trial must be statistically sound.

The final stage of a clinical trial is the **statistical analysis** of data obtained. Relatively simple tests like the **Student's t-test**, or the **Chi-square test** may be sufficient to determine the **significance** of results.

1.10 DENTAL PHARMACOLOGY

Dentifrices and Mouthwashes

Dentifrices (Latin. *dens*, tooth; *fricare*, to rub) are *pastes* or *powders* or *gels* used with a tooth brush for cleaning the teeth. Their function is to remove bacterial *plaque; prevent dental caries* and *gingivitis*; and to *desensitize the exposed dentine.*

Mouthwashes or mouthrinses are liquid preparations used for the maintenance of oral hygiene.

The usual ingredients of toothpastes/powders are:

1. **Abrasives**
2. **Thickening/Binding agents**
3. **Humectants**
4. **Solvents**
5. **Detergents (Surfactants)**
6. **Flavouring agents**
7. **Sweeteners**
8. **Colouring agents**
9. **Antiseptics and preservatives**
10. **Special therapeutic additives**

1. **Abrasives:** These are substances used for *abrading, grinding*, or *polishing* the teeth. The

degree of abrasivity depends on the *hardness*, *morphology* of particles, and the *concentration* of the abrasive in the paste.

These abrasives are less hard than the *enamel*, but as hard or harder than the *dentine*. The amount and type of the abrasive in the paste gives it a creamy consistency. Transparent toothpastes (gels) are obtained by mixing abrasives. The abrasive effect is measured on the RDA (Radioactive Dentine Abrasion) scale, and ranges from 40-80 on the RDA scale.

Examples: Hydrated silica, alumina, and calcium carbonate. Other agents include dicalcium phosphate, calcium pyrophosphate, and chemically inert plastic particles.

2. **Thickening/Binding agents:** These agents bind water and prevent the toothpaste from drying. Binders control the viscosity and give the paste a creamy consistency. They have an emulsifying effect preventing solids and liquids separating out. *Examples*: Carboxymethylcellulose is commonly used, and forms an adhesive gel by imbibing water. Other agents include glycerol, sorbitol, polyethylene glycol, and propylene glycol.

3. **Humectants:** These short-chained polyalcohols are hygroscopic, and keep the paste soft and creamy when exposed to air. *Examples:* Glycerine and sorbitol.

4. **Solvents:** Water is the most common solvent used in toothpastes. Alcohol is used as a solvent and taste enhancer in mouth rinses.

5. **Detergents (Surfactants):** These surface active agents possess both hydrophobic and hydrophilic properties. They exert a cleaning and antibacterial effect. *Example:* Sodium lauryl sarcosinate (SLS) is preferred to soaps used in the past.

6. **Flavouring agents:** These agents are used to provide a sensation of 'tingling freshness' to toothpastes and mouthwashes. *Examples:* Essential oils like spearmint, peppermint, eucalyptus, and menthol.

7. **Sweeteners:** Sodium saccharine, sorbitol and glycerine are used to improve the taste. Xylitol is a sweetener with an anti-caries activity.

8. **Colouring agents:** Titanium dioxide is used to give a white opaque colour. For *red* colour liquor azorubri or liquor caramini is used. For blue colour methylene blue is used.

9. **Antiseptics and preservatives:** Antiseptics in toothpastes have a mild and transient action. Commonly used agents are thymol, eugenol, cinnamon, benzoic acid, and myrrh. *Chlorhexidine* is claimed to inhibit plaque formation. Antacids like *magnesium hydroxide* may be used to neutralize the acid produced on the surface of the teeth inhibiting tooth decay. But plaque is resistant to momentary changes in pH. *Preservatives* prevent the growth of micro-organisms. *Examples:* Sodium benzoate, methylparaben, and ethylparaben.

Special Therapeutic additives

One or more therapeutic agents may be added to toothpastes and mouthwashes, namely, *anti-caries; anti-plaque; anti-calculus, anti-dentine hypersensitivity; anti-aphthous ulcer; whitening agents;* and *anti-halitosis.*

Anti-caries agents

Fluoride is considered to be the most effective caries-inhibiting agent. Commonly used fluorides are sodium fluoride, monofluoro-phosphate, and stannous fluoride. The fluoride amount in the toothpaste is between 0.01 to 0.15%.

Xylitol is a sugar alcohol, and exerts *cariostatic* effect by inhibiting carbohydrate metabolism in many oral micro-organisms. Reduction in acid formation from glucose, leads to reduction in plaque formation.

Calcium phosphate addition in toothpastes and mouthwashes improves the remineralisation and fluoride uptake by the teeth.

Sodium bicarbonate increases the pH of saliva and creates a hostile environment for the growth of *acid-forming bacteria,* and suppresses their virulence. In addition it prevents caries by reducing enamel solubility and increasing remineralisation of enamel.

Anti-plaque agents

Sodium Lauryl Sulphate (SLS): The enzymes *glucosyltransferase* and *fructosyltransferase* sythesise *glucan in situ* from *sucrose* which provides a surface for colonization of *Streptococcus mutans*. This bacterium is responsible for growth of *plaque*. SLS inhibits these enzymes and checks the regrowth of plaque.

Triclosan: It is a synthetic non-ionic chlorinated phenolic compound with antiseptic properties. Triclosan has broad-spectrum efficacy against *Gram +ive,* and *most Gram –ive bacteria, mycobacteria, anaerobic bacteria*, and *fungi (Candida species)*. By its action on the cytoplasmic membrane it causes *lysis* of micro-organisms. It also has an anti-inflammatory action and inhibits both *cyclo-oxygenase (COX) and lipoxygenase (LOX)*. This in turn inhibits the production of *prostaglandin* and *leukotrienes.* It also reduces oral mucosal irritation caused by SLS.

Metal ions: Widely used metal ions in dental preparations are zinc as *zinc chloride*, and stannous-ions as *stannous fluoride.* These metals limit bacterial growth and plaque formation, and exert a *cariostatic* activity.

Essential oils: Thymol, menthol, eucalyptol, and methyl salicylate have antibacterial activity. Mouth rinses containing these active ingredients inhibit plaque formation and gingivitis.

Chlorhexidine: Chlorhexidine preparations are considered to be "gold standards" for antiplaque mouthwashes due to their prolonged broad-spectrum antimicrobial activity. It is retained in the oral cavity for 24 hours by binding to phosphate, sulphate, and carboxyl groups in bacteria, plaque, saliva, and on the enamel surface. Local side effects include taste disturbance, and staining of teeth and tongue. Its use must be restricted to a short-term measure.

Anti-calculus Agents

Anti-calculus agents delay dental plaque calcification, and promote plaque removal by tooth brushing.

Pyrophosphate: It inhibits the formation of supragingival dental calculus. The salts used are *tetrasodium, tetrapotassium*, or *disodium pyrophosphate.* Pyrophosphate has a high affinity for hydroxyapatite (HA) surfaces by interaction with ionic calcium. This interaction on the enamel surface inhibits calcium phosphate (tartar) formation.

Zinc: It has an anti-calculus effect due to its anti-plaque activity. In addition, it inhibits calculus formation by inhibiting crystal growth.

Anti-aphthous ulcer Agents

Aminoglucosidase and Glucose oxidase: A dentifrice containing a combination of these two enzymes reduces the frequency of recurrent aphthous ulcers. The ulcers become smaller, and the healing time is shorter. Ultimately the frequency of aphthous ulcer episodes is decreased.

Whitening Agents

Whitening toothpastes prevent stain formation, remove surface stains with abrasives, and polish the teeth.

Abrasives: These agents effectively remove the *discoloured pellicle,* which is a brown to black coating that forms near the gingival margin of the teeth as a result of improper brushing. *Examples* include *hydrated silica, alumina,* and *calcium carbonate.*

Dimethicones: These substances chemically range from low molecular weight *polydimethyl-siloxane* fluids to high molecular weight polymers which are gum-like in nature. They smoothen the tooth surface thereby prevent stain formation.

Papain: It is sulfhydryl protease consisting of a single polypeptide chain extracted from *Carica papaya* plant. It possesses a proteolytic action, and is used as a non-abrasive whitening agent.

Sodium bicarbonate: It is effective in removing *intrinsic* tooth stains.

Anti-halitosis Agents

Bad breath or *halitosis* originates mainly from the mouth. The unpleasant smell is due to the retention of anaerobic Gram –ive bacteria in the mouth. These bacteria use sulphur-containing amino acids as substrates and produce *fowl-smelling volatile sulphur-containing compounds* (VSC). Lately, it has been found that *Solobacterium moorei* is the organism largely responsible for chronic bad breath.
Zinc inhibits the production of VSC in the mouth by interacting with sulphur in the amino acids or their metabolites. It is retained in the mouth for 2-3 hours after tooth brushing.

Tooth Bleaching (Whitening) Agents

Tooth bleaching is a fairly common procedure in dentistry, especially in the field of *cosmetic dentistry.* Deciduous teeth in children are generally whiter than the adult teeth. Genetics plays a role in the colour of teeth. As a person ages adult teeth become darker due to changes in the mineral structure of the teeth. Other causes for *dicoloured teeth include injury, medications (tetracycline), dental restorations, excessive fluoride, tobacco, coffee, tea, soft drinks, red wine*, and *deposits of tartar.*

Tooth whitening can be achieved by two ways: (i) *Peroxide-containing bleaching Agents* which remove surface (extrinsic) and deep (intrinsic) stains; and (ii) *Non-bleaching whitening toothpastes* (dentifrices) which work by physical or chemical action and remove surface stains by polishing or chemical chelation respectively. These products are available over-the-counter (OTC).

Peroxide-containing bleaching agents

A. Home-Use Whiteners

Carbamide peroxide: Dentist-dispensed products usually contain 10% carbamide peroxide (equivalent to about 3% hydrogen peroxide). It is the most commonly used Ingredient in home-use bleaching products.

Mode of action: In a water-based solution carbamide peroxide breaks down into *hydrogen peroxide* and *urea.* Hydrogen peroxide is the active ingredient. Other ingredients of peroxide-containing whiteners include glycerin, carbopol, sodium hydroxide and flavouring agents. Commonly observed side effects are *temporary tooth sensitivity* and *irritation of the oral mucosa* and *gums.* Rarely irreversible tooth damage may occur.

B. In-office Whiteners

Hydrogen peroxide: Professionally applied bleaching products contain *hydrogen peroxide* in concentrations from 15 to 35%, and may be combined with ultraviolet light, or laser which speeds up the whitening process. In the process soft tissues have to be protected by a *rubber dam* or *gel.*

Non-bleaching whitening toothpastes

Many whitening toothpastes (dentifrices) are available OTC. They contain chemical agents to polish and improve tooth appearance by removing surface stains. These pastes contain particles of silica, aluminium oxide, calcium carbonate, or calcium phosphate to grind off surface (extrinsic) stains. They have no effect on intrinsic stains. Dentifrices do not provide whitening levels as attained with bleaching products. Bleaching products should only be used after consultation with a dentist. Newly whitened teeth may more readily absorb stains. Beverages like tea, coffee, and cola drinks should be avoided for several days. Tobacco smoking, and stain-producing foods must be avoided. Brushing twice daily, and flossing once daily is advisable.

Demulcents, Astringents & Caustics

Demulcents

Demulcents are substances which protect the mucous membranes and lessen irritation. They relieve minor pain and inflammation of the mucosa. Demulcents consist of colloidal solutions of gums or proteins which are adsorbed on to the mucosal surface, forming a protective layer.

Gum Acacia: It is the dried exudate from the branches and stems of *Acacia senegal,* and several other species of *Acacia*. As a gummy mucilage it provides a protective coating over the oral mucosa, and is incorporated in antiseptic pastilles for catarrhal infections of the mouth. In addition, gum acacia is used to emulsify oils and suspend powders in water.

Gum Tragacanth: It is the dried gummy exudation obtained by incision from *Astragalus gummifer* and allied species. It forms viscous mucilage with water in concentrations as low as 1 per cent. In dental practice it is a useful demulcent when applied over mucous abrasions caused by dentures. Powdered tragacanth dusted upon the moistened palatial surface of an upper denture forms a valuable fixative, as the gelatinous mass under pressure minimizes air leakage and increases the adhesion by suction.

Glycerol (Glycerine): Glycerine is hygroscopic, absorbs moisture, and is a mild irritant. Thus it is generally hydrated with rose water (2 parts) and used as a protective for the skin and mucosa. Some useful combinations are:

Borax (sodium borate) Glycerine: A 12 per cent by weight solution is used to paint the tongue and throat for *mouth infection.*

Boroglycerine (Glyceryl borate): It is obtained by heating glycerine and boric acid, and used as an demulcent-antiseptic in stomatitis.

Phenol Glycerine: A 16 per cent by weight solution is used as an antiseptic in *ulcerative stomatitis* and *tonsillitis.*

Tannic acid Glycerine: A 15 per cent by weight solution is used as an astringent paint for *infections of the mouth and throat.*

Glycerine may also be used as a sweetening agent in liquid dosage forms, and is a diuretic in high concentrations when taken systemically. *Starch glycerine* is used as an emollient. In the form of a *rectal suppository,* due to its irritant action, it causes evacuation of the bowels.

Astringents

Astringents are chemicals that tend to shrink body tissues when applied topically. Locally they precipitate the proteins which adhere to the surface and offer protection to the underlying mucosal cells. **Styptics** are agents which precipitate surface proteins and arrest capillary oozing of blood. At times these two terms are used interchangeably.

Astringents may be considered under two heads: (i) *Metallic astringents;* and (ii) Vegetable astringents.

Metallic Astringents

Zinc chloride (5 to 10%): It is used to treat *aphthous ulcers* and *ulcerative gingivitis.*

Zinc sulphate (0.5 to 1%): It is used as a mouthwash for *stomatitis* and *chronic alveolar abscess.*

Alum (1 to 2%): It is used as an astringent mouthwash to harden the gums. As a haemostatic powder it may be applied to the gum for *shrinking the ulcerated gum.*

Copper sulphate (0.5 to 2%): It is used as a mouthwash for *indolent ulcers,* and to *clean pyorrhoeal pockets.*

Silver nitrate (10%): The solution is used for the local treatment of *aphthous ulcers.*

Vegetable astringents

Tannic acid: It has an astringent and mild antiseptic action. It hardens the superficial layers of the mucosa, and decreases the absorption of toxins, and checks inflammation. As a 3 to 5 per cent solution it is used as a *mouthwash, dentifrice,* and an *obtundent.* It may also be used as a *styptic* and *mummifying agent.*

Catechu: It is the dried extract obtained from *Oak galls* which are formed by the invasion of wasps and insects on the leaf buds of *Uncaria gambier* which swells up into globular masses. It contains tannic acid, and may be used to harden gums as a mouthwash.

Caustics

Caustics (corrosives) are protoplasmic poisons which cause local necrosis and death of tissues, and at times cause liquefaction. *Eschcharotics (cauterizants)* cause local destruction of tissues and precipitate proteins. Most caustics are also escharotics. Some *acids, alkalies,* and *metallic salts* are used as caustics. Some useful caustics are detailed below:

Trichloracetic acid: It causes dehydration of cells, and dissolution of cellular proteins. In dental practice it is used to cauterize granulation and small *polyps* or *gum growths* as a 50 per cent solution. Also used for aphthous ulcers and pyorrhoeal pockets as a 5 to 20 per cent solution. A dilute solution is used to remove tobacco stains from teeth.

Lactic acid: In suitable dilutions it is used to treat gingivitis, aphthous ulcers, leukoplakia, and pyorrhoeal pockets.

Silver nitrate: It is a clear, colourless, crystalline substance, freely soluble in water, and rapidly darkens on exposure to light. As a 10 per cent solution it is used to treat *infected aphthous ulcers.* As toughened silver nitrate it is used for *cauterization of wounds*, and for *removing granulation tissue* and *warts.*

Zinc chloride: It can be used as a substitute for silver nitrate. As a 5 to 10 percent solution it is used to desensitize exposed dentine.

Copper sulphate: It is an astringent and fungicide, and used to remove unhealthy granulations from pyorrhoeal pockets.

Carbolic acid (Phenol): Locally it is an escharotic and anaesthetic as a 3 to 4 per cent solution. It has antiseptic, obtundent, caustic, and styptic properties. It is used to remove pieces of *hypertrophied gums*, and to *control gingival seepage during cavity preparation.* Phenol should be used with care as it can produce internal and external *white burns.*

Dental Protectives & Dressings

Dental protectives and dressings comprise of material used as protective lining for cavities, to prevent staining or chemical irritation of the dentine, and as varnishes applied over synthetic filling material to protect them until setting is complete over time. They also help in the healing process. Some commonly used dental protectives are detailed below:

Zinc oxide: It is a white, colourless, tasteless powder, insoluble in water. It is an astringent and antiseptic on topical application. As a protective it provides a base for ointments and cements. Internally it acts as an *antiseptic* and *adsorbent*. *Uses:* (i) used with *carbolised resin* as a dressing in cavities, and for bleeding sockets after tooth extraction; (ii) for treating *dry socket*; and (iii) used with *eugenol* as an *obtundent* for sensitive teeth.

Resin: It is an amorphous, brittle residue left after distillation of turpentine oil. Resin is applied to *exposed dentine*, and for *sealing the tubules*, whereby it acts as a mechanical barrier to external stimuli.

(a) Carbolised resin: It contains resin (4 parts), carbolic acid (4 parts), and chloroform (3 parts). *Uses:* (i) as an *obtundent* dressing in cavities; (ii) as a *haemostatic* (styptic) plug for bleeding sockets; and (iii) as an *emollient* dressing to treat 'dry socket'.

(b) Cavity varnish: It has its base as resin dissolved in a volatile solvent like ether, chloroform, or acetone. When applied to *silicate fillings*, it protects the gel formation from moisture during the primary setting period. Later the volatile solvent evaporates, leaving the resin as a cover over the filling.

Calcium hydroxide: It is a soft, white, odourless, alkaline salt, bitter in taste. In dental practice it is used as a *bland capping material*. As it is alkaline in reaction, it stimulates odontoblastic activity. *Uses*: It is used as a paste in sterile water for *capping* pulp exposure, and results in complete pulp healing in about 4 weeks. Internally it can be used as an *antacid* and *astringent*.

Petrolatum (Vaseline): Petrolatum (yellow or white soft paraffin, petroleum jelly, paraffin jelly) is a yellow or white substance obtained as an intermediate product on distillation of petroleum. It is a mixture of softer members of paraffin or methane series of hydrocarbons. *Uses:* (i) as an *emollient* application on cracked lips; (ii) applied on discs or strips to protect silicate and cement fillings while *polishing* them; (iii) for applying to the matrix band before inserting a cement filling; (iv) to vaseline instruments before placing a carbolised resin dressing; and (v) to vaseline instruments to prevent rusting. In addition, Vaseline is used as a soothing agent on burns and abrasions of the skin, and as a base for ointments.

Glycerine (Glycerol): It is a clear, colourless syrupy liquid with a sweet taste, miscible with water and alcohol. It is prepared synthetically or obtained as a by product in soap manufacture. It is extensively used as a *solvent* or *vehicle* for many topical drugs. Along with starch it is used as an *emollient* known as *glycerite,* and 50% glycerol in an aqueous solution is a good antiseptic. *Uses:* In dentistry (i) as a solvent for borax (one part borax and 6½ parts of glycerine) applied to the oral mucosa for the treatment of *thrush*, and *stomatitis*; (ii) as a vehicle for pumice for *polishing teeth* and *fillings*; (iii) in the manufacture of *toothpaste*; (iv) it is applied to *carbolic acid burns* in the mouth; and (v) applied to *cracked* or *dry lips* before dental procedures.

Gutta-percha: It is the coagulated milky juice obtained from certain species of rubber trees. Purified gutta-percha is a white, odourless, tasteless, inert mass which readily softens on heating and hardens on cooling. It is soluble in oil of eucalyptus and chloroform. *Uses:* It is used as a *cavity dressing,* and to maintain *optimal space between teeth.*

Obtundents & Mummifying Agents

Obtundents are agents used to dull, diminish or eliminate the sensitivity of the dentine. They can be used to make excavation of the tooth almost painless. *Obtundents* act by: (i) *Paralysing sensory nerve endings*, e.g., phenol, camphor, menthol, thymol, creosote, clove oil, etc.; (ii) *Destruction of nerve tissue*, e.g., alcohol; (iii) *Precipitating proteins*, e.g., zinc chloride, silver nitrate; and (iv) *Blocking action potential in intradermal nerves*, e.g., potassium salts.

Ideal obtundents are those which cause least of irritation, do not stain the dentine, and are potent enough to diminish its sensitivity. The drawback is that they may shrink the pulp. Some major agents are detailed below:

Sensory nerve paralysers

Phenol (Carbolic acid): It has colourless crystals, liquefied by addition of water (10%). Locally it has a rapid obtundent action, and does not stain healthy dentine. It is a protoplasmic poison by nature, but does not penetrate deeply. Numbness is preceded by mild irritation. Penetrability can be increased by combining it with potassium hydroxide and glycerin.

Camphor, Thymol, Menthol: The three are combined in a proportion of 1:2:1 respectively, and used to produce a rapid action in cases of *dry dentine*.

Creosote: It is a mixture of phenols, obtained by fractional distillation of wood. Its action is similar to phenol, with a better penetrability. Like phenol it has antiseptic, deodorant and mild local anaesthetic action.

Clove oil: It is a volatile oil obtained from the dried flower buds of *Eugenia caryophyllum*. Eugenol is its active ingredient, and it has local anaesthetic, antiseptic, and rubefacient action. It is non-irritant, but can stain the dentine yellow. Dressing of zinc oxide and clove oil may be used to relieve pain of an infected dry socket.

Destruction of nerve tissue

Alcohol: Ethyl alcohol as a 70% solution has optimal penetrability into tissues. It does not stain the dentine, is non-toxic to the pulp, and does not penetrate very deeply. It acts by precipitating protein in the dentine, and painless excavation is possible. *Benzyl alcohol* can also be used as it has a local anaesthetic activity.

Protein precipitation

Zinc chloride: Its local application in a concentrated form leads to precipitation of dentinal proteins, and desensitization. It does not penetrate deeply, and does not stain teeth.

Silver nitrate: It is a clear, colourless, crystalline substance, freely soluble in water, and rapidly darkening on exposure to air. Locally it acts as a protein coagulant, astringent, antiseptic, and caustic. Contact with gums has to be avoided. With the advent of local anaesthetics the use of obtundents has declined. *Xylocaine* is now used by hypodermic injection or topical application.

Nerve action potential blockers

Potassium salts: Potassium ions block action potential generation in intradermal nerves. They increase the concentration of potassium ions around pulpal nerves, and depolarize the nerves. Thus potassium desensitizes the dentine, but its inclusion in toothpates is controversial.

Mummifying agents

These agents are used to harden the pulp tissue and root canal so as to maintain aseptic conditions, especially when it is not possible to remove the pulp and the contents of the root canal completely. These agents have *astringent* and *aseptic* properties, as outlined below:

Paraformaldehyde: It acts by slow liberation of formaldehyde. The action is slow and painless without any staining. Sometimes it may penetrate the pulp and cause inflammation.

Iodoform: It acts by slow liberation of iodine, and has both *antiseptic* and *anodyne* properties. It may be mixed with other agents like tannic acid, eugenol, cinnamon oil and glycerin to form a paste.

Tannic acid: It is an *astringent* and hardens the tissues, which avoids infection. The advantage is that it causes shrinkage of tissues. But if absorbed in large amounts it may cause liver damage.

Root Canal Filling Materials

Root canal treatment is an "endodontic treatment" to treat the inside of the tooth, and is carried out by *endodontists*. It is indicated when the pulp in the root canal becomes inflamed or infected due to tooth decay. If left untreated, it causes severe pain and leads to abscess formation.

In the root canal procedure the inflamed or infected pulp is removed, the inside of the canal is cleaned and smoothened, and then the space is filled and sealed with *temporary filling material*. It is essential that the root canal before filling is made aseptic. After 6-8 weeks the space is filled with permanent filling material, and the dentist places a *crown (cap)*, or other restoration on top, and then the tooth becomes functional. *Filling materials* used to fill the root canal must be *biocompatible*. The most popular material used is *gutta-percha*, a rubber-like material.

Gutta-percha: In the Malay language *gatah* means gum; *percha* means a tree. Gutta-percha is the coagulated, purified, dried milky juice (latex) of several trees belonging to the Sapotaceae family. It is used as a filling material in the form of *semisolid cones* or *points* and *zinc oxide*. Gutta-percha is placed with an adhesive cement to completely seal the root canal. Temporary filling material is removed before final restoration. Other materials used for filling include *silver amalgam* and *silver points*.

Dental Caries

Dental caries is an infectious disease which damages the tooth structures, leading to *tooth decay* or *dental cavities*. These three terms are often used as synonyms. If untreated, it leads to pain, infection, periodontitis, and tooth loss.

Tooth decay is caused by certain acid-producing bacteria, mainly *Lactobacillus* and *Streptococcus mutans*, which cause damage in the presence of fermentable carbohydrates like *glucose, fructose*, and *sucrose*. The resultant high levels of *lactic acid* in the mouth damage the teeth. Normally there is a constant state of *demineralisation* and *remineralisation* between the tooth and the surrounding saliva, but when the pH at the tooth surface drops below 5.5 (acidic), demineralization proceeds faster. This leads to loss of mineral structure and tooth decay. Acid-producing bacteria, food debris, and saliva combine in the mouth to form a sticky substance called *plaque*. It adheres to the teeth just above the gum line, and at the edges of fillings. If the plaque is not removed regularly by tooth brushing, it mineralizes into *tartar*, which irritates the gums and results in periodontitis. The acid in the plaque dissolves the enamel surface and creates holes (cavities), which are initially painless. When these cavities reach deep into the pulp of the tooth, there is extreme pain ultimately leading to *tooth loss*.

Depending on the location there are two types of caries: (i) *Pit and fissure caries* located on the chewing surfaces of the molars; and (ii) *Smooth surface caries* which involves the roots and other smooth surfaces of the tooth. Depending on the depth of involvement of the hard tooth tissue, it may be labeled as *"dentinal caries"* or if deeper, *"cementum caries"*.

Prevention of Dental Caries

The main factors responsible for development of caries include *cariogenic bacteria, bacterial plaque, dietary sugar* for acid production, *stagnation of food* material in the mouth, and *susceptible dental tissues*.

Oral hygiene and *dietary modification* are necessary to prevent caries. *Brushing* of teeth twice, and *flossing* once daily, with regular dental checkup is advisable. In addition, minimise snacking, and sipping of sugary drinks. Dental sealants and fluoride are recommended to protect against caries.

Fluorides

Fluoride is the most effective caries-inhibiting agent, and many *toothpastes* and *mouthwashes* today contain fluoride in some form or the other. The most common form is *sodium fluoride,* but *mono-fluoro-phosphate,* and *stannous fluoride* are also used. The fluoride content in *toothpastes* is between 0.10 to 0.15%. Fluoride *rinses* are also available.

Mechanism of action: There are *three* main theories about the action of fluoride in the prevention of caries:

(i) Fluoride is incorporated into the enamel during tooth development, and replaces hydroxyl groups to form *calcium fluorophosphate.* Fluoroapatite is more resistant to acid than hydroxyapatite. This provides *"caries resistance",* which once attained lasts always, and mineralization of teeth is more effective. A caution is that too much fluoride during tooth development age can cause dental fluorosis.

(ii) Fluoride has *antibacterial* action. The *hydrogen fluoride* formed penetrates the bacterial cell membrane, and kills the bacteria.

(iii) Fluoride is incorporated into the bacterial plaque, and on the enamel surface as *calcium fluoride.* This diffuses with acid from the plaque into the enamel pores and forms *fluoroapatite,* which is more resistant to subsequent acid attacks. Thus fluoride decreases the demineraisation and increases remineralisation of the enamel.

When fluorides are to be applied topically, the plaque should be removed beforehand, so that adequate concentrations reach the enamel surface.

Methods of use: Fluorides act on teeth both on *systemic* or *local* administration:

***Fluorides in drinking water*:** They are most effective when ingested during the period of dental development. According to the WHO drinking water supply should ideally maintain a fluoride concentration of one part per million (ppm). For example, in certain geo-environmental areas in southern Rajasthan the ground water fluoride level ranges from 1.5 to 4.0 ppm. Such high levels lead to dental and skeletal fluorosis.

***Fluoride tablets*:** These contain 0.25 to 1.0 mg of fluoride in lactose base. Mottling of enamel can be a complication, specially if a fluorinated dentifrice is also being used. Fluoride tablets may be used where fluoride content in drinking water is less than 0.3 ppm.

***Fluoride toothpastes*:** Dentifrices are an effective method of using fluoride. When the teeth are brushed regularly the fluoride salt comes in contact with the enamel. Fluoride toothpastes contain *sodium fluoride,* or *sodium monofluorophosphate* with a mild abrasive. These toothpastes can reduce caries by 20 to 30%. It is doubtful whether it is safe for infants to use fluoride toothpastes, as a lot of fluoride can be swallowed resulting in '*mottling*' of teeth.

***Fluoride mouthwashes*:** Best results have been obtained by daily use of *0.05% sodium fluoride solution* rinsed round the mouth for 1 or 2 minutes under supervision.

Fluorides for topical application:

1. **Sodium fluoride:** It is usually applied as a 2% solution. It is chemically stable, has to be stored in plastic containers, is not irritating to the gums, and does not stain teeth.

2. **Stannous fluoride:** It is used as 2 to 8% solution, and is more effective than sodium fluoride. Its disadvantage is that it is unstable in water, has an unpleasant taste, and causes gingival irritation.

3. **Acidulated phosphate fluoride (APF):** It is a solution of sodium fluoride in weak phosphoric acid. It increases the uptake of fluoride by enamel more compared to sodium fluoride or stannous fluoride. APF gels are applied to the teeth in trays, in caries-prone children under supervision. Undue ingestion of the gel may lead to nausea.

Adverse effects of Fluorides:

Ingestion of an overdose of sodium fluoride can cause *acute poisoning* manifested as nausea, vomiting, diarrhoea, and bleeding from gums. *Chronic endemic fluorosis* affects the teeth, bony skeleton, and other organs.

Dental fluorosis*:** The enamel is *mottled* when the fluoride content of drinking water exceeds 2 to 4 ppm. In early stages the teeth have chalky white patches, which later become brownish. In advanced stages the enamel is 'pitted' and 'brittle'. ***Skeletal fluorosis: It develops when the fluoride content of drinking water is between 4 and 14 ppm, as in certain geographic belts in North India. Its main feature is *excessive calcification.* The *osteophytes* formed at the margins of joints, tendons, and ligaments lead to fusion of joints. The vertebral column becomes rigid. The neural canal is narrowed, and compresses the spinal cord, leading to *paraplegia.*

In conclusion, the fluorides have serious toxic effects, manifested after many years in life. Fluorides undoubtedly increase the resistance of teeth to caries. Use of *fluoridized toothpastes* has caused a striking decline in the prevalence of caries. In addition, *dietary modification* also has a role to play in the prevention of caries.

Treatment:

Destroyed tooth structure does not regenerate. But the progression of cavities can be checked by treatment to preserve the tooth, and prevent complications like *tooth abscess, fractured tooth, pain*, and *tooth hypersensitivity*.

Restorative materials: For filling tooth cavities the decayed material is removed by drilling, and replaced by restorative material like *silver alloy, gold, porcelain,* or *composite resin.* Porcelain and composite resin can be made to match the natural appearance of the tooth, specially for the front teeth. *Alloy* (amalgam) and *gold* are stronger and used on back teeth. If the decay is extensive, a covering jacket or "cap" (crown) is fitted over the affected tooth. Crowns are often made of *gold, porcelain*, or *porcelain with fused metal.*

Silver-coloured metal dental fillings contain *mercury* that can cause health problems, and neurotoxic effects on the CNS of pregnant mothers, and fetuses. In this connection the US FDA has issued an 'alert' notice, and caution has to be exercised.

Dental sealants: These are thin plastic-like coatings applied to the worn out chewing surfaces of molars for *prevention of accumulation of plaque.*

Root canal therapy: This is recommended if the pulp in the tooth dies due to infection and decay, or trauma. The centre of the tooth, including the nerve and blood vessels (pulp) is removed along with decayed portion of the tooth. The clean canal is then filled with a rubber-like material called *gutta-percha,* and a crown can be fixed over it. If all efforts fail to save the tooth, an extraction has to be done.

SPECIAL TOPICS

Use of Steroids in Dentistry

Adrenal corticosteroids have potent *anti-inflammatory, antitoxic,* and *antiallergic* activity **(Chap. 7.5)**. Specific use in dentistry is summarized below:

Oral mucosal lesions: Steroids are used to treat oral ulceration and mucosal lesions like *erosive lichen planus, erythema multiforme,* and *pemphigus*. Both topical and systemic steroids may have to be administered. In severe cases steroids have to be injected into and around the lesion. Topical steroid preparations are: *triamcinolone acetonide* 0.1%; *hydrocortisone succinate* 2.5 mg; and *betamethasone 17-valerate* spray. Intralesional steroids are *triamcinolone hexacetonide* and *hydrocortisone acetate.* For systemic use *prednisolone* is employed.

Temporomandibular joint pain: Intra-articular injections of *hydrocortisone* or *prednisolone* are used for pain relief.

Bell's palsy: It is a unilateral facial paralysis of one or more branches of the facial nerve (VII cranial), usually thought to be viral in aetiology. Initially high dose treatment is started within 5 days of onset, and tapered off over 10-12 days.

Postoperative pain and swelling: To reduce the pain and swelling after operations like removal of an *impacted third molar*, a short course of *methylprednisolone* or *betamethasone* is helpful.

Anaphylactic and hypersensitivity reactions: Treatment outline is detailed in Chapter 4.6.

Use of Analgesics in Dentistry

Morphine and related analgesics are used as potent analgesics for relieving moderate to severe pain, but their application in dentistry is limited. Dental pain like *in pulpitis, dry socket, or perichondritis* is effectively treated by local measures.

Pain after dental surgical procedures has an inflammatory component. Opioids are devoid of any anti-inflammatory activity. Thus, analgesics like the NSAIDs are more effective than opioids.

Use of Local Anaesthetics in Dentistry

The pharmacology of local anaesthetics is detailed in Chapter 3.8. In dental practice the following factors have to be kept in mind:

Cocaine HCl: It is used as a 10% solution and has a rapid onset of action. Because of its *sympathomimetic* properties and *strong stimulant action on the CNS,* and potential to produce *dependence*, its use is restricted to topical application.

Benzocaine: It is an insoluble and stable compound, and is used topically in the form of *lozenges*, with or without *menthol.* It helps patients unable to tolerate dentures. Occasionally used to relieve pain of severe oral ulceration.

Procaine HCl: Procaine with adrenaline is seldom used these days. But it is useful in patients sensitive to lignocaine as an infiltration anaesthetic.

Lignocaine HCl (Lidocaine): It is used as an infiltration anaesthetic when use of procaine with adrenaline is dangerous, e.g., in patients with cardiovascular disease or hyperthyroidism.

Prilocaine HCl with felypressin: Prilocaine is used as an infiltration anaesthetic when procaine with adrenaline is contraindicated, e.g., in patients with cardiovascular disease or hypertension. It is combined with *felypressin* when a long duration of anaesthesia is required.

Mepivacaine HCl: It is available as a 3% (1.8 ml cartridge) for infiltration anaesthesia. It is a short-acting agent.

Bupivacaine HCl (Marcain): It is used as an injection with adrenaline, and has a fairly rapid onset of action (4 minutes), with a long duration of action (6-7 hours). It also reduces postoperative analgesic requirements.

Dental uses of Antiseptics and Disinfectants

Antiseptics are substances which inhibit the growth of micro-organisms at the site of application, i.e., they are *bacteriostatic.* Whereas, the term *disinfectant* is usually applied to substances used for destruction of pathogenic organisms on inanimate objects, and are *bactericidal* in nature. Disinfectants are used on objects like surgical equipment for which heat sterilization is not possible. These *local anti-infective agents* are detailed in **Chapter 10.**

Dental applications of some agents are outlined below:

Alcohols: *Ethyl alcohol* and *isopropyl alcohol* (50 to 70% by weight) are used for disinfection of the skin. Alcohol is a *protoplasmic poison.*

Aldehydes

Formaldehyde: It has bactericidal activity against bacteria, fungi, and viruses. But the action is slow. In 2 to 8% concentrations it is used to disinfect inanimate objects. In vapour form it is used to sterilize blankets, and rooms.

Glutaraldehyde: It is superior to formaldehyde and acts on all micro-organisms, including *hepatitis B virus.* It is used in 2% concentrations for cold sterilization of surgical instruments. Exposure should be for at least 1 hour or preferably up to 12 hours.

Chlorhexidine gluconate: It is a strong bactericidal compound, non-irritant to tissues, and used to treat superficial infections by Gram +ive bacteria. In dentistry it is used as a mouthwash for treatment of *aphthous ulcers* and *prophylaxis of dental caries.* It acts by adsorbing on to the enamel and dentine. *Side effects* include skin sensitivity, tissue damage, and bleeding from mucosal surfaces. Taste disturbance, staining of teeth, and swelling of the parotid gland may occur. Many preparations (solutions, creams, gels, mouthwashes) are available, depending on the use.

Dyes

All dyes are derivatives of coal tar. The *aniline dyes* include *gention violet*, and *brilliant green*, and the *acridine dyes* include acriflavine, and *proflavine.*

Gention violet: It is a fungicide, and may be used in the treatment of *oral thrush* (Candidiasis). However antifungal antibiotics are preferred.

Acriflavine and **proflavine** are active against Gram +ive and Gram –ive organisms. They are used for application to superficial wounds.

Halogens

Sodium hypochlorite: A 2% solution is used as an antiseptic irrigant of *root canals,* and is an effective solvent of necrotic tissue. In the process chlorine is liberated which combines with the proteins of tissues and bacteria, exerting a cleansing effect. There is a rapid loss of activity when chlorine liberation ends.

Iodoform, Iodophores (Povidone Iodine), Metacresol acetate, and Camphorated paramonochlorphenol are agents used for the irrigation and sterilization of root canals.

Hexachlorophene: it is very effective against Gram +ive cocci, and is an excellent surface disinfectant. It is used on the skin prior to surgery, and as a pre-surgical hand cream.

To summarize, dental uses of antiseptics are: *(i) pre-operative skin or oral mucosa preparation; (ii) as an ingredient of dentifrices; (iii) inhibition of dental plaque; (iv) irrigation of root canals; 'cold' sterilization of instruments and equipment; (vi) storage of sterilized surgical equipment; (vii) cleaning of the operative field; and (viii) pre-operative preparation of the surgeon's hands.*

Emergencies in Dental Practice

Most of the emergencies considered here are likely to be rare, if proper precautions and pre-procedure evaluation of the patient is done. But the dentist must be able to recognize and manage them, if they occur. He must maintain an *emergency kit of drugs* for immediate use, if needed. Some of the hazards are detailed below:

1. Fainting
2. Angina pectoris/myocardial infarction
3. Cardiac arrest
4. Acute allergic (anaphylactic) reactions
5. Adrenal crisis
6. Epilepsy
7. Hypoglycaemia/hyperglycaemia
8. Drug reactions/interactions
9. Anaesthetic accidents
10. Haemorrhage

1. **Fainting:** The attack is precipitated by anxiety and stress, and the symptoms include nausea, sweating, and dizziness followed by unconsciousness. It is due to transient hypotension, and cerebral ischaemia. These attacks can be terminated by putting the patient flat to improve cerebral circulation. If it fails then *aromatic spirits of ammonia* can be held under the nostril for short inhalation. A *glucose drink* may be provided. In anxious patients sedation with *diazepam* (5 mg, orally) may be administered on the night before, and 1 hour before the procedure. These fainting attacks must be distinguished from other causes of syncope like hypoglycaemic coma, cardiovascular disturbances like heart blocks and bradycardia.

2. **Angina pectoris/myocardial infarction:** Patients with a history of coronary heart disease must be evaluated for their cardiovascular status prior to any dental surgical procedure. Recurrent anginal attacks may lead to *acute myocardial infarction.* Drug management of angina pectoris and myocardial infarction is detailed in **Chapter 4.5.**

3. **Cardiac arrest:** Causes of cardiac arrest include myocardial infarction, anaesthetic accidents, acute anaphylactic reactions, and adrenal crisis. *Cardio-pulmonary resuscitation* (CPR) has to be immediately initiated, as the blood supply cut-off to the brain for 3 minutes or over is likely to cause brain death. Urgent procedures include: (i) thump the patient's chest mid-sternum; (ii) start *external cardiac massage*; (iii) start *artificial ventilation*; and (iv) take measures to increase venous return. These measures are to be taken before the management is taken over by the *Intensive Care Unit* (ICU) staff.

4. **Acute allergic (anaphylactic) reactions:** The main features are bronchospasm with wheeze, circulatory collapse due to widespread vasodilatation and increased capillary permeability. Later, consciousness is lost, and the patient becomes cyanosed. The drug management is outlined in **Chapter 4.6.**

5. **Adrenal Crisis:** Response of patients on long-term steroid therapy is unpredictable, and an *acute circulatory collapse* may occur even after a simple dental extraction. Due to an inadequate response to "stress", some special precautions must be taken: (i) major surgery must be done in a hospital; (ii) minor operations should preferably be done under local anaethesia, and intravenous steroids should be given prophylactically; and (iii) even if brief general anaesthesia is to be given, hydrocortisone hemisuccinate 100 mg IV should be given pre-operatively. These patients should be kept under observation for at least 1 hour after operation. Further details are given in **Chapter 7.5.**

6. **Epilepsy:** If the patient has an attack during dental surgery, they must be prevented from injuring themselves. All appliances should be quickly removed from the mouth. Recovery is fairly rapid. In case *status epilepticus* (seizures in rapid succession) occurs, it has to be managed in a hospital. The drug of choice is *diazepam* (10 mg) intravenously **(Chap. 2.6).**

7. **Hypoglycaemia/hyperglycaemia:** Diabetic patients due to lack of proper control may pass into hypoglycaemia or hyperglycaemic ketosis. It has to be treated as an emergency **(Chap. 7.4).**

8. **Drug reactions / interactions:** These have to be kept in mind during all dental procedures, and a complete drug history of the patient must be obtained prior to all further medication **(Chap. 1.8).**

9. **Anaesthetic accidents:** Use of general anaethetics may cause serious accidents in dental surgery. Overdosage of *intravenous anaesthetics* and anaphylactic reactions has to be guarded against **(Chap. 2.3).**

10. **Haemorrhage:** When there is persistent bleeding from the site of operation without any systemic cause, systemic fibrinolysis-inhibitors like *tranexamic acid* may be used. Locally *haemostatic (styptic) agents* like *gelatin sponge, oxidized cellulose,* or *fibrin foam* may be used **(Chap. 5.2).**

Emergency kit

The "emergency kit" for dental practice should include:

1. **Hydrocortisone sodium succinate:** 100 mg IV or IM, For *anaphylactic shock.*
2. **Adrenaline HCl (I:1000 soln):** o.5 ml IM (must never be given IV). *For anaphylactic shock.*
3. **Chlorpheniramine:** 10 to 20 mg IM or IV. For *allergic reactions.*
4. **Dextrose (10 ml ampoules of 50% solution):** 5 to 20 ml IV. For *hypoglycaemia.*
5. **Glucagon injection:** 0.5 to 1.0 mg IM or SC. For *acute hypoglycaemia.*
6. **Diazepam:** 10 mg IV for adults; for children over 7 years, 5mg; for infants, 2.5 mg/kg body weight IV. For *epilepsy.*
7. **Morphine sulphate injection:** 8 to 20 mg IM or IV. For *myocardial infarction.*
8. **Pethidine HCl injection:** 75 mg IM or IV. For *myocardial infarction.*

Such an "emergency kit" must always be at hand to meet any untoward eventuality.

Drugs Acting on the Central Nervous System

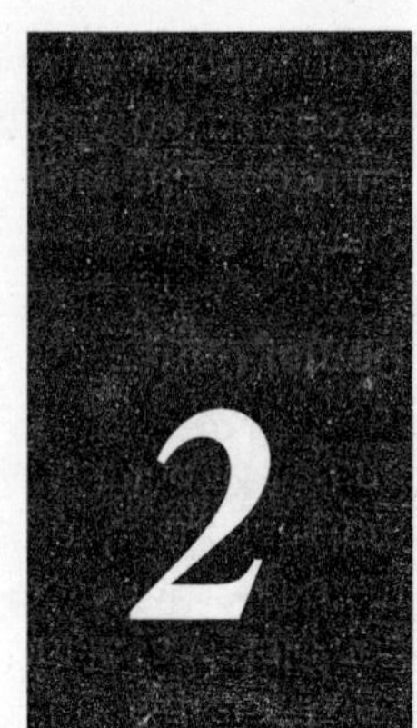

2.1 GENERAL CONSIDERATION

The human nervous system is an extremely complex structure, having more than 12 billion nerve cells or **neurones**. With the **endocrine system,** it coordinates and regulates the functioning of all body organs. Transmission of information in the endocrine system is by circulating **hormones**, and this provides for a slowly developing but long-lasting control, i.e., it functions as a **slow communication system.** In contrast, the **nervous system** can evoke rapid changes in body function as transmission of information is through **electrical** conduction of impulses along nerve fibres, and chemical transmission of impulses by **neurotransmitters** between nerve fibres, resulting in a moment-to-moment control, i.e., it functions as a **rapid communication system.**

DIVISIONS OF THE NERVOUS SYSTEM

The basic organisation of the nervous system is as under:

1. **Central Nervous System**
   i. Brain
   ii. Spinal cord.
2. **Peripheral Nervous System**
   i. Somatic system
   ii. Autonomic system
      a. Parasympathetic division
      b. Sympathetic division.

CENTRAL NERVOUS SYSTEM

The central nervous system (CNS) consists of the brain and spinal cord, and serves to coordinate and direct all body functions. It enables the organism to adapt to a constantly changing environment, thereby maintaining **homeostasis.**

Impulses to the brain (afferent) from sensory receptors, and from the brain (efferent) to the skeletal muscle, are conveyed by a sequence of electrical and chemical means. The sensory and motor branches in combination comprise the somatic system, and the nature of the response is **voluntary.** The ANS is **involuntary** in nature and controls the vegetative functions in the body. Its two divisions maintain a balance of opposing effects on the body's smooth muscle, myocardium, viscera and glands.

The brain has a complex collection of nerve cells and their processes, which are functionally interconnected, but anatomically independent. Information in the form of an impulse originating in a single neurone can propagate throughout the CNS. The transmission process is predominantly a chemical phenomenon in the majority of mammalian synapses.

The brain has three major divisions–the **hindbrain** (myelencephalon, metencephalon), the **midbrain** (mesencephalon), and the **forebrain** (diencephalon, telencephalon). The hindbrain runs from the top of the spinal cord into the midbrain, and includes the **medulla oblongata** and the **pons.** These form the **brainstem** on which the

cerebrum seems to be balanced. Above and behind the brainstem is the **cerebellum.**

FUNCTIONS OF THE CNS

Cerebral Cortex

The cerebrum contains about 9 billion neurones, and is the site for *consciousness.* On removal of the cerebrum the human being becomes totally blind, extensively paralysed, and although primitive vegetative functions can be carried out, death soon follows.

The cerebral cortex contains *sensory, motor* and *association areas* that receive information, which is processed and signals are transmitted to appropriate parts of the body along effector neurones. The **association areas** are responsible for the highest mental activities, namely, **memory, reasoning, judgement** and **imagination**.

Basal Ganglia

The **basal ganglia** comprise three areas in the forebrain–the *caudate nucleus, putamen* and *globus pallidus*–as well as several areas in the midbrain, such as the *substantia nigra, red nucleus* and *subthalamic nucleus.* These structures are responsible for the **integration and regulation of locomotor activity,** and **postural reflexes.** Pathologic changes in these ganglia result in the appearance of movement disorders like **parkinsonism.**

Limbic System

The main group of brain structures controlling emotional behaviour is collectively termed as the **limbic system.** It consists of several subcortical areas **(thalamus, hypothalamus, olfactory** and **pyriform lobes, hippocampus, amygdala, septum, preoptic area** and **portions of the basal ganglia),** and a surrounding ring of cortical tissue on the **medial** and **ventral surfaces of each cerebral hemisphere** (**Fig. 2.1**). The limbic system regulates many aspects of behaviour, like feelings of **pleasure**, **anger**, **rage** and **fear**. It also regulates **biological rhythms, sexual activity, feeding** and **learning.**

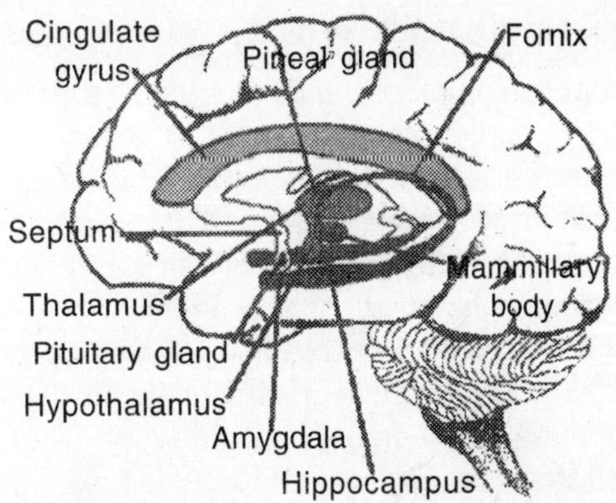

Fig. 2.1: *The limbic system (see text).*

Reticular Formation

The **reticular formation** is a diffuse network of cells and nuclei scattered throughout the brainstem and extending upwards into the midbrain. These **bridge portions** of the CNS contain most of the nuclei of the cranial nerves, as well as the inflow and outflow tracts from the cortices and the spinal cord. The term ascending **reticular activating system** (RAS) is often used with reference to these structures.

Functionally, the RAS serves to arouse the cortex and maintain a state of **alertness** or **arousal.** The function of the RAS is very susceptible to many classes of drugs like **barbiturates, anaesthetics** and **antipsychotics.**

Thus, the **basal ganglia, limbic system** and the **reticular formation** function as integrated systems to control certain aspects of behaviour.

ELECTROENCEPHALOGRAM (EEG)

The EEG is a tracing of changes in voltage that are generated by the brain. Many studies of the effect of drugs on the CNS have made use of the EEG, and in man it is often the only method available for monitoring the level of excitation of the brain.

BASIC NEUROSCIENCE

The functional unit of the CNS is the **neurone**. Most neuropharmacological agents act on the neurone, thereby altering its normal function.

Synaptic transmission between neurones can be affected by altering the levels of the neurotransmitter in the presynaptic neurone. This can be achieved by agents which:(i) block or enhance the *biosynthesis* of the neurotransmitter; (ii) block or enhance the metabolic *degradation* of the neurotransmitter; or (iii) alter the *re-uptake* and *re-utilisation* of the neurotransmitter in the presynaptic terminals.

CNS NEUROTRANSMITTERS

A large number of CNS neurotransmitters have been either tentatively or positively identified. Some of the more important neurotransmitters are considered in greater detail hereunder.

Acetylcholine (ACh) is mainly excitatory in the brain. It was the first compound to be identified as a transmitter in the CNS.

Cholinergic neurones are particularly abundant in the *basal ganglia*, and others are involved in cortical *arousal* responses, and in *memory*. Hence, atropine-like drugs can impair memory.

Gamma-aminobutyric acid (GABA) is present in all areas of the CNS, mainly in *local inhibitory interneurones*. It promptly inhibits central neurones when applied locally.

Drugs which are thought to act by modifying GABAergic synaptic transmission include the **benzodiazepines, barbiturates, alcohols, valproate** and **general anaesthetics.**

Glycine is another inhibitory CNS neurotransmitter. Whereas, GABA is primarily located in the brain, glycine is found predominantly in *spinal interneurones* (ventral horn). Glycine is antagonized by **strychnine,** and its release is prevented by **tetanus toxin,** thereby both substances cause convulsions.

Neuropeptides form a big group of possible central transmitters, but little is known yet about their functions.

The most widely studied of these putative peptide neurotransmitters (or neuromodulators) are the **endorphins** which exhibit pharmacological properties similar to morphine, and can bind to **"morphine receptors"** in the brain.

MONOAMINES

The **catecholamines** generally have **inhibitory** effects when applied locally onto central neurones.

Dopamine among the catecholamines, is the most important neurotransmitter in the CNS, while *noradrenaline* and *adrenaline* are important amine neurotransmitters in the peripheral sympathetic nervous system. Dopamine pathways project from the **substantia nigra** in the midbrain to the **basal ganglia**, and from the midbrain to the limbic cortex and other limbic structures.

Noradrenaline containing cell bodies are located in the *brainstem*. Fibres from these nuclei innervate a large number of cortical and subcortical areas. Functions ascribed to noradrenergic neurones include **learning** and **memory, sleep-wake cycle** and **a role in affective disorders.**

Adrenaline is found only in very low concentration in the mammalian CNS. It is of minor importance in the brain.

Serotonin (5-hydroxytryptamine) is localized in the **raphe nuclei**, and considerable amounts are also present in the **hypothalamus,** the **limbic system,** the **brainstem** and the **pituitary gland**. Current evidence indicates that serotonin is involved in the regulation of several aspects of behaviour, **sleep/wake cycle, temperature control, pain perception, depression, sexual activity, aggressiveness** and **hypothalamic control** of the release of pituitary hormones.

Histamine occurs in the brain, particularly in certain **hypothalamic neurones,** and evidence is strong that histamine is a neurotransmitter. A possible role of histamine in **regulation of food and water intake, thermoregulation, and hormone release** has been suggested.

BLOOD-BRAIN BARRIER

It has been long known that not all substances present in the bloodstream can readily gain entry into the brain. However, this apparent barrier to drugs is **relative** rather than **absolute.** In fact, there are several barriers to substances entering the brain from the systemic circulation.

The term **blood-brain barrier (BBB)** is usually applied to the lack of passage of certain drugs, or other exogenously administered chemicals into the brain.

2.2 ALCOHOL AND ALCOHOLISM

Production of alcohol needs only a few basic ingredients: these are **sugar, water, yeast** and a **warm atmosphere.** It is formed naturally by yeast fermentation of starch and sugar in fruits, grains, potatoes or sugarcane. **Alcoholic beverages** have been used as nutritious food, medicines and for religious ceremonies. The therapeutic value of ethanol is limited, but alcohol abuse is a major problem.

ALCOHOLS AND ALCOHOLIC BEVERAGES

The **aliphatic** alcohols form a homologous series beginning with **methanol** (methyl alcohol); **ethanol** (ethyl alcohol); **n-propanol; isopropanol** etc. In this chapter when the term **alcohol** is used, it indicates ethyl alcohol (ethanol).

Alcoholic beverages mainly contain ethanol (concentration varies with the type of preparation). The term **beverage** stands for a liquor for drinking. All alcoholic beverages are produced by the process of **fermentation.** In the presence of water, yeast converts the sugar (glucose) of plants into alcohol as under:

$$\underset{\text{(Glucose)}}{C_6H_{12}O_6} + \xrightarrow{\text{Yeast}} \underset{\text{(Ethanol)}}{2C_2H_5OH} + \underset{\text{(Carbon dioxide)}}{2CO_2}$$

Distillation can further increase the alcohol concentration greatly, and the law sets limits on the content which may be sold.

ETHANOL (ETHYL ALCOHOL)

Pharmacokinetics

Absorption

Ethanol (C_2H_5OH) is a water soluble molecule, and is rapidly and almost completely absorbed throughout the gastrointestinal tract. About 80 percent is absorbed from the small intestine. Eating food before or during drinking retards absorption. Individuals show great variation in the speed of absorption.

Distribution

The distribution of alcohol is throughout the body water. The rate of distribution to specific parts depends on the degree of vascularization. In organs of high blood flow, like the **brain, liver, lungs,** and **kidneys,** equilibrium occurs rapidly. Tests for drunkenness generally involve an analysis of blood, the **expired air;** or the urine for their alcohol content. Alcohol readily crosses the placental barrier.

Metabolism

Over 90 percent of the alcohol consumed is completely oxidized in the liver, the remainder being eliminated through the lungs, and in small amounts in the urine. It requires about 1 hour to metabolize the alcohol contained in 10 to 12 ounces of **beer,** 3 to 4 ounces of **wine,** or 1 ounce of **whisky.**

An increase in alcohol oxidation is observed in chronic alcoholics due to an **induction** of microsomal ethanol oxidation activity.

Mode of Action

Ethanol exerts its action on the brain by dissolving in **neuronal plasma membranes.** Once ethanol dissolves in lipid membranes, it disturbs the function of ion channels and other proteins embedded therein. The movement of chloride ions, specially that stimulated by gamma-aminobutyric acid (GABA), is enhanced by ethanol.

Pharmacological Properties

Local Actions

When applied topically, it cools the skin through evaporation; acts as an **astringent** (precipitates protein); **counter-irritant,** or **rubifacient** (produces mild burning); and helps prevent bedsores in bedridden patients.

Ethanol is **bactericidal** to most common pathogens. Concentrations of 70 percent ethanol will kill upto 90 percent of surface bacteria within 2 minutes.

Systemic Actions

Central nervous system: Alcohol is primarily a CNS depressant, and the degree of depression is directly proportional to the quantity of ethanol consumed. The "**stimulation**" which is noted in the initial stages of alcohol consumption is the result of a depression of the brain areas which ordinarily exert inhibitory control over psychomotor activity and behaviour. Progressive depressant effects of alcohol range from sedation, ataxia, slurred speech, altered judgement, coma and death.

Cardiovascular system: In moderate amounts, alcohol causes vasodilation, specially of the cutaneous vessels. Myocardial contractility is reduced, and excessive ingestion can lead to **congestive heart failure. Elevated triglyceride levels** are noted in chronic alcoholics, however, small to moderate amounts can elevate the levels of **high-density lipoproteins** (HDL), which have a protective action.

Gastrointestinal system: Small amounts of alcohol stimulate secretion of gastric juice and hydrochloric acid. High concentrations of alcohol on prolonged consumption result in inflammation of the gastric mucosa and development of **gastritis.** Impaired absorption of nutrients and vitamins (specially water-soluble vitamins) can lead to **malnutrition**. Chronic alcohol ingestion leads to hepatitis and cirrhosis. Malnutrition and vitamin deficiencies contribute to **alcoholic liver damage.**

Endocrine system: Gynaecomastia and testicular atrophy have been noted in alcoholics. It is a popular belief that alcohol is an **aphrodisiac.** Aggressive sexual behaviour is often evident after alcohol, as a result of loss of inhibition and restraint. However, objective measurements reveal that alcohol significantly decreases sexual responsiveness in both men and women. *Impotence* and *sterility* are consequences of prolonged alcohol consumption.

Musculoskeletal system: Alcohol significantly impairs psychomotor performance, and blunts reflex motor activity.

Other systems: Alcohol has a **diuretic** effect, presumably due to inhibition of release of the antidiuretic hormone (ADH) from the posterior pituitary.

Chronic alcohol ingestion increases the risk of certain types of cancer, notably *oropharyngeal, laryngeal, oesophageal, hepatic* and *possibly pancreatic.*

Excessive alcohol consumption during pregnancy, specially during the first trimester, can lead to foetal abnormalities (teratogenesis).

Therapeutic Uses

External uses: Application of alcohol to the skin has a cooling effect with evaporation, and alcohol sponges are sometimes used to **lower fever.** Alcohol solutions may be used as rubbing agents to prevent **decubitus ulcers** in bedridden patients. As **skin disinfectant** prior to injection, blood sampling and other invasive needle procedures (optimal strength for this purpose is 70 percent by volume); and as an ingredient of **anhidrotic** and **astringent** lotions to decrease sweating.

Local uses: Injection of dehydrated alcohol around the nerves or ganglia is used for relief of chronic intractable pain, e.g., pain of **trigeminal neuralgia,** or **inoperable carcinoma.** Inhalation of **ethanol mist** has been used as an **anti-foaming agent** to collapse the foam obstructing the tracheobronchial tree in **acute pulmonary oedema** secondary to **left heart failure.**

Adverse Reactions

Acute Ethanol Intoxication

Most patients recover with only residual **hangover**. Usually the person lapses into **coma,** which prevents further intake of ethanol. An additional feature of intoxication is **hypothermia,** specially in the elderly. The skin is cold and clammy, pupils normal or dilated, and the respiration is depressed and noisy.

Treatment: The treatment is essentially **supportive** and consists of maintaining respiration; blood pressure; and body temperature until the ethanol has been removed by metabolism or by **haemodialysis.** Administer **hypertonic mannitol** solution intravenously, if intracranial pressure is raised, and start **artificial respiration,** if necessary. Regulate **fluid** and **electrolye balance.**

Chronic Ethanol Abuse

Why *alcoholism* develops readily in some individuals than in others is not known. There is evidence that alcoholism may be, partly, *genetically* determined.

Tolerance with repeated use is a complex process, involving several mechanisms like **accelerated metabolism,** and central **neuronal receptor adaptation** to the continued presence of alcohol. Both, **psychological** and **physical dependence** can occur. The **withdrawal syndrome** may begin within 6 to 8 hours. Ethanol causes **chronic gastritis** and **constipation.** Other pathological findings include **pancreatitis, peripheral neuropathy,** and **gonadal failure** in both men and women.

Treatment of alcoholism: The immediate concern is often **detoxification** and management of the **withdrawal syndrome. Multivitamin supplements** are helpful in combating dietary deficiencies. **Benzodiazepines** are the drugs of choice for suppressing the withdrawal syndrome. Additional treatment requires complete **abstinence, psychiatric treatment** and support from organisations like the **Alcoholics Anonymous** (AA). The use of **disulfiram, phenothiazines, butyrophenones, phenytoin** and **propranolol** is helpful.

Disulfiram

Disulfiram (tetraethylthiuram disulphide) is an antioxidant which blocks the oxidative metabolism of ethanol at the acetaldehyde stage. Thus when ethanol is ingested even in small amounts by an individual who has previously taken disulfiram, there is a 5- to 10-fold increase in blood **acetaldehyde levels,** and this leads to unpleasant symptoms known as the **disulfiram reaction** or **acetylaldehyde syndrome** or **mal rouge.**

Therapeutic use: Disulfiram is used in the adjunctive treatment of **chronic alcoholism** with proper motivation and behavioural therapy.

Dosage: Administered orally in a single daily dose of 500 mg for 1 to 2 weeks. Once the patient has fully recovered, a maintenance dose of 125 to 500 mg per day may be used until the patient feels no compulsion to drink.

Adverse reactions: Usual side effect encountered in the absence of alcohol is *transient drowsiness*. Other adverse effects include *headache, restlessness, skin eruptions, optic* or *peripheral neuritis, metallic taste, impotence, fatigue, tremor* and *occasionally psychosis.*

Contraindications and interactions: Disulfiram is absolutely contraindicated in the presence of severe myocardial disease, coronary occlusion, psychoses, and pregnancy. Notable interactions are: disulfiram potentiates the effects of diazepam, chlordiazepoxide, oral anticoagulants and phenytoin.

Naltrexone

Naltrexone is a pure *opioid receptor antagonist.* Presumably it blunts the "pleasurable" effects of alcohol drinking, and has been approved by the FDA for treatment of alcohol dependence.

Naltrexone is administered in a dose of 50 mg once a day for treatment of alcoholism. Common *adverse effects* are nausea, dizziness, and headache. *Contraindications* are acute hepatitis and liver failure. Combination of naltrexone with disulfiram should be avoided as both drugs are hepatotoxic.

Newer drugs used for managing alcoholism are: **Topiramate** (anti-seizure drug); **Acamprosate** and **Triapride.**

METHANOL

Methanol (methyl alcohol, wood alcohol, CH_3OH) is the simplest aliphatic alcohol. It has no therapeutic use, but is widely used commercially as an industrial **solvent;** as an ethanol **denaturant;** and as a **fuel.** Methanol has pharmacological properties similar to ethanol. It is sometimes consumed accidentally or as a substitute for ethanol, often with disastrous results (**blindness**, **coma** and **death**).

Methanol is readily absorbed and distributed throughout the body. It is metabolized at about one-seventh the rate of ethanol and is largely oxidized to **formic acid.** Methanol toxicity appears to be primarily due to the formation of formic acid, and direct toxic action of **formaldehyde.**

Methanol is a generalized CNS depressant, but less potent than ethanol. A severe **acidosis** then develops, and is followed by optic damage that can lead to **partial** or **total blindness.**

Treatment of methanol poisoning involves counteracting the acidosis by infusion of **sodium bicarbonate** (about 3 gm/hr) until the urine pH reaches 7.5. Retinal damage and blindness are caused by **formic acid.** *Ethanol administration* has been used in the treatment of methanol poisoning. This reaction prevents the formation of the toxic metabolites of methanol, thereby allowing time for methanol to be excreted unchanged.

2.3 GENERAL ANAESTHETICS

It was in the middle of 1800s that the first demonstrations of drug-induced general anaesthesia using volatile liquids **chloroform** and **diethyl ether** were reported. Later, the anaesthetic properties of **nitrous oxide gas,** originally suggested by Priestley in 1776, were revealed. The modern age of anaesthesia began with the introduction of the intravenous barbiturate, **thiopental** in the 1930s, and the skeletal muscle relaxant **d-tubocurarine** about a decade later.

OBJECTIVES OF GENERAL ANAESTHESIA

General anaesthetics are CNS depressants that are used to bring about a **reversible loss of pain sensation and consciousness.** Their use permits painful surgical procedures to be performed without the patient being aware of it, or even reacting reflexly. The goals of general anaesthesia are: (i) **analgesia;** (ii) **loss of consciousness,** in which the patient is unaware of what is going on, and is later totally unable to recall what took place, i.e., amnesia; (iii) **loss of reflexes** to minimize laryngospasm, cardiac arrhythmias, salivation, vomiting, and postoperative abdominal distension; and (iv) **skeletal muscle relaxation**, which is desirable during abdominal surgery.

STAGES OF GENERAL ANAESTHESIA

Classical pattern described by Guedel in 1920 applies to **diethyl ether.** In modern anaesthesiology, however, the distinctive signs of each stage are frequently obscured, because many newer agents have a very **rapid onset of action,** and quickly bypass the early stages.

Stage I: Analgesia.

Stage II: Excitement.

Stage III: Surgical Anaesthesia. **Stage III** is further divided into **four** planes.

Stage IV: Apnoea. **Stage IV** begins with complete respiratory paralysis, and ends with failure of circulation. It is considered as the stage of overdosage, and the medullary centres are completely paralyzed.

During **recovery** from deep anaesthesia, the patients reflexes return in reverse order from that in which they were lost.

MECHANISMS OF GENERAL ANAESTHESIA

The general anaesthetics produce a **progressive depression** of the CNS. The degree of depression depends on the concentration of the drug in the CNS.

General anaesthetics preferentially depress the **ascending reticular activating system** (RAS), which is concerned in maintaining alertness and wakefulness. By reducing the number of impulses transmitted to the cerebral cortex, these drugs progressively **reduce sensory awareness,** and when a sufficient concentration of the anaesthetic is reached, consciousness is lost.

ADJUNCTIVE ANAESTHETIC MEDICATION

Preanaesthetic medication: Premedication is defined as the administration of drugs before the anaesthetic is given. The main aims are: (i) **Relief of anxiety** (anxiolytics, e.g., diazepam, midazolam); (ii) **Reduction in salivary and mucous secretions** (anticholinergics, e.g., atropine, hyoscine); and (iii) **Inhibition of undesirable side effects** (e.g., bradycardia and muscle spasms) occurring reflexly in response to the anaesthetic agent.

Medication during anaesthesia: Neuromuscular blocking agents are administered during the operation while the patient is still at a light level of anaesthesia.

Postoperative medication: The main indications for the use of drugs postoperatively are to relieve: (i) nausea and vomiting by **antiemetics** (e.g. prochlorperazine); (ii) abdominal distention and urinary retention by **cholinergics** (e.g. bethanechol); (iii) pain by **analgesics** (e.g. pethidine); and (iv) constipation by **laxatives** and stool softeners (e.g., docusate, bisacodyl). **Anticholinesterase drugs** may be used postoperatively to antagonize neuromuscular blockade induced by drugs like d-tubocurarine.

CLASSIFICATION

I. **Inhalation anaesthetics**
   a. Gases (Nitrous oxide).
   b. Volatile liquids (Ether, Halothane, Enflurane, Isoflurane, Desflurane, Sevoflurane).

II. **Intravenous anaesthetics**
   a. Ultrashort-acting barbiturates (Thiopental, Methohexital, Thiamylal).
   b. Non-barbiturate hypnotic (Etomidate).
   c. Dissociative agents (Ketamine, Fentanyl/Droperidol).

INHALATION ANAESTHETICS

The inhalation anaesthetics enter the circulation on absorption from the alveoli of the lungs. From the blood the agent is transferred to the brain. Eventually most inhalation agents are returned to the lungs and excreted in exhaled air mostly unchanged.

Gases

Three gases (nitrous oxide, cyclopropane, ethylene) are available for use, and of these nitrous oxide is used most extensively. A total anaesthetic regimen includes other anaesthetics, sedatives, narcotics, anxiolytics and muscle relaxants. Such a regimen, termed **balanced anaesthesia,** produces rapid induction with minimal adverse effects, and allows a significant reduction in the amount of each drug required.

Nitrous Oxide (N_2O): Nitrous oxide (laughing gas) is an inorganic general anaesthetic commonly used as a component of "balanced anaesthesia".

Volatile Liquids

Other than nitrous oxide, the most commonly used inhalational anaesthetics are the volatile liquids. They are administered by inhalation of the vapours with adequate amounts of oxygen. The **depth of anaesthesia** can be controlled fairly well by varying the concentration.

Ether (Diethyl Ether): Diethyl ether was the first clinically useful volatile liquid anaesthetic. As the disadvantages outweigh the advantages ether is *rarely* used currently.

Halothane: Halothane is a potent, non-flammable, pleasant smelling volatile liquid anaesthetic, and is one of the most widely used anaesthetics. Skeletal muscle relaxation is only fair.

Enflurane: Enflurane is a potent anaesthetic, widely used today for many surgical procedures. Induction and recovery are rapid, and the drug is non-flammable. Enflurane produces better muscle relaxation, and less myocardial sensitization to catecholamines than halothane.

Isoflurane: Isoflurane is structurally similar to enflurane, but with several advantages. It has a rapid onset and quick recovery. It does not sensitize the heart to catecholamines and produces good muscle relaxation.

INTRAVENOUS ANAESTHETICS

The general anaesthetics administered IV include: (i) three **ultrashort-acting barbiturates** (methohexital, thiamylal, thiopental), mainly used for **induction** of anaesthesia and as sole anaesthetics for **short surgical procedures;** (ii) a rapid-acting non-barbiturate hypnotic, **etomidate** used for induction, and for supplementing other anaesthetics like nitrous oxide; and (iii) two **dissociative anaesthetics** which can be administered IV or IM to induce a **neuroleptic-like** state, characterized by analgesia, quietude, and detachment from the environment without loss of consciousness (**ketamine**, **fentanyl/droperidol**).

Ultrashort-acting Barbiturates

Thiopental/Methohexital/Thiamylal: The IV barbiturates depress the CNS, producing hypnosis and anaesthesia without analgesia. Muscle relaxation is inadequate, even with deep anaesthesia.

Uses: The main uses are: (i) *induction* of anaesthesia; (ii) *supplementation* of other general anaesthetics; (iii) production of anaesthesia for short surgical procedures with minimal pain; (iv) induction of *hypnosis*; (v) control of convulsive state during and following general or local anaesthesia; and (vi) for *narcoanalysis* and *narcosynthesis* in psychiatric disorders (thiopental).

Fate: Induction is smooth and rapid. Onset occurs within 30-60 seconds of IV injection. They quickly cross the blood-brain barrier, and are then rapidly redistributed to other parts of the body.

Adverse reactions: A dose-dependent respiratory depression occurs. Other side effects are laryngospasm, coughing, and yawning.

Precautions: Absolute contraindications include latent or manifest porphyria, and absence of suitable veins for IV administration. Thiopental is contraindicated in status asthmatics.

Nonbarbiturate Hypnotics

Etomidate: Etomidate produces rapid hypnosis following IV injection, but is not an analgesic. Cerebral blood flow is slightly reduced. Respiratory depression is minimal.

Uses: Etomidate is used for induction of general anaesthesia; and for prolonged sedation of critically ill patients.

Fate: Onset is within 1 minute, and effect persists for 3 to 5 minutes. It is rapidly metabolized in the liver, and primarily excreted by the kidneys.

Adverse reactions: Hypotension, tachycardia, cardiac arrhythmias, laryngospasm, hiccups, postoperative nausea and vomiting can occur.

DISSOCIATIVE AGENTS

Two drugs, ketamine and fentanyl/droperidol are used in certain situations when an anaesthesia-like state is desired, but unconsciousness would be disadvantageous.

Ketamine: Dissociative anaesthesia is a state in which the anaesthetized patient feels totally dissociated from the surroundings. Ketamine is a rapid-acting anaesthetic producing a state of **dissociation**, with profound analgesia, normal skeletal muscle tone and laryngeal reflexes, and variable cardiovascular and respiratory reflexes. The patient appears to be awake, but does not respond to pain and does not recall the experience on recovery (amnesia). Ketamine has a wide margin of safety.

Uses: Diagnostic and short surgical procedures not requiring muscle relaxation, e.g., treatment of burns. For induction of anaesthesia.

Adverse reactions: Emergence reactions (detailed above) can be minimized by giving diazepam or a short-acting barbiturate.

Fentanyl/Droperidol: Innovar is a drug combination containing a **narcotic analgesic** fentanyl, and a **neuroleptic** droperidol. The two are often used together to produce **neuroleptanalgesia,** a state in which consciousness is not lost, but the anxiety of the patient is allayed, and the ability to perceive pain is reduced or abolished. The addition of nitrous oxide to this combination produces **neuroleptanaesthesia.**

Uses: Innovar is used: (i) production of *tranquilization* and analgesia for diagnostic and minor surgical procedures; (ii) *anaesthetic premedication* and induction of anaesthesia; and (iii) *adjunct for general anaesthesia* in combination with nitrous oxide and oxygen.

Adverse reactions: Muscle rigidity, hypotension, slight respiratory depression and drowsiness have been reported. The neuroleptic droperidol can induce extrapyramidal reactions.

2.4 SEDATIVE-HYPNOTICS AND ANXIOLYTIC DRUGS

The primary use of **sedative-hypnotics** and **anxiolytics** is to induce calmness (anxiolytics), or to produce sleep (sedative-hypnotics). **Insomnia** is a common problem. It includes a wide variety of sleep disturbances, like difficulty in falling asleep, early or frequent awakenings, and remaining unrefreshed after sleep.

SLEEP PATTERNS

Normal sleep consists of two major phases, **REM** (rapid eye movement) and **non-REM** sleep, which occur cyclically over an interval of about 80 to 90 minutes. REM sleep covers about 20 to 25 percent of total sleep time, and during this most dreaming occurs.

Non-REM sleep comprises 75 to 80 percent of total sleep time. Children spend more time than adults in deep sleep, whereas the elderly spend relatively little time in deep sleep.

SEDATIVE-HYPNOTICS

The sedative-hypnotics are classified into **barbiturates** and **non-barbiturate.**

Barbiturates

Barbiturates are derivatives of malonylurea (barbituric acid). Barbituric acid itself has no depressant action on the CNS.

Table 2.1 : *Classification of barbiturates*

Drug	Onset of action (min)	Peak effect (hrs)	Elimination Half-life (hrs)	Adult Oral Dose (mg)	
				Sedative	Hypnotic
Long-acting					
Mephobarbital	60-90	10-12	60-120*	15-30 bid/tid	100-200
Phenobarbital					
Intermediate-acting					
Amobarbital	45-60	6-8	15-40	15-50 bid/tid	100-200
Aprobarbital				40 tid	40-160
Short-acting					
Pentobarbital	10-15	3-4	18-42	20 tid/qid	100
Secobarbital				30-50 tid/qid	100
Ultrashort-acting					
Methohexital	0-1	3-5 min	3-8	For IV general anaesthesia	
Thiopental				–	–

* Values are for phenobarbital.

Barbiturates are valuable as *anaesthetics* and *anticonvulsants*. However, the benzodiazepines have replaced the barbiturates as hypnotics, sedatives and anxiolytics.

Classification: Barbiturates have been traditionally classified as **long-acting**, **intermediate-acting, short-acting** and **ultrashort-acting** compounds **(Table 2.1)**.

The ultrashort-acting barbiturates are primarily used as intravenous general anaesthetics (**Chap. 2.3**).

Pharmacological Actions: The barbiturates exert many pharmacologic effects, such as sedation, hypnosis, anaesthesia, anticonvulsant activity, respiratory depression and enzyme induction. In addition, on chronic use, they have a potential for inducing *habituation* and *dependence*.

1. **Sedation:** In low doses, barbiturates produce mild drowsiness, accompanied by decreased motor activity and a sense of well-being. This sedative action results from a non-specific depression of the **reticular activating system** (RAS) in the brainstem.
2. **Hypnosis:** An indication for most barbiturates is the *relief of temporary insomnia*. They induce sleep in a dose 3 to 4 times higher than the sedative dose. Barbiturate use also has **"hangover"** effects such as daytime drowsiness, psychomotor impairment, and depression.
3. **Anaesthesia:** The highly lipid-soluble, rapid-acting derivatives (methohexital, thiopental) are administered IV for induction of anaesthesia (**Chap. 2.3**).
4. **Anticonvulsant activity:** The long-acting compounds, **phenobarbital,** and **mephobarbital** are indicated in the therapy of **grand mal epilepsy** and **cortical focal seizures.** These drugs appear to have selective anticonvulsant activity. Phenobarbital is the preferred anticonvulsant.
5. **Respiratory depression:** Barbiturates exert a dose-dependent respiratory depression.
6. **Enzyme induction:** Barbiturates, specially phenobarbital, can accelerate the functioning of hepatic microsomal enzymes, a process called **enzyme induction.** Barbiturates, in fact, accelerate their own metabolism, and thus *tolerance* develops.

Other actions: Amnesia (forgetfulness) may follow barbiturate use. **Aggressive behaviour** is sometimes observed in barbiturate abusers.

Mode of Action: The most sensitive area of the CNS to the action of the barbiturates is the **midbrain reticular formation,** where they elevate the threshold for electrical stimulation. Neuronal activity in the limbic system and hypothalamus is also reduced by barbiturates. Facilitation of GABA (gamma-aminobutyric acid) activity in the brain, has been observed with barbiturates.

Pharmacokinetics: Barbiturates are absorbed to varying degrees from the stomach, small intestine, rectum and IM sites. The duration of action of a barbiturate depends on: (i) *its rate of hepatic degradation*; (ii) *its degree of lipid solubility*; and (iii) t*he degree of binding to serum proteins.*

Long-acting barbiturates are metabolized mainly in the liver. Ultrashort-acting barbiturates are highly lipid-soluble, and have a rapid onset and short duration of action.

Barbiturates and their metabolites are mainly excreted via the kidneys.

Therapeutic Uses

1. A**cute convulsive states** (IV or IM).
2. **Grand mal epilepsy** (phenobarbital).
3. **Induction of anaesthesia,** and brief minor surgical procedures (ultrashort-acting barbiturates).
4. Aid in **psychoanalysis.**
5. **Kernicterus:** Barbiturates raise bilirubin binding Y protein. Phenobarbital has been used in *hyperbilirubinaemia* and *kernicterus*.

Adverse Reactions:

1. **Hangover** and drowsiness occur in the morning after barbiturate use.
2. **Respiratory depression.**
3. **Paradoxical excitement:** In some patients (particularly in the elderly and debilitated) barbiturates produce restlessness, excitement and delirium paradoxically.

4. **Drug automatism:** It is a state of amnesia in which the patient takes repeated doses of barbiturates leading to acute poisoning.
5. Hypersensitivity reactions.
6. Barbiturate dependence. On chronic use **psychological** and **physical dependence** can occur.
7. **Acute barbiturate overdosage:** Acute poisoning results in marked respiratory depression (Cheyne-Stokes breathing), lowered body temperature, tachycardia, hypotension, oliguria, circulatory collapse and coma. **Treatment** consists of supporting respiration and circulation. With longer-acting barbiturates, alkalinizing the urine promotes excretion of the drug and diuresis. **Haemodialysis** or **peritoneal dialysis** is often needed. **Fluid replacement** should be undertaken.

Contraindications: Barbiturates should be given cautiously in the presence of **hepatic** and **pulmonary insufficiency.** They are contraindicated in patients with **chronic emphysema,** myxoedema, renal failure, intermittent porphyria, and in patients with suicidal tendencies.

Drug Interactions: Barbiturates cause induction of the hepatic microsomal enzymes (**Chap. 1.8**). Thus they increase their own metabolism leading to **tolerance.** Barbiturates potentiate the CNS depressant effects of **alcohol**, **narcotic analgesics, antihistamines, anaesthetics, anxiolytics, central muscle relaxants** and other **sedative-hypnotics**.

Nonbarbiturate Sedative-Hypnotics

The **benzodiazepine hypnotics** have several advantages over barbiturates, like absence of enzyme induction, little effect on REM sleep, and smaller abuse potential, and thus have become the most widely prescribed hypnotics.

Benzodiazepine hypnotics: The three benzodiazepines, namely, **flurazepam, temazepam,** and **triazolam** are solely used for the short-term management of insomnia, and termed as **benzodiazepine hypnotics.**

The benzodiazepine hypnotics have several advantages: (i) wider margin of safety; (ii) minimal REM sleep time reducing effect; and (iii) absence of enzyme-inducing effects. Thus, the **benzodiazepines are the preferred hypnotics** in most patients. However, the incidence of psychological dependence on benzodiazepines is increasing with their rising usage.

Mode of Action: The basic mode of action of benzodiazepines is **facilitation** of the action of the inhibitory neurotransmitter GABA. The site of

Table 2.2 : *Dosage and characteristics of benzodiazepine hypnotics*

Drug	Preparation	Adult Dosage Range (Oral)	Clinical Characteristics
Flurazepam	Capsules -15, 30 mg	15-30 mg at bedtime	*Long-acting benzpdiazepine*; residual effects persist for days after stoppage, not recommended for children under 15 years.
Temazepam	Capsules-15, 30 mg	15-30 mg at bedtime	*Intermediate acting benzodiazepine*; transient sleep disturbances after discontinuation; not recommended in children under 18 years.
Triazolam	Tablets-0.125, 0.25, 0.5 mg	0.25 to 0.5 mg at bedtime	*Short-acting hypnotic*; minimal hangover, not recommended in children under 18 years; rebound insomnia may occur.

action in the CNS appears to be the **limbic system, thalamus,** and the **midbrain reticular formation.** REM sleeptime remains unaltered, and there is no microsomal enzyme induction.

Use: Short-term (maximum 4 weeks) treatment of insomnia.

Pharmacokinetics: The oral absorption of all the hypnotic benzodiazepines is good; sleep usually occurs within 15 to 45 minutes. The drugs and their metabolites are excreted in the urine.

Dosage: The usual dosages are presented in **Table 2.2.**

Adverse reactions: Hypnotic doses of benzodiazepines frequently cause daytime drowsiness, lightheadedness, headache, dizziness, ataxia, and slight motor incoordination. Flurazepam causes "hangover" on repeated administration, and interferes with psychomotor performance like driving. Serious adverse reactions are rare. **Paradoxical reactions** like nervousness, irritability, tachycardia, sweating and nightmares have been recorded. **Tolerance** can occur. Benzodiazepine **dependence** is less severe than with barbiturates. Benzodiazepines are contraindicated in pregnant women as foetal damage has been reported.

Zolpidem: Zolpidem is a **nonbenzodiazepine sedative-hypnotic.** Modulation of the *GABA receptor chloride channel macromolecular complex* is responsible for its *sedative*, *anticonvulsant*, *anxiolytic*, and *myorelaxant* properties. On stoppage of zolpidem administration the beneficial effects on sleep persist for up to a week. *Tolerance* and *physical dependence* occurs rarely. Currently zolpidem is approved only for *short-term treatment of insomnia.*

Zolpidem is readily absorbed from the gut. Its plasma half-life is about 2 hours. In therapeutic doses (10-20 mg orally) zolpidem rarely produces daytime sedation or amnesia.

ANTIANXIETY DRUGS

Antianxiety drugs or **anxiolytics** are agents used to relieve stress, tension and anxiety, generated by the complex and hectic modern daily life. **Anxiety** is defined as an exaggerated feeling of apprehension, uncertainty, and fear. **Acute anxiety** is generally transient. The **somatic** manifestations of anxiety include fatigue, dizziness, palpitation, indigestion, headache, muscle aches, insomnia, and excessive perspiration.

The main advantage of anxiolytics over the barbiturates is their significantly **higher sedative-to-hypnotic ratio**, i.e., the margin between their calmness producing dose and the hypnotic dose is much greater than that of the barbiturates.

Classification

Antianxiety drugs can be classified into *three* groups:

1. **Benzodiazepines:** Chlordiazepoxide, Diazepam, Clorazepate, Alprazolam, Halazepam, Lorazepam, Midazolam, Oxazepam, Prazepam.
2. **Miscellaneous:** Buspirone, Hydroxyzine, Propranolol, Chlormezanone

Benzodiazepines: The benzodiazepines are the most commonly prescribed antianxiety agents. They are primarily used for relief of **situational anxiety**.

Pharmacological actions: These agents produce sedation, hypnosis, **anxiolytic activity, skeletal muscle relaxation** and **anticonvulsant activity.**

Antianxiety effects: The benzodiazepines exert a ***more specific effect on the limbic system***, and therefore reduce anxiety in doses which do not produce drowsiness or sleep.

Anticonvulsant effects: The benzodiazepines raise the threshold for electrically-induced seizures in experimental animals. Clinically, **diazepam, clonazepam, lorazepam** and **nitrazepam** are used as antiepileptics (**Chap. 2.5**).

Skeletal muscle relaxant effect: The benzodiazepines induce voluntary muscle relaxation (hypotonia) without affecting normal locomotion in therapeutic doses.

Hypnotic effect: The Benzodiazepines can be used as hypnotics, and in therapeutic doses they do not suppress REM sleep, but markedly suppress stage 4 sleep. Most benzodiazepines *decrease sleep latency*, and reduce the number of awakenings.

Cardiovascular system: The cardiovascular effects are minor, except in severe intoxication in which the blood pressure falls.

Analgesic action: Diazepam causes transient analgesia in man on intravenous administration.

Mode of Action: The benzodiazepines act selectively on the **polysynaptic neuronal pathways** throughout the CNS. Their main site of action is the ***midbrain reticular formation***, which is the region responsible for maintenance of wakefulness. The benzodiazepines facilitate the action of gamma-aminobutyric acid (GABA). The benzodiazepine receptors are closely associated with the receptors for GABA, which is the major inhibitory neurotransmitter in the brain.

Pharmacokinetics: Benzodiazepines are generally well absorbed orally, but the rates differ widely. Thus, there is variability in the onset of action following a single dose (**Table 2.3**). IM absorption of **lorazepam** is rapid and complete, but that of chlordiazepoxide and diazepam is erratic.

The benzodiazepines are quite lipid-soluble and distribute widely throughout the body. Protein binding is high (80%-90%). These drugs are mainly metabolized in the liver, and excreted largely through the urine.

Therapeutic Uses: The benzodiazepines are widely used drugs, and quite often overused. Their main uses are detailed below:

1. Symptomatic relief of **anxiety.**
2. **Insomnia:** For this condition nitrazepam, flurazepam and temazepam are used.
3. **Epilepsy:** The agents clonazepam and diazepam are useful in *status epilepticus*.
4. **Preoperative sedation:** Midazolam, a short-acting agent is used parenterally.
5. **Spasticity:** Diazepam reduces spasticity associated with upper motor neurone lesions.
6. **Muscle spasm.**
7. **Tetanus:** A continuous IV infusion of diazepam 3-10 mg/kg/24 hours, or intermittent IV doses of 0.1-0.3 mg/kg may be used to control spasms.
8. **Alcohol withdrawal** manifestations are best controlled by diazepam or chlordiazepoxide.
9. **Adjunctive treatment** prior to cardioversion or endoscopic procedures to lessen anxiety.
10. **Miscellaneous:** Used for relieving anxiety

Table 2.3 : *The pharmacokinetic parameters and dosage of some selected benzodiazepines*

Drug	Daily Dosage Range (mg)	Onset of Action (Oral)	Peak Plasma Levels (hrs.)	Activity of Metabolities	Elimination Half-life (hrs)
Alprazolam*	0.75-3.0	Fast	1-2	Active*	12-15
Chlordiazepoxide	15-100	Moderate	0.5-4	Active	5-30
Chlorazepate	15-60	Fast	1-2	Active	30-90
Diazepam	4-40	Very fast	0.5-15	Active	20-50
Halazepam	60-160	Fast	1-3	Active	12-15
Lorazepam	2-8	Moderate	1-4	Inactive	10-15
Nitrazepam	5-10	Moderate	1-3	Inactive	18-28
Oxazepam	30-120	Slow	1-4	Inactive	5-15
Prazepam	20-60	Slow	2-6	Active	30-100

* Alprazolam has two metabolites, one of which is inactive.

in disorders like *peptic ulcer*, *hypertension*, *angina pectoris*, and *rheumatic disorders*.

Adverse Reactions

Transient drowsiness, ataxia, confusion, fatigue and lethargy occur in the initial phase of therapy. Other adverse reactions are less commonly seen during short-term therapy.

CNS—Confusion, disorientation, agitation, slurred speech, headache, syncope, vertigo.

Gastrointestinal—Dry mouth, constipation, nausea, anorexia, vomiting.

Cardiovascular/Haematologic - Bradycardia, hypotension, palpitation, oedema, agranulocytosis, neutropenia.

Hypersensitivity—Skin rash, urticaria, angioneurotic oedema, bronchial spasm.

Miscellaneous—Changes in libido, menstrual irregularities, nasal congestion, hiccups, diplopia, nystagmus, hepatic dysfunction, thrombophlebitis on IV injection, pain on IM injection. **Drug dependence** can occur.

Overdosage symptoms include drowsiness, confusion, ataxia, and hypotension, but rarely significant circulatory or respiratory depression is seen. **Treatment** is mainly supportive, and includes IV fluids, pressor agents and osmotic diuretics. Haemoperfusion through an activated charcoal column may be useful.

Drug Interactions

1. Benzodiazepines enhance CNS-depressant effects of alcohol, barbiturates, antihistamines, phenothiazines and opiates.
2. The effects of phenytoin may be potentiated by benzodiazepines.
3. The effects of benzodiazepines are lessened in individuals who smoke.
4. Increased muscle relaxant effect with other centrally or peripherally acting muscle relaxants.
5. Oral contraceptives and valproic acid reduce the metabolism of diazepam.

Miscellaneous Antianxiety Drugs

Buspirone: Buspirone is the first member of a new class of anxiolytic agents that can relieve symptoms of anxiety in doses that do not cause sedation. The **mode of action** of buspirone is not completely established, but it appears to have an affinity for certain **serotonin** and **dopamine receptors.**

Buspirone lacks the muscle-relaxant and anticonvulsant actions of the benzodiazepines, and does not exhibit a significant sedative effect.

Uses: Buspirone is used in the **short-term management of anxiety disorders.** The recommended initial dose in 5 mg 3 times daily.

Pharmacokinetics: On oral administration absorption is rapid and peak plasma levels occur within 45 to 90 minutes. It is metabolized in the liver, mainly to hydroxylated inactive metabolites excreted largely in the urine. Elimination half-life is 2-3 hours.

Adverse reactions: Like the benzodiazepines, buspirone appears to be safe even in very high doses. Common side effects are dizziness, headache, nervousness, fatigue, excitement and insomnia.

Hydroxyzine: Hydroxyzine is an antihistamine (H_1-receptor antagonist) that exhibits a mild CNS-depressant action, exerted at subcortical brain levels. It possesses a number of other pharmacologic actions like **anticholinergic**, **bronchodilator, analgesic, antispasmodic, antiemetic** and **skeletal muscle relaxant activity.** This drug displays a good safety margin.

Mode of action is incompletely known. It interferes with the action of histamine, acetylcholine, and serotonin.

Uses: (i) Symptomatic treatment of **psychoneurotic states;** (ii) To relieve symptoms of **anxiety;** (iii) Management of pruritus, associated with dermatoses; (iv) Adjunctive treatment of **alcohol withdrawal** or **delirium tremens;** and (v) **Pre- and postoperative sedation.** The usual dosage for adults is 50 to 100 mg orally 3 to 4 times daily.

Propranolol: The beta-blocker propranolol has been widely used in the treatment of cardiovascular diseases. It is also useful in some forms of *anxiety*, particularly characterisized by somatic symptoms, or by *performance anxiety* (stage fright).

2.5 ANTIEPILEPTICS

Epilepsy is a chronic disorder of the central nervous system (CNS). The term **primary** or ***idiopathic epilepsy*** includes those cases where no cause for the seizure can be identified. **Secondary** or **symptomatic epilepsy** designates the disorder when factors like *trauma*, *neoplasm*, *infection*, *poisoning*, *fever*, *cerebrovascular disease*, or *withdrawal of certain drugs*, cause the disease.

CLASSIFICATION OF EPILEPTIC SEIZURES

The term "Epilepsy" is used to describe the occurrence of sudden, recurring discharges from abnormally functioning brain cells, leading to **motor**, **sensory, autonomic,** and **psychic** manifestations. Such abnormal brain discharges are called **seizures.**

Seizures can be broadly categorized into **generalized** and **partial** (localized) types. The more common generalized seizures are: (i) tonic-clonic convulsions or **grand mal epilepsy;** (ii) simple absence seizures or **petit mal epilepsy;** (iii) **myoclonic jerking;** (iv) **atonic/akinetic;** and (v) **infantile spasms** (hypsarrhythmia). Generalized seizures are bilateral and symmetric. Partial seizures originate in a specific part of the brain and may be subdivided into: (i) **simple** or **focal seizures** in which there is minimal spread of the discharge; limited to the extremities; and (ii) **complex seizures** in which the discharge becomes widespread and behavioural aberrations are seen, referred to as **temporal lobe** or **psychomotor epilepsy.** A simplified classification of the common epilepsies is presented.

From the clinical standpoint, subdivisions of epileptic seizures are **grand mal, petit mal, psychomotor, focal** or **Jacksonian seizures** and **status epilepticus**. Recording of the electrical activity of the brain by placing electrodes on the scalp (EEG) is a standard diagnostic procedure.

CLASSIFICATION OF ANTIEPILEPTICS

The antiepileptic drugs may be classified according to their chemical structure:

1. **Anticonvulsant barbiturates:** *Phenobarbital*, mephobarbital, metharbital.
2. **Hydantoins:** *Phenytoin*, ethotoin, mephenytoin.
3. **Oxazolidinediones:** *Trimethadione*, paramethadione.
4. **Succinimides:** *Ethosuximide*, methsuximide, phensuximide.
5. **Iminostilbines:** *Carbamazepine.*
6. **Benzodiazepines:** *Clonazepam, diazepam*, clorazepate, nitrazepam.
7. **Valproic acid derivatives:** *Valproic acid*, valproate sodium, divalproex sodium.
8. **Chemically unrelated anticonvulsants:** Acetazolamide, primidone, phenacemide, lidocaine, magnesium sulphate.

Anticonvulsant Barbiturates

Phenobarbital, Mephobarbital, Metharbital

Phenobarbital is the most commonly used compound. Dose is 50-100 mg bid or tid.

Mode of action: The exact role of gamma-aminobutyric acid (GABA) is unclear, but **potentiation of GABA-ergic activity** may be playing a role.

Pharmacokinetics: The antiepileptic barbiturates are well absorbed orally. These drugs are widely distributed in the body; unchanged drug and the metabolic products are excreted in the urine.

Therapeutic Uses

1. Treatment of *grand mal seizures.*
2. Generalized *myoclonic jerks* and *cortical focal seizures.*
3. Control of *status epilepticus.* (IV phenobarbital used).

Adverse reactions: *Drowsiness, lethargy* and *dizziness* are the most frequently noted side effects. Less common adverse reactions are *bradycardia, hypotension, hypoventilation, bronchospasm, skin rash*, confusion, ataxia, and *aggressive behaviour.*

Hydantoins

Phenytoin, Ethotoin, Mephenytoin

Phenytoin is the most frequently prescribed drug. Dose is 100 mg tid.

Mode of action: The hydantoins **inhibit the spread** of seizure activity. The motor cortex is the primary site of action. Increased release, or activity of GABA is an additional mechanism of action.

Pharmacokinetics: Phenytoin is slowly absorbed from the small intestines. Phenytoin is erratically absorbed on IM injection. It is metabolized in the liver, and excreted largely as conjugated metabolites in urine.

Therapeutic Uses

1. Control of **grand mal seizures.**
2. **Psychomotor epilepsy.**
3. **Trigeminal neuralgia**, and **alcohol withdrawal syndrome.**
4. **Status epilepticus**, and seizures occurring during neurosurgery.
5. **Jacksonian seizures.**
6. Termination of digitalis-induced cardiac arrhythmias.

Adverse reactions: Frequent side effects are sluggishness, ataxia, slurred speech, nystagmus and confusion. Other adverse reactions include gingival hyperplasia, osteomalacia and bone marrow depression.

Oxazolidinediones
Trimethadione, Paramethadione

The oxazolidinediones are effective drugs for the control of simple absence (*petit mal*) seizures. The two available drugs, **trimethadione** and **paramethadione,** only differ slightly in their pharmacologic properties.

Mode of action: They **elevate** the **seizure threshold** in the thalamus, and interfere with the propagation of seizure activity.

Pharmacokinetics: Oxazolidinediones are readily absorbed from the GI tract, and peak plasma concentrations occur in 30-60 minutes. Both compounds are metabolized in the liver to an active metabolite, which is slowly excreted by the kidneys. Trimethadione dose is 300 mg tid.

Therapeutic use: Simple **absence (petit mal)** seizures refractory to other drugs.

Adverse reactions: Common side effects are drowsiness, GI distress, hiccups and photophobia. Other adverse effects are: nausea, vomiting, anorexia; vertigo, irritability, personality changes, precipitation of grand mal seizures.

Succinimides
Ethosuximide, Methsuximide, Phensuximide

The three succinimides currently available have little differences amongst them. Dose: 500 mg/day.

Mode of action: The succinimides resemble the oxazolidinediones in that they suppress absence seizures.

Pharmacokinetics: Succinimides are well absorbed orally, and peak serum levels are attained in 2-4 hours. They are **not** bound to plasma proteins. They are metabolized in the liver, and are excreted in the urine.

Therapeutic use: They are drugs of choice for **simple absence (petit mal) seizures.**

Adverse reactions: Common side effects are GI distress, drowsiness, ataxia and dizziness. Other adverse effects include: nervousness, euphoria, aggressiveness, confusion, depression, night terrors and sleep disturbances.

Iminostilbines

Carbamazepine

Carbamazepine is structurally related to tricyclic antidepressants, and has actions similar to phenytoin.

Mode of action: Carbamazepine increases latency, decreases responsivity, and suppresses after-discharges in polysynaptic pathways associated with cortical and limbic function.

Pharmacokinetics: Oral absorption is slow but complete, peak plasma levels are attained in 4 to 6 hours; widely distributed and highly protein bound (75%). It is metabolized in the liver, and excreted by the kidneys.

Therapeutic Uses

1. Treatment of **psychomotor seizures.**
2. **Grand mal seizures.**
3. **Mixed seizures** or **complex partial seizures.**
4. **Trigeminal neuralgia.**

Dosage: Carbamazepine is used orally as 200 mg tablets, and 100 mg chewable tablets.

Adverse reactions: Common side effects are drowsiness, dizziness, ataxia, nausea and diplopia.

Benzodiazepines

Clonazepam

Clonazepam, a long-acting benzodiazepine, is used primarily in **absence (petit mal) seizures.** It causes significant CNS depression and results in **psychological dependence.** Tolerance limits the usefulness of clonazepam for chronic therapy.

Mode of action: The precise mode of action is not well established. Clonazepam potentiates inhibitory mechanisms in subcortical brain structures.

Pharmacokinetics: Onset of action on oral administration is within 30 to 60 minutes; maximum levels occur in 1 to 2 hours; and effects persist for 6 to 12 hours. It is metabolized in the liver and excreted in the urine.

Therapeutic Uses

1. Petit mal variant (**Lennox-Gestaut syndrome**).
2. **Myoclonic** and **akinetic** seizures.
3. **Simple absence seizures** refractory to succinimides.

Dosage: Clonazepam is administered orally as 0.5, 1.0 or 2.0 mg tablets. In **adults,** initial dose is 0.5 mg tid. In children, initially 0.01 mg/kg to 0.03 mg/kg/day.

Adverse reactions: Common side effects are drowsiness, ataxia and abnormal behaviour. Other adverse reactions include confusion, depression, insomnia, slurred speech, nystagmus, psychosis, ankle oedema, blood dyscrasias and lymphadenopathy. Dependence and tolerance can develop.

Diazepam

Diazepam is useful as an adjunct in the management of **convulsive disorders,** specially **minor motor seizures.** Its main indication is parenterally (IV) for the treatment of **status epilepticus** (see later). It is also used for convulsions accompanying **acute alcohol withdrawal. Oral dosage** for adults ranges from 2 to 10 mg bid to qid.

Clorazepate

Clorazepate is used as an adjunct in the treatment of **partial seizures.** The initial dose is 7.5 mg tid in adults, and bid in children from 9 to 12 years of age.

Valproic Acid Derivatives

Valproic acid, Valproate Sodium, Divalproex Sodium

Valporic acid, its sodium salt, and divalproex sodium (composed of equal parts of valproic acid and valproate sodium) provide improved seizure control when added to drug regimens of patients with **multiple seizure types,** refractory to other treatments.

Mode of action: Valproic acid induces an elevation in the functional levels of GABA in the CNS. The **metabolic acidosis** caused by valproic acid may also have some protective action against seizures.

Therapeutic uses: (i) For treatment of **simple and complex** absence seizures, including petit mal seizures; (ii) used as adjunct in the treatment of **multiple seizure types.**

Dosage: The recommended initial dose is 15 mg/kg/day which may be increased by 5 to 10 mg/kg/day at 1-week intervals till optimal control is obtained or side effects occur. Maximum daily dose is 60 mg/kg.

Adverse reactions: Common side effects are nausea, vomiting and indigestion. In addition, sedation, abdominal cramps, and minor elevations of transaminases (SGOT, SGPT) and LDH may occur. Lenticular opacities, nystagmus, diplopia, dizziness, acute pancreatitis and blood dyscrasias may occur. **Fatal hepatic failure** can occur.

OTHER UNRELATED ANTICONVULSANTS

Acetazolamide

Acetazolamide is a carbonic anhydrase inhibitor used as an adjunct to control **petit mal,** and other **absence** or **non-localized** seizures. This drug has also been employed as a **mild diuretic,** for relief of **migraine,** and for the treatment of **chronic open-angle glaucoma.**

The beneficial effect largely is due to the mild **acidosis** produced by acetazolamide.

The usual starting dose of acetazolamide is 250 mg/day, and the maintenance range is 375 to 1000 mg/day, generally in combination with another antiepileptic. It is **contraindicated** in patients with **sulphonamide allergy.**

Primidone

Primidone is not a true barbiturate, but is structurally related to phenobarbital, and has a similar action profile. Its **mode of action** is similar to phenobarbital. It is used to treat **grand mal seizures**; **psychomotor seizures;** complex and partial motor seizures (Jacksonian).

Phenacemide

Phenacemide is a structural analogue of hydantoins, and is useful in **severe epileptic states,** specially mixed forms of **psychomotor seizures refractory to other medications.** It is employed as a last resort, because of its extreme toxicity.

Lidocaine

Lidocaine is used as an alternative to general anaesthesia in the treatment of **status epilepticus.**

Magnesium Sulphate

Magnesium, in the form of magnesium sulphate, is an effective anticonvulsant in seizures associated with **toxaemia of pregnancy**, and other conditions with abnormally low plasma magnesium.

Magnesium controls convulsions possibly by *blocking the release of acetylcholine (ACh) from the motor nerve ending.* It also has a depressant effect on the CNS. **Adult IM doses** range from 1 to 5 g of a 25 to 50 percent solution, up to 5 times a day, if necessary. **Adverse effects** include sweating, hypotension, sedation, confusion, hypothermia, flaccid paralysis, respiratory depression, and circulatory collapse.

Lamotrigine, Gabapentin, Vigabatrin, and **Felbamate** are *four* newer antiepileptics under evaluation.

Drug Therapy of Status Epilepticus

Status epilepticus is a medical emergency, resulting from continuous or repetitive grand mal seizures. Serious brain damage is likely, and the degree of danger is related to the duration of seizures. The essential principle of therapy is to administer adequately large doses of an appropriate anticonvulsant by the IV route.

The management of status epilepticus is directed towards *securing airway, protection from injury, maintenance of fluid and electrolyte balance and drug therapy*:

1. **Diazepam:** Intravenous diazepam is the drug of choice, and should be administered immediately. The usual adult dose is 10 mg (children over 7 years, 5 mg; infants 0.25 mg /kg body weight). The injection may be repeated after 15 minutes. Continuous IV infusion (1 mg / minute) may be given.
2. **Phenobarbital:** In an adult a slow IV injection of up to 250 mg of phenobarbital over a period of 2-3 minutes is given. This dose may be repeated after 30 minutes, if necessary.
3. **Phenytoin:** IV infusion of phenytoin is given not exceeding 50 mg / minute in adults.
4. **Paraldehyde:** It is given in a dose of 0.1 ml / kg body weight by deep IM injection (plastic syringes must not be used).

5. **Lidocaine:** As a last resort, and an *alternative to general anaesthesia*, lidocaine is sometimes infused IV when all other drugs have failed.

To sum up, **diazepam** is the drug of choice. If it fails **paraldehyde** is given. Barbiturates are best avoided because of the risk of respiratory depression.

2.6 NARCOTIC ANALGESICS

Narcotic analgesics are a group of **naturally occurring** and **synthetic agents** which interact with specific **opioid receptor sites** in the CNS to relieve pain in conscious persons.

TERMINOLOGY

Drugs used in the management of severe pain have been designed as **"narcotic analgesics".**

The term **"opiate"** has been loosely applied to morphine derivatives, thus comprising the **natural** and **semisynthetic** compounds. Currently, the term "opioid" is preferred to designate all such substances, **natural**, **semisynthetic**, or **synthetic** that activate opioid receptors.

NEUROPHYSIOLOGY OF PAIN

Peripheral mechanisms: Pain is produced by damage to tissues that leads to the liberation of chemicals near the nerve endings. There is evidence indicating that locally produced chemicals like **bradykinin** and **prostaglandins** are associated with production of pain. Other chemicals like **histamine, acetylcholine, lactic acid, serotonin** and **potassium** are also involved in the initiation of pain impulses.

Visceral pain is primarily conducted by sympathetic nerves, and is dull, aching and vaguely localized. Pain of visceral origin is sometimes felt on certain cutaneous areas of the body surface at some distance from the involved viscera (**referred pain**).

Central neural mechanisms: Although the appreciation of pain is complicated and complex in nature, the **"gate control" theory,** which essentially is an input control mechanism, has proved useful in explaining some aspects of it.

TYPES OF ANALGESICS

Analgesia denotes relief of pain. The term "analgesic" covers those agents only, which provide **nonspecific relief** from the pain, without loss of consciousness.

Analgesic drugs are divided into **two** main groups:

i. **Narcotic analgesics:** These agents are capable of relieving *severe* pain, but are also moderately or strongly **addictive.** This group includes the **opioids,** which bind to the **opioid receptors in the CNS.**
ii. **Non-narcotic analgesics:** These agents relieve *mild* to *moderate* pain, and are **non-addictive.** This group includes **aspirin,** and other analgesic-antipyreptics, and their site of action is peripheral.

OPIUM AND ITS ALKALOIDS

The poppy plant, ***Papaver somniferum,*** is the source of opium. The poppy plant is found in India, Turkey, China, South-east Asia, Russia, and Mexico.

Opium is obtained by incising the unripe seed capsule of the poppy plant. The milky juice that oozes out is dried in air and forms a brown gummy mass. After further drying, it is powdered. This **powdered opium** contains over 20 alkaloids. The useful alkaloids of opium are **morphine, papaverine** and **noscapine** (see below).

These alkaloids have **two** distinct chemical forms:

1. **Phenanthrene derivatives:** These are analgesic alkaloids consisting of **morphine; codeine** and **thebaine.**
2. **Benzylisoquinoline derivatives:** These include **papaverine** which is a spasmolytic and vasodilator; and **narcotine** or **noscapine** which is an antitussive.

CLASSIFICATION OF NARCOTIC ANALGESICS

1. **Narcotic Agonist Analgesics**
   A. *Phenanthrenes*
      i. *Naturally occurring* opium alkaloids (*morphine, codeine*).
      ii. *Semisynthetic derivatives* of morphine (*hydromorphone, oxymorphone*).
      iii. *Semisynthetic derivatives* of codeine (*hydrocodone, oxycodone*).
   B. *Methadones* (methadone, propoxyphene).
   C. *Morphinan* (levorphanol).
   D. *Phenylpiperidine (pethidine).*
2. **Narcotic Agonist-Antagonist Analgesics**
   A. *Phenanthrene (buprenorphine, nalbuphine).*
   B. *Morphinan (butorphanol).*
   C. *Benzomorphans (phenazocine, pentazocine).*

OPIOID RECEPTORS

Opioid receptors were first isolated by Pert and Snyder in 1973. The opioids exert their effect by combining with the opioid receptors in the CNS. These receptors appear to be the site of action of the endogenous opioids—the **enkephalins, dynorphins,** and **endorphins.**

ENDOGENOUS OPIOIDS

The CNS sites that contain opioid receptors also contain **endogenous** morphine-like peptides that interact with the opioid receptors to elicit effects similar to those of exogenous narcotic agonists. **Three** groups of endogenous opioid peptides have been isolated, and termed **endorphins**, **enkephalins** and **dynorphins.** Their further consideration is beyond the scope of this text.

Pharmacologic Actions of Narcotic Analgesics

The pharmacologic effects of opioids involve many systems in the body, and are outlined in **Table 2.4.**

Table 2.4: *Major pharmacologic effects of narcotic analgesics*

System	Effects
Central nervous system (CNS)	Analgesia, Sedation, Euphoria, Emesis Depressed cough reflex Respiratory depression
Cardiovascular system (CVS)	Orthostatic hypotension (depression of medullary vasomotor centre, and peripheral vasodilation)
Gastrointestinal tract (GIT)	Decreased peristalsis and stomach motility Delayed gastric emptying Constipation
Smooth muscle	Increased tone of most nonvascular smooth muscles (e.g., GI, urinary and biliary tracts)
Urinary system	Urinary tract spasm Contraction of urinary sphincter Release of antidiuretic hormone (ADH)
Eye	Miosis

NARCOTIC AGONIST ANALGESICS

Phenanthrenes

Morphine

Morphine is the prototype narcotic analgesic.

Pharmacological Actions

Central nervous system: The most important action of morphine is relief from pain, and it relieves nearly all types of pain. Morphine **elevates the pain perception threshold**, and modifies the patient's subjective awareness of pain. **Euphoria** may also occur. **Tolerance** and **dependence** develop to the analgesic effect of morphine.

Other **suppressant central effects** produced by morphine include drowsiness, and with larger doses sleep. Morphine depresses the **respiratory centre**. The **cough centre** is also *depressed.*

Central stimulating actions: Morphine causes vomiting in 10-15 percent of patients by stimulation of the **chemoreceptor trigger zone**. **Epileptic fits** may be provoked. Morphine causes **pupillary constriction**.

Gastrointestinal and urinary tracts: Morphine increases the muscle tone throughout the gastrointestinal tract, which is combined with decreased peristalsis, leading to **constipation**.

Cardiovascular system: In therapeutic doses in the supine position, there is no major effect on blood pressure or heart rate.

Respiratory system: Morphine depresses the respiratory centre in the brainstem. The **cough reflex is depressed**. It causes constriction of the bronchial smooth muscle.

Pharmacokinetics: Morphine is irregularly absorbed from the gastrointestinal tract, and is rarely administered orally for pain relief. Morphine undergoes a considerable hepatic first-pass metabolism, and only 30 percent of an oral dose reaches systemic circulation. The oral route is useful in the *management of cancer pain*. Morphine and its congeners are well absorbed by diffusion from parenteral sites, and can be given by SC, IM or IV injection. The major route of elimination of metabolites is by glomerular filtration into the urine.

Therapeutic Uses

1. **Pain:** For acute pain following injury, myocardial infarction, or in the immediate postoperative period, the average adult dose is 10 mg SC or IM repeated 4-6 hourly. Morphine may be given intravenously when rapid relief is required.

   Morphine or one of its congeners may be used for **relief of pain in terminal illness** due to cancer.
2. **Left ventricular failure:** Morphine is effective in the relief of *acute left ventricular failure* and *dyspnoea* due to associated pulmonary oedema.
3. **Cough:** The cough reflex is suppressed by the opioids. Codeine is preferable.

Adverse Reactions

Nausea, vomiting, constipation, respiratory depression, histamine release, cardiovascular effects (hypotension and bradycardia), increased intracranial pressure, bronchial spasm, spasm of biliary and urinary tracts, and urinary retention. On repeated administration tolerance and dependence occurs.

Contraindications and precautions: To sum up, morphine and other opioids are to be used with caution, or are contraindicated in:

i. Head injuries, delirium tremens, increased intracranial pressure;
ii. Severe bronchial asthma, emphysema, and other diseases with a limited pulmonary reserve;
iii. Metabolic disorders like myxoedema, Addison's disease, hepatic cirrhosis, and also renal failure; and
iv. Prostatic hypertrophy, hypovolaemic shock and hypersensitivity.

Preparations and dosage: Morphine is available in the form of **morphine sulphate** and **morphine hydrochloride.** It is usually administered by IM or SC injection in a dose of 10 mg / 70 kg body weight (range 5 to 20 mg). It may also be given IV in a dose of 2.5 to 15 mg in 4 to 5 ml of water for injection, administered slowly over 4 to 5 minutes.

Drug interactions: The CNS-depressant effects of opioids may be potentiated or prolonged by concurrent use of other CNS depressants like barbiturates, alcohol, anaesthetics, and phenothiazines.

Acute Opioid Poisoning (Acute Toxicity)

Acute opioid poisoning may result from *clinical* overdosage, *accidental* overdosage usually in addicts, or attempts at *suicide*.

Symptoms and signs: The triad of **coma, pinpoint pupils** and **depressed respiration** strongly suggest poisoning. With large overdosage there is profound coma, and the patient cannot be aroused. The respiratory rate is slow (at times 2 to 4/minute). **Cyanosis** may be present. The blood pressure progressively falls. The pupils are symmetrical and pinpoint.

Treatment: The first step is to establish a patent airway and ventilate the patient. In opium overdosage, it is desirable to administer a **charcoal mixture,** or to wash the stomach (gastric lavage) with solutions of **alkaloidal precipitants** (e.g., tannic acid), or oxidizers (i.e., **potassium permanganate** 1: 5,000 dilution).

Immediate steps should be taken to combat advancing respiratory depression. For this **opioid antagonists** like **naloxone** can produce a dramatic reversal of severe respiratory depression. Naloxone is administered in small doses of 0.4 mg IV, repeated after 2 to 3 minutes. **Pulmonary oedema** may be countered by **positive pressure respiration.**

Chronic toxicity (Opioid addiction): The nature of opioid dependence has been discussed in **Chapter 2.10.**

Codeine

Codeine is the second most important alkaloid of opium poppy. It is widely used as an **analgesic, antidiarrhoel** and **cough suppressant.** Analgesic potency is considerably lower than morphine. Codeine 120 mg IM is equivalent to 10 mg of parenteral morphine. It produces slight *sedation, practically no euphoria*, and *no noticeable respiratory depression* in therapeutic doses. **Tolerance** develops far less rapidly than with morphine and dependence occurs rarely. **Dosage** of codeine phosphate for **analgesia** in adults ranges from 15 mg to 60 mg qid orally, SC, IM or IV. For **cough suppression** the dose is 10 to 20 mg every 4 to 6 hours to a maximum of 120 mg/24 hours.

Hydromorphone

Hydromorphone is a clinically used semisynthetic derivative of morphine. It is *10 times more potent* than morphine as an analgesic, and so also its respiratory depressant effect is greater. It produces less sedation, vomiting and nausea. It has a *high abuse potential* and is a popular "street drug". **Dose:** 2 mg to 4 mg orally, SC, IM every 4 to 6 hours.

Heroin

Heroin is another semisynthetic derivative of morphine. It is 3 times more potent than morphine as an analgesic. It causes less sedation, less constipation, and less nausea and vomiting compared to morphine. It produces **marked euphoria** and has a very high addiction liability. Hence, it is not available as a drug for routine use. It may be used for the management of **terminal illness due to cancer.**

Oxycodone

Oxycodone is used for relief of moderate to severe pain, and possesses good **antitussive** action. Oxycodone hydrochloride is usually administered orally in a dose of 5 mg every 6 hours.

Methadone

Methadone may be used to relieve **severe pain** in a dose of 2.5 to 10 mg IM, SC or orally. For **chronic pain** relief it is administered in a dose of 5 mg every 12 hours to 20 mg every 5 hours. Methadone is also used for **detoxification** and maintenance of opioid (morphine or heroin) addicts. It acts in two ways: (i) **suppress the withdrawal syndrome,** and (ii) **maintains patients** who have been withdrawn from narcotics, and are in a stage of minimal craving for the narcotic (**Chap. 2.10**).

Propoxyphene

Propoxyphene is a **very weak analgesic,** structurally related to methadone, and has little antitussive activity. Its addiction liability equals that of codeine. Propoxyphene (dextropropoxyphene) is superior to codeine as it does not produce constipation, and the incidence of nausea, vomiting and dizziness is lower. It may be used to treat myalgia, neuralgia, migraine, backache, and arthritic pain. In high doses it produces *euphoria* and *dependence*. The oral dose of dextropropoxyphene hydrochloride is 65 to 130 mg every 4 hours.

Phenylpiperidines

Pethidine

Pethidine was introduced in 1939 as t*he first synthetic narcotic analgesic*. It is the most frequently prescribed opioid. Pethidine is a moderately potent analgesic (1/10 morphine), with weak antitussive activity.

Pethidine is used for treating **moderately severe pain,** and the usual dose is 25-100 mg IM, SC and occasionally by slow IV drip. It may also be given orally in a dose of 50-150 mg. It is useful for relief of pain of **coronary occlusion**, **biliary** or **renal colic.** It is used preoperatively as an adjunct to anaesthesia, and for **obstetrical analgesia** at 1-3 hours intervals.

Adverse effects include dizziness, tachycardia, nausea, vomiting, orthostatic hypotension, and excitement. Respiratory depression occurs with higher doses.

NARCOTIC AGONIST-ANTAGONIST ANALGESICS

Phenanthrenes

Buprenorphine

Buprenorphine is a narcotic agonist-antagonist. It is a semisynthetic derivative of thebaine. Its **antagonist** activity is equal to that of naloxone. Buprenophine is 20 to 30 times more potent than morphine as an analgesic.

Buprenorphine is used in the treatment of **moderate to severe pain,** after **myocardial infarction** and in **terminal care.** The usual dose range is 0.3 to 0.6 mg IM, or slow IV every 6 hours, as needed.

Nalbuphine

Nalbuphine possesses both **agonistic** activity, and weak **antagonistic** activity. It may precipitate withdrawal symptoms in narcotic addicts. The usual dose is 10 mg / 90 kg body weight SC, IM or IV, repeated every 3-6 hours, as necessary. Maximum dose is 160 mg/day.

Morphinan

Butorphanol

Butorphanol is a potent analgesic, about 4 to 7 times more potent than morphine on weight basis. Respiratory depression is more marked than with morphine. It possesses weak narcotic antagonistic activity, and withdrawal symptoms can occur in narcotic dependent patients. The usual dose is 2 mg IM every 3-4 hours, or 1 mg IV every 3-4 hours. It is ineffective by month.

Benzomorphans

Phenazocine

Phenazocine is one of the most potent narcotic analgesics on a weight basis. It is claimed that phenazocine does not cause spasm of the sphincter of Oddi, and thus is useful in treating **biliary** and **pancreatic** pain. It is used as an analgesic in **terminal care** of cancer patients in doses of 5 mg (20 mg if needed). Phenazocine can also be given, for **postoperative pain** and for **obstetrical analgesia.**

Pentazocine

Pentazocine possesses some narcotic antagonistic activity also, and can produce withdrawal symptoms in narcotic dependent patients. Pentazocine is used for relief of **chronic intractable pain.** The usual dose is 50 mg every 3-4 hours orally (maximum dose 600 mg/day).

NARCOTIC ANTAGONISTS

Considering the **agonist-antagonist ratios** of various opioids and opioid antagonists, morphine is a **pure agonist** while **naloxone** and **naltrexone** are **pure antagonists.**

Drugs capable of reversing the effects of narcotic agonists are termed **narcotic antagonists.** Both the drugs currently in use in this category–**naloxone** and **naltrexone**—are viewed as "pure"

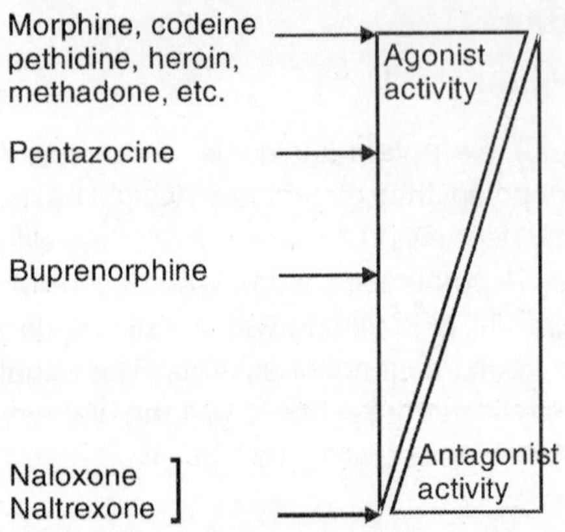

Fig. 2.2 : *The agonist:antagonist ratios of some opioids and opioid antagonists (see text).*

Naloxone

Mode of action: Naloxone exhibits a very high affinity for the (mu) μ receptors, and is capable of displacing narcotic drugs from these sites, reversing their effects. No tolerance or dependence has been reported.

Therapeutic uses: Naloxone is used for: (i) **Reversal of respiratory depression** and other adverse effects induced by overdosage of opioids; and (ii) **Diagnosis of acute opioid overdosage**.

Dosage: To treat known or suspected overdosage in adults an initial dose of 0.4 mg to 2 mg IV wiith additional doses repeated at 2 to 3 minute intervals, as needed upto 3 doses.

Adverse reactions: The main adverse reactions include nausea, vomitting, sweating, tachycardia, and increased blood pressure. Excessive dosage can result in excitement.

Naltrexone

Mode of action: Naltrexone blocks the effects of opioids by a **competitive binding** at opioid receptors. It is a **pure antagonist.** When given concurrently with opioids to a properly motivated individual, it provides an adjunctive means for maintaining an opioid-free state.

Therapeutic use: Used as adjunctive therapy in the maintenance of an opioid-free state in detoxified former addicts.

Dosage: Naltrexone is available as 50 mg tablets. The initial dose is 25 mg and the patient should be observed for 1 hour. If no withdrawal signs occur, an additional 25 mg is given. Thereafter, 50 mg once daily will provide effective blocking action.

Adverse reactions: Major side effects are due to the precipitation of a withdrawal syndrome, and include nervousness, headache, insomnia, cramps, nausea, vomiting, muscle pain and nasal congestion.

ANTITUSSIVES

Most drugs used for the suppression of cough act by **blocking the central component of the cough reflex.** Narcotics are particularly effective in this respect. **Codeine** is the most widely used agent. Other agents are:

Dextromethorphan

Dextromethorphan has **antitussive activity,** but no analgesic activity. It acts centrally to **elevate the cough threshold.** The usual dose is 15-30 mg every 4 to 6 hours.

Noscapine

Noscapine has **antitussive** properties It has minimal other effects on the CNS. Noscapine is the principal antitussive in several proprietary preparations. The usual dose is 15-30 mg every 4 to 6 hours.

2.7 NONSTEROIDAL ANTI-INFLAMMATORY AGENTS (DRUGS FOR GOUT, RHEUMATOID ARTHRITIS AND MIGRAINE)

There are two main classes of pain: **superficial** (integumental), and **deep.** Some pain receptors in the body are **chemoreceptors,** as compounds like **bradykinin** and **prostaglandins** can elicit pain.

TERMINOLOGY

The **non-narcotic analgestics** are a large group of drugs which have **analgesic, antipyretic** and **anti-inflammatory actions.** They have been variously named–**analgesic-antipyretics**; **aspirin-like drugs;** and **nonsteroidal anti-inflammatory drugs (NSAIDs).**

CLASSIFICATION

The nonsteroidal anti-inflammatory drugs may be classified as under:

Nonsteroidal Anti-inflammatory Drugs (NSAIDs)

1. **Salicylates:** Aspirin, methyl salicylate, salicylic acid, sodium salicylate, sufasalazine.
2. **Para-aminophenol:** Paracetamol.
3. **Pyrazolones:** Phenylbutazone, oxyphenbutazone, sulfinpyrazone
4. **Indole derivative:** Indomethacin.
5. **Propionic acid derivatives:** Ibuprofen, fenoprofen, ketoprofen, naproxen, flurbiprofen.
6. **Fenamate:** Mefenamic acid.
7. **Phenylacetic acid derivative:** Diclofenac, aceclofenac.
8. **Oxicams:** Piroxicam, tenoxicam.
9. **Sulfonanilide:** Nimesulide.
10. **Coxibs:** Celecoxib, valdecoxib, etoricoxib.
11. **Miscellaneous:** Hydroxychloroquine, penicillamine.
12. **Gold compounds:** Auranofin, aurothioglucose, gold sodium thiomalate.
13. **Nutraceuticals:** Glucosamine and Chondroitin sulphate.
14. **Antigout drugs:** Colchicine, probenecid, sulfinpyrazone, allopurinol.

Salicylates

The salicylates are derivatives of salicylic acid. Aspirin is the most popular analgesic. It is one of the oldest drugs in use.

Aspirin (Acetylsalicylic Acid)

The **prototype** synthetic salicylate, aspirin, was introduced as a substitute for sodium salicylate.

Pharmacological Actions and Mode of Action

The salicylates act both **centrally** and **peripherally** to produce their therapeutic and toxic effects. Aspirin exhibits analgesic, antipyretic and anti-inflammatory action.

Analgesic/anti-inflammatory action: The analgesic action is mainly a peripheral effect, in the form of a ***blockade of pain impulse generation.*** They exert some action on subcortical sites like the **thalamus** and **hypothalamus.**

The **prostaglandins** are released on tissue damage, and are present in the inflammatory exudates. The final step in prostaglandin synthesis is governed by the enzyme **prostaglandin synthetase,** and aspirin inhibits its activity. Prostaglandins play a part in the **erythema, oedema, pain** and **fever** associated with inflammation. The analgesic anti-inflammatory drugs inhibit **cyclo-oxygenase,** and **reduce prostaglandin production.** They also have an **anti-bradykinin** action.

Antirheumatic action: The mechanism of antirheumatic action is unclear. The salicylates and other antirheumatic drugs prevent the release of **lysosomal enzymes** which destroy the cartilage of rheumatic joints.

Antipyretic action: Body temperature is controlled from a hypothalamic integrating centre (thermostat). Fevers caused by bacterial endotoxins or viruses, are caused by *endogenous pyrogens* which act directly upon the thermoregulatory neurones in the hypothalamus to increase the set point temperature.

Salicylates have a marked antipyretic action, and reduce elevated body temperature. This is accompanied by profuse sweating, and is due to inhibition of the synthesis and release of PGE_2 in the **hypothalamus.** PGE_2 has a strong pyrogenic action.

Respiration and acid-base balance: The salicylates cause serious acid-base imbalances. As a secondary effect **respiratory alkalosis** occurs.

Gastrointestinal effects: The gastric mucosa shows *gastritis* with *superficial gastric ulceration.*

Cardiovascular effects: Therapeutic doses of salicylates have no important direct cardiovascular action. The peripheral vessels dilate after large doses, due to a direct effect on the smooth muscle.

Hepatic and renal effects: Salicylates elevate enzyme activities in the plasma which indicate hepatic dysfunction (SGOT, SGPT, alkaline phosphatase), and occasionally *hepatomegaly* occurs.

Prolonged salicylate dosage can cause *permanent renal damage.*

Platelet anti-aggregatory action: Platelet aggregation is inhibited by aspirin, but not to a significant extent by other salicylates. Low doses of aspirin (40 to 80 mg/day) are more effective in reducing platelet aggregation than high doses.

Endocrine effects: The plasma levels of adrenocorticosteroids transiently increase, mainly by displacement from plasma proteins. In diabetes mellitus, **aspirin lowers the blood glucose level.**

Uricosuric effect: In suitable doses the salicylates increase the urinary excretion of urates.

Salicylates and pregnancy: There is no evidence that salicylates cause foetal damage in humans.

Local effects: Salicylic acid is an irritant to the skin and mucosa and destroys epithelial cells. This **keratolytic action** of salicylic acid is used for the local treatment of corns, warts, fungal infections, and certain types of eczematous dermatitis. **Methyl salicylate** (oil of wintergreen) is irritating both to the skin and mucosa. It is used externally, in liniments as a **counterirritant.**

Pharmacokinetics

Orally ingested salicylates (aspirin and sodium salicylate) are absorbed rapidly, partly from the stomach, but mostly from the upper small intestine. Appreciable plasma concentrations are reached within 30 minutes, after a single dose. The pharmacokinetics of salicylate elimination is complex.

Therapeutic Uses

1. **Analgesia:** Aspirin is used for the relief of mild to moderate pain of musculoskeletal origin, e.g., **headache, myalgia, neuralgia, toothache, dysmenorrhoea,** and **backache.**
2. **Antipyresis:** Aspirin lowers elevated body temperature (pyrexia). The antipyretic response is non-specific and offers only a symptomatic relief. Use of aspirin should be avoided in cases of very high fever (hyperpyrexia), as it may produce a *shock-like state* due to profuse sweating, and a sudden fall in body temperature.
3. **Anti-inflammatory activity:** Salicylates may be used for various inflammatory conditions, e.g., **rheumatoid arthritis, osteoarthritis, bursitis,** and **acute rheumatic fever.** Large doses of aspirin (3 g to 7g/day) are usually necessary.
4. **Prophylaxis** of thromboembolic complications like **venous emboli,** and **cerebral ischemia** associated with cardiovascular disorders. Aspirin reduces the **risk of transient ischemic attacks** (TIA).
5. **Prevention of re-infarction** in patients with previous history of *acute myocardial infarction* or *unstable angina.*

Contraindications and Precautions

Salicylates are contraindicated in cases of **salicylate hypersensitivity, haemophilia, bleeding ulcers** and **other baemorrhagic states.** The **Reye's syndrome,** has been linked with the use of aspirin in children under the age of 12 years who have **influenza** or **chickenpox.**

Preparations and dosage of salicylates: The various preparations and usual dosages of salicylates are listed in **Table 2.5.**

Table 2.5 : *Preparations and dosage of salicylates*

Drug	Preparations	Dosage range	Comments
Aspirin	Tablets, gum tablets, Enteric-coated tablets, Timed release tablets, Enteric coated capsules, suppositories	Adults: Pain, fever-325 to 650 mg. Transient ischaemic attacks-40-130 mg/day; prevention of myocardial infarction - 325 mg/day	Keep aspirin in a cool, dry place; use suppositories for a vomiting patient
Methyl salicylate (oil of winter green)	10% to 50% in Ointment or liniment	Applied topically as a counterirritant to relieve muscular and rheumatic pain	Significant absorption can occur through skin and produce untoward effects; very toxic if ingested orally.
Salicylic acid	Cream - 2.5, 10% Ointment - 25,40, 60% Gel- 6,17% Soap - 3.5% Liquid- 13.6 Plaster - 40%	Applied to the affected area at night, and wash off in the morning	Used topically as a keratolytic agent for psoriasis, acne, keratosis, fungal infections or other conditions requiring removal of dead skin.

Adverse Reactions

The most frequent side effects with salicylates are **heartburn, nausea** and **gastric distress.** These can be overcome by taking the drug with food, a full glass of water, an antacid or in one of the enteric-coated dosage forms.

1. **Salicylism:** Large doses of salicylates result in headache, dizziness, tinnitus, confusion, sweating, deafness, palpitation and hyperventilation.
2. **Haemorrhage:** Major G.I. bleeding occurs in chronic users of aspirin.
3. **Hypersensitivity reactions.**
4. **Reye's syndrome:** Use of salicylates, specially aspirin in children with *influenza* has been associated with Reye's syndrome, a life threatening conditions marked by severe vomiting, lethargy, delirium, coma and death.
5. Other adverse reactions include renal dysfunction, delirium, hallucinations, acid-base disturbances, hyperthermia, petechial haemorrhages, hypokalaemia, convulsions, respiratory failure, coma and death.
6. **Drug interactions:** The metabolites of aspirin enhance the actions and toxicity of **oral anticoagulants, heparin, naproxen, oral antidiabetics, phenytoin, thiopental, indomethacin, methotrexate,** and **valproic acid.**

Salicylate Poisoning

Because of the easy availability of salicylates in the household, salicylates are a frequent cause of intoxication in children. In adults the intoxication is generally **accidental** or **suicidal. Acute intoxication** is manifested by early signs of CNS stimulation including hyperventilation; later complex acid-base imbalances, and petechial haemorrhages occur.

Treatment: The patient should be hospitalized. **Gastric lavage, alkalinization, diuresis** and **intensive supportive measures** are necessary. **Activated charcoal** reduces the absorption of salicylate from the gut. Hyperthermia and dehydration need sponging with tepid water or alcohol provides quick relief. **Bicarbonate solutions** must be infused intravenously to maintain alkaline diuresis. **Plasma transfusion** may be beneficial. Haemorrhagic phenomena may necessitate **whole blood transfusion** and vitamin K. In very severe intoxication, measures like **exchange transfusion, peritoneal dialysis, haemodialysis, or haemoperfusion** are effective in removing the salicylate from the system.

Sulfasalazine

It was originally introduced for the treatment of *ulcerative colitis,* but was later shown to be effective also in patients of *rheumatoid arthritis.* This drug is approved by the FDA, USA for use in **rheumatoid arthritis.** *Dosage* is 2 g/day in 4 divided doses. ***Adverse reactions*** include dizziness, rashes, photosensitivity, anorexia, nausea and vomiting. Rarely neutropenia, hypersensitivity pneumonitis and sterility may occur.

NON-SALICYLATES

Para Aminophenol

Paracetamol (Acetaminophen)

Paracetamol is the major *metabolite of phenacetin* and has similar analgesic-antipyretic actions, but it does not possess any anti-inflammatory or antirheumatic activity. It has no effect on platelets or blood clotting mechanisms. Paracetamol is a *weak inhibitor of perpheral prostaglandin synthetase, and is as potent as aspirin in inhibiting the brain prostaglandin synthetase.*

Pharmacokinetics: The absorption rate and relative bioavailability of paracetamol are increased by concomitant administration of *metoclopramide.* It is evenly distributed throughout the body. The major metabolites are excreted in the urine.

Therapeutic uses: Paracetamol is a mild analgesic-antipyretic. It does not irritate the gastric mucosa, and has therefore been employed as a **substitute for aspirin.** The usual dose is 0.5 to 1 g (1-2 tablets) repeated 4-6 hourly to maintain analgesia.

Adverse effects include drug rashes, methaemoglobinaemia and blood dyscrasias occasionally. On prolonged usage, or overdosage or abuse, **paracetamol liver damage** may occur.

Analgesic Nephropathy

High consumption of non-narcotic analgesics increases the incidence of chronic renal disease manifested as **papillary necrosis, interstitial fibrosis** and **tubular atrophy.** This problem is still incompletely resolved.

Indole Derivative

Indomethacin

Indomethacin is used in **rheumatoid arthritis**, and **ankylosing spondylitis** for its anti-inflammatory, and antipyretic effects. Indomethacin *inhibits prostaglandin* E_2.

Pharmacokinetics: Indomethacin is rapidly and completely absorbed from the gut following oral administration. Indomethacin and its metabilities are excreted in the urine.

Dose: Indomethacin is available for oral use in capsules containing 25 or 50 mg of the drug. The **initial dose** is 25 mg twice daily, and can be increased by 25 mg increments weekly to a total daily dose of 100 to 200 mg taken with food or after meals.

Toxicity: The most common adverse effects are headache, light headedness, confusion or hallucinations. Gastric bleeding is not common but can occur. Haemopoietic reactions like neutropenia, thrombocytopenia, and rarely aplastic anaemia may occur.

Propionic Acid Derivatives

Ibuprofen

Like aspirin, ibuprofen has analgesic, *anti-inflammatory* and *antipyretic* action. It is rapidly absorbed from the gastrointestinal tract and peak plasma concentrations are reached in 1 to 2 hours. It is rapidly metabolized and eliminated in the urine.

Clinically it is used in the treatment of **rheumatoid arthritis, osteoarthritis, ankylosing**

spondylitis, dysmenorrhoea, cervical spondylosis, and **ophthalmic, dental** and **ENT inflammation.** The adult dose is 400 mg tid or 300 mg qid. *Side effects* include gastrointestinal disturbances, headache, dizziness and fluid retention.

Fenoprofen: Fenoprofen is chemically and pharmacologically similar to ibuprofen. **Dosage** ranges between 1.2 and 1.8 g per day in three to four divided doses.

Ketoprofen: It is virtually completely absorbed from the gut. The recommended daily dose is 100 to 150 mg per day in divided doses.

Naproxen

Like aspirin, it has *analgesic-antipyretic* and *anti-inflammatory* actions. It is fully absorbed when administered orally. It is almost completely bound (98 to 99%) to plasma proteins following therapeutic doses. Clinically it is used in the treatment of **rheumatoid arthritis, osteoarthritis** and **ankylosing spondylitis.** The dosage is 250 mg given twice daily with meals if gastric discomfort is experienced.

Flurbiprofen

Flurbiprofen is considered to be one of the potent inhibitors of prostaglandin synthesis. Flurbiprofen also is a potent **inhibitor of leucocyte migration** into inflamed tissues.

Flurbiprofen is well absorbed orally; peak blood levels occur 0.5 to 4.0 hours after administration. The elimination half-life is 5-7 hours. No accumulation of the drug occurs. It is highly bound (99%) to plasma proteins, and excreted in the urine.

Flurbiprofen is used in the treatment of **rheumatoid arthritis, osteoarthritis** and **ankylosing spondylitis,** and the daily dosage is 200 to 300 mg in 2 to 4 divided doses. **Adverse reactions** include GI disturbances like diarrhoea, dyspepsia, and vomiting. GI bleeding and ulceration is rare.

Fenamate

Mefenamic Acid

It is absorbed rather slowly from the gut, reaching peak concentrations in 2-4 hours. It is 98.5 percent bound to plasma proteins. It has the property of *inhibiting cyclo-oxygenase.*

Gastrointestinal symptoms are the most common adverse effects. **Diarrhoea** occurs in a large number of patients. Other infrequent side effects include dizziness, rashes, haemolytic anaemia, agranulocytosis and megaloblastic anemia.

Phenylacetic Acid Derivative

Diclofenac

Diclofenac has analgesic, antipyretic and anti-inflammatory activities. It is an **inhibitor of cyclo-oxygenase** and its potency is appreciably greater than that of indomethacin, naproxen and several other NSAIDs.

Diclofenac is approved for long-term treatment of **rheumatoid arthritis, osteoarthritis** and **ankylosing spondylitis.** Also used in short-term treatment of acute musculo-skelatal injury, acute painful shoulder, postoperative pain, and dysmenorrhoea. The daily dosage is 100 to 200 mg bid or tid. **Adverse reactions** include GI disturbances and headache, and a reversible elevation of serum transaminases. Skin rashes, allergic reactions, fluid retention, oedema, and impairment of renal function can occur.

Aceclofenac

Aceclofenac has actions and side effects similar to naproxen. Like diclofenac it is used in the management of **rheumatoid arthritis, osteoarthritis** and **ankylosing spondylitis.** Unlike diclofenac it stimulates the synthesis of *glucosaminoglycans* (GAG), and thereby helps in the healing process. Dose: 100 mg bid.

Oxicams

Piroxicam

Piroxicam possesses anti-inflammatory, analgesic, and antipyretic activity. It is the NSAID offered for once-a-day treatment of **rheumatoid arthritis** and **osteoarthritis** and this helps patient compliance.

Piroxicam is an *inhibitor of prostaglandin biosynthesis*, comparable to indomethacin. It also *inhibits activation of neutrophils*, which is an additional mode of its anti-inflammatory action. It is well absorbed on oral administrations and peak plasma levels are attained in 3 to 4 hours. Piroxicam is extensively metabolized to inactive compounds and excreted in urine (two thirds) and faeces (one third). *Adverse GI reactions* are common, but oedema, dizziness, headache, rash and haematological changes can occur. Serious GI toxicity in the form of bleeding, peptic ulceration, and perforation have been reported. The dose is 20 mg daily as a single dose. Maximal therapeutic response should not a expected before 2 weeks.

Tenoxicam

Tenoxicam is an orally effective anti-inflammatory agent, and a *potent inhibitor of prostaglandin synthesis by blocking the enzyme cycloxygenase.* Additionally, it inhibits leucocyte function including phagocytosis and chemotaxis and scavenging of free oxygen radicals. It has an exceptionally long half-life (70 hrs) and steady-state levels are reached in about 2 weeks. It is effective in ***rheumatoid arthritis, osteoarthritis,*** short-term treatment of ***soft tissue injuries, gout,*** and nonarticular conditions like ***tendinitis, bursitis*** and ***backache.***

Dosage: Usual dose is 20 mg once daily. For ***gout*** it is given in a dose of 40 mg/day for 2 days. Followed by 20 mg/day for 5 days.

Sulfonanilide

Nimesulide

Nimesulide is a sulfonanilide compound. Its action is rather different than that of the classic NSAIDs. It is a relatively *weak* inhibitor of prostaglandin synthesis, but has a *potent anti-inflammatory action.* The safety of nimesulide as an NSAID is debatable.

Coxibs

Celecoxib, Valdecoxib and Etoricoxib

Celecoxib, Valdecoxib and Etoricoxib are **selective inhibitors of cyclo-oxygenase-2** (Cox-2). Their effects are similar to diclofenac, and they also share the side effects of other NSAIDs. Risk of upper GI lesions is lower than the aspirin-like drugs. But they offer no protection against ischaemic cardiovascular diseases.

Celecoxib

Celecoxib is a nonsteroidal anti-inflammatory drug. **Indications:** Pain and inflammation in **osteoarthritis** and **rheumatoid arthritis. Contraindications:** Sulphonamide sensitivity, renal impairment, inflammatory gut disease, and severe congestive heart failure. **Side effects:** Insomnia, pharyngitis, flatulence, stomatitis, palpitation, depression, anxiety, alopecia, taste alteration. *Dose*: 200 mg daily in 2 divided doses, increased to a maximum of 200 mg bid. Lately, **Cox-3 selective inhibitors** are under development.

Miscellaneous Anti-inflammatory Agents

Hydroxychloroquine

Hydroxychloroquine, an antimalarial has also been employed in the treatment of **rheumatoid arthritis** and **systemic lupus erythematous.**

Penicillamine

Pencillamine is a **chelating agent** used to remove excess copper in patients with **Wilson's disease** (hepatolenticular degeneration). It is also approved for the treatment of **severe forms of rheumatoid arthritis,** but the use is restricted to patients unresponsive to other less toxic agents.

In rheumatoid arthritis, pencillamine is administered initially in a dose of 125 to 250 mg/day orally for 4 weeks. *Adverse reactions* include stomatitis, pruritus, loss of taste, nausea and proteinuria. Bone marrow depression may occur.

Gold Compounds

Auranofin , Aurothioglucose, Gold Sodium Thiomalate

Aurothioglucose and **gold sodium thiomalate** contain 50 percent gold and are used intramuscularly (IM). **Auranofin** is an orally effective compound containing 29 percent gold. These gold compounds can temporarily **arrest the progression** of bone destruction in the involved joints.

Aurothioglucose: Weekly IM injections (preferred site is intragluteal); first week, 10 mg; second and third weeks, 25 mg; thereafter 50 mg/ week.

Gold sodium thiomalate: Weekly IM injections, first week, 10 mg, second week, 25 mg thereafter 25-50 mg/week until clinical improvement or toxicity occurs.

Auranofin: Administered orally 6 mg a day, as a single or 2 divided doses.

Gold is well distributed in the body and major sites of localization are bone marrow, liver, skin and bone. *Arthritic joints appear to concentrate more gold than non-involved joints.*

Adverse reactions: Most common side effects are dermatitis, stomatitis, pruritus, metallic taste, flushing, sweating, and proteinuria. Other adverse reactions include alopecia, grayish blue skin pigmentation, gingivitis, vaginitis, blood dyscrasias (rarely), glomerulitis, tubular necrosis, and anaphylactic shock. *Thus, gold compounds are potentially highly toxic substances.*

Glucosamine sulphate plus Chondroitin sulphate

Glucosamine sulphate (up to 1500 mg/day) plus *Chondroitin sulphate* (up to 1200 mg/day) have been used for the treatment of **osteoarthritis**. They act synergistically and stimulate the production of *proteoglycans* and *glycogen*, restore cartilage matrix, normalize cartilage metabolism, and stimulate the synthesis of synovial fluid. It is claimed that these agents halt the degeneration, and promote the regenerative process in the osteoathritic joint. Further studies are in progress. This class of agents has been labelled as **nutraceuticals** or **dietary supplements.**

Antigout Drugs

Gout is a ***purine metabolism disorder*** resulting from an excess of uric acid in the blood (hyperuricaemia) due to either its overproduction or faulty elimination. Crystals of **monosodium urate** begin to precipitate, and get deposited in joints, skin, kidney and other tissues. **Gouty arthritis** usually involves a single joint (monoarticular), but may involve many joints (polyarticular). Blood ordinarily contains uric acid in a concentration of 3 to 7 mg/ dl of serum.

Classification

Three types of drugs are employed in the treatment of gout:

1. Drugs used in **acute gout: Colchicine, naproxen, sulindac, indomethacin, corticotrophin, corticosteroids.**
2. Drugs used for long-term control of gout, acting by **increasing** the excretion of uric acid by the kidneys, i.e., **uricosuric agents: Probenecid, sulphinpyrazine.**
3. Drugs for prevention of urate synthesis in the body: **Allopurinol.**

Colchicine

Colchicine is an alkaloid derived from the corm and seeds of ***Colchicum autumnale.*** It has *no anti-inflammatory or analgesic activity*, but is very effective in suppressing inflammation and pain in gouty joints. It does not enhance renal excretion of uric acid.

Mode of action: The mechanism of action of colchicine in acute gout is incompletely understood.

Pharmacokintics: Colchicine is rapidly absorbed from the gastrointestinal tract. Its plasma $t\frac{1}{2}$ is 30 minutes. It is partly metabolized and a major portion is excreted via the bile.

Therapeutic uses: Acute gouty arthritis.

Dosage: For acute attacks 0.5 or 0.6 mg is

administered orally every hour until pain subsides, or nausea, vomiting and diarrhoea develop.

Toxicity: Colchicine causes nausea and vomiting or abdominal pain in about 80 percent of patients. Diarrhoea is considered as the *therapeutic end point* and as soon as it occurs, administration should be stopped irrespective of the symptoms. Black tarry stools or light red blood in stools indicates gastrointestinal bleeding. **Bone marrow depression**, perpheral neuritis, myopathy, renal damage, hepatocellular failure and alopecia may occur.

Uricosuric Drugs

Probenecid

Since 1950, probenecid has been known to be a very useful uricosuric agent in gout.

Mode of action: Probenecid acts by inhibiting renal tubular reabsorption of uric acid, thereby greater amount of uric acid is eliminated in the urine.

Pharmacokinetics: After oral administration, probenecid is rapidly absorbed within an hour, and peak plasma levels are attained in 2 to 4 hours. About 90 to 95 percent of the metabolites are also lost in the urine.

Therapeutic uses: Probenecid is used for the **prophylaxis of gout;** hyperuricaemia; and for the reduction of tubular excretion of penicillins and cephalosporins.

Dosage: For uricosuric therapy, initially 250 mg twice daily orally, is administered preferably after meals, increased after a week to 500 mg twice daily, then upto 2 g daily.

Toxicity: Occasionally nausea, vomiting, urinary frequency, headache, flushing, dizziness and rashes may occur. Rarely hypersensitivity reactions, nephrotic syndrome, hepatic necrosis and aplastic anaemia occur.

Xanthine Oxidase Inhibitor

Allopurinol

Allopurinol inhibits the enzyme xanthine oxidase, reducing the formation of uric acid from xanthine and hypoxanthine.

Pharmacokintics: Allopurinol is rapidly and completely absorbed from the intestine. Its plasma t½ is about 3 hours. It is largely converted to oxypurinol, which itself is a weak xanthine oxidase inhibitor.

Therapeutic uses: Allopurinol is used for **gout prophylaxis** and for **long-term treatment of hyperuricaemia and its complications.**

Dosage: Initially, 100 mg as a single dose is given after meals, gradually increased to 300 mg daily. Usual maintenance dose is 200-600 mg daily.

Toxicity: Gastrointestinal disorders, drowsiness and hypersensitivity reactions may occur. Rarely it may also cause myelosuppression.

ANTIRHEUMATIC DRUGS

Rheumatic diseases are inflammatory or degenerative disorders that affect mainly the musculoskelatal system, i.e., the joints, muscles, ligaments, tendons and bursae. The primary aim of treatment is reduction of **pain** and **inflammation, maintenance of joint mobility, and prevention of deformity.**

Classification

The antirheumatics may be broadly grouped into two (i) the **non-steroidal anti-inflammatory drugs** (NSAIDs) and (ii) the **slow-acting antirheumatic drugs** (SAARDs). The latter group includes **gold sodium thiomalate, penicillamine, hydroxychloroquine**, the **immunosuppressives,** and the **corticosteroids.**

Drug Therapy

Non-steroidal anti-inflammatory drugs (NSAIDs). Aspirin is still an important agent in the medical management of rheumatoid arthritis. For full anti-inflammatory effectiveness, aspirin must be taken in much larger amounts than for ordinary analgesia. To avoid gastrointestinal irritation the dose of aspirin (4-5 g/day) should be taken after meals, or with milk.

Gold compounds: Chrysotherapy, i.e., treatment with gold salts, sometimes suppresses the rheumatic process in patients.

Pencillamine: It has a similar action to gold. Comparative studies indicate that pencillamine is as effective as gold or azathioprine. Because of its hazardous adverse effects, pencillamine is reserved for patients with long-standing disease refractory to standard therapy.

Antimalarials, Chloroquine and **hydroxychloroquine** may be used in active **rheumatoid arthritis, systemic lupus erythematous,** and **discoid lupus erythematous.** They have a similar action to gold and are better tolerated than either gold or penicillamine, but their use is limited by their ocular toxicity.

Adrenocorticosteroids and ACTH are *held in reserve* and used when absolutely necessary to keep the patient from being incapacitated.

Intra-articular steroid therapy: In inflammatory conditions of the joints particularly in rheumatoid arthritis corticosteroids are given by intra-articular injection to relieve pain, increase mobility or reduce deformity in one or a few joints. Full aseptic precautions are essential. *Hydrocortisone acetate* 5-50 mg, according to the joint size is injected intra-articularly. *Triamcinolone acetonide, triamcinolone hexacetonide, dexamethasone sodium phosphate,* and *methylprednisolone acetate* may be used intra-articularly.

Corticotrophin (ACTH) has also sometimes been employed in rheumatoid arthiritis. Its advantages are that it stimulates the production and release of steroids; and there is less of osteoporosis and muscle weakness.

Immunosuppressants: These agents are useful alternatives in cases that have failed to respond to gold, penicillamine and chloroquine. **Azathioprine** (1.5 to 2.5 mg/kg) per day in divided doses and **chlorambucil** (5 mg/day) may be used.

ANTIMIGRAINE DRUGS

Headache is the most common complaint of patients seen by the physician. They may be of two types: (i) **tension or muscle contraction headaches;** and (ii) **vascular headaches.** The tension headaches are difficult to manage, but respond to non-narcotic analgesics like *aspirin* or *paracetamol.*

Vascular headaches are the result of dilatation of the intracranial and extracranial arteries, and are sometimes classed as **migraine** and **non-migraine** types. Hypertensive vascular headaches are best dealt by controlling blood pressure by antihypertensive agents. Migraine headaches are classified as: (i) classic migraine; (ii) common migraine; and (iii) cluster headache (a unilateral vascular headache).

Drug Therapy

Drugs used to treat migraine may be discussed under two heads: (i) treatment of an **acute migraine attack;** and (ii) **prophylaxis of migraine.**

Acute migraine attack: Most migraine headaches respond to analgesic like **aspirin** and **paracetamol.** Alternatively **ergotamine tartrate;** ergotamine tartrate 1 mg, plus caffeine 100 mg or dihydroergotamine mesylate.

Other drugs include **metoclopramide** or the **phenothiazine** and **antihistamine** antiemetics. **Diazepam** or other anxiolytics may be useful adjuncts to counteract muscle spasm and anxiety which is often present in a migraine attack.

Prophylaxis of migraine: The drugs which are helpful in preventing attacks are: (i) **Clonidine** in a dose of 50 mcg bid, increased after 2 weeks to 75 mcg bid, if necessary; (ii) **Propranolol** 20-40 mg bid or tid for prevention of severe recurrent migraine; (iii) **Prochlorperazine** in a dose of 5 mg tid; (iv) **Methysergide** an *antiserotonergic* drug, in a dose of 1.0 mg at bedtime; (v) **Pizotifen** another *antiserotonergic* drug in a dose of initially 500 mcg daily, increased to 3 mg/day in divided doses, if necessary; (vi) **Cyproheptadine** an older *antihistamine-antiserotonergic* drug, in a dose of 4-20 mg/day in divided doses, and (vii) **Topiramate** is a broad-spectrum anticonvulsant which inhibits central neurotransmission by facilitating the effects of *gamma-aminobutyric acid* (GABA). It also has been licensed for *migraine prophylaxis* in a dose of 50 mg bid orally.

DRUGS FOR CENTRAL PAIN SYNDROMES

Central pain syndromes are caused by diseases or injuries affecting portion of the CNS, e.g., **tabes dorsalis,** and **postherpetic neuralgia.** The aetiology of others, e.g., **trigeminal neuralgia** remains unexplained.

Carbamazepine is the drug of choice for the treatment of **trigeminal** and **glossopharyngeal neuralgia,** and **tabes dorsalis.** It is usually administered in a dose of 200 mg to a maximum of 1.2 g daily.

Phenytoin: It is sometimes used in the treatment of **trigeminal neuralgia.** Phenytoin is also reported to be effective in several other pain syndromes, e.g., **peripheral neuralgia, phantom limb pain, thalamic pain** and **postherpetic neuralgia.** It is employed in a dose of 300-400 mg daily.

In this Chapter mainly the nonsteroidal anti-inflammatory drugs have been discussed. They cause reduction of oedema, erythema and resulting tissue damage associated with inflammatory conditions and may also induce analgesia and antipyresis.

2.8 PSYCHOPHARMACOLOGICAL AGENTS (ANTIPSYCHOTICS, ANTIDEPRESSANTS, ANTIMANICS AND HALLUCINOGENS)

Clinical psychopharmacology made major advances with the introduction of **chlorpromazine** and reserpine. Today, **reserpine** is no longer used because of its toxicity.

TERMINOLOGY

In general, drugs primarily used for treating psychoses are called **antipsychotics;** those used for treating depressive illness ***antidepressants;*** those used to control mania–**antimantics**; and those used for treating anxiety neuroses - **antianxiety agents.** The antianxiety drugs have been discussed in **Chapter 2.4.** Lysergic acid diethylamide (LSD) and drugs with similar activity are called **hallucinogens** (psychotominetics).

ANTIPSYCHOTICS (NEUROLEPTICS)

The antipsychotic agents are highly effective in excited or **agitated psychotic states.**

Nature of Psychoses

The chief characteristic of psychotic individuals is a persistent inability to recognize reality. Their personality and behaviour become severely disorganized.

It is believed that **noradrenaline** and **dopamine** in particular are involved in the schizophrenic process.

CLASSIFICATION

They are listed with their pharmacological profile in **Table 2.6.**

Phenothiazines

Chlorpromazine is the most commonly employed phenothiazine.

Pharmacological Actions

Chlorpromazine blocks **nonadrenaline, dopamine, serotonin, acetycholine,** and **histamine** receptor sites.

Behavioural effects: In man, there is drowsiness and a tendency to fall asleep, but 'arousal' can be produced by moderate stimulation. It exerts a central **antihallucinatory** and **calming** activity.

Other central effects include (i) inhibition of the **chemoreceptor trigger zone** and thereby exerting an **antiemetic effect;** and (ii) inhibition of hypothalamic function, causing loss of temperature control (**hypothermia**), galactorrhoea, amenorrhoea, delayed menstruation, and weight gain. Many phenothiazines have powerful **extrapyramidal effects.**

To sum up, the antipsychotic drugs share two novel pharmacological actions: (i) their ability to **ameliorate schizophrenia;** and (ii) their ability to evoke **extrapyramidal syndromes.** Both of these are mediated through the **postsynaptic**

Table 2.6 : *The classification, dosage and pharmacological profile of antipsycotics*

Classification Generic Name	Total daily dose (mg; oral)	Sedative Effects	Extra-pyramidal Effects	Hypoten-sive Effects	Anticholinergic Effects
1. **Phenzpthiazines**					
(a) *Aliphatics*					
Chlorpromazine	50-1500	++++	++	++++	++
Promazine	50-1000	+++	+	+++	++
Triflupromazine	50-200	++++	++	+++	++
(b) *Piperdines*					
Thioridazine	50-800	++++	+	++++	++++
(c) *Piperazines*					
Prochlorperazine	10-150	++	+++	+	++
Trifluoperazine	5-30	++	+++	+	++
2. **Butyrophenones**					
Haloperidol	2-15	+	++++	+	++
3. **Dibenzoxazepine**					
Loxapine	20-250	++	+++	++	++
4. **Dibenzodiazepine**					
Clozapine (atypical antipsychotic; minimal central antidopaminergic activity)					
5. **Diphenylbutylpiperidine**					
Pimozide	1-20	+	++	++	+
6. **Benzisoxazole**					
Risperidone	4-16	+	+	+	+
7. **Thienbenzodiazepine**					
Olanzepine	5-20	++	+	+	+

dopamine receptor blockade. In addition, they also affect the functioning of the *three* main integrating systems, namely, the **reticular activating system, limbic system,** and **hypothalamus.**

Pharmacokinetics

Most studies have been carried out on chlorpromazine. When given orally, it is incompletely absorbed with a bioavailability of about 30 percent. Peak plasma levels are reached in 2-3 hours.

Metabolism is primarily by hepatic microsomes. With chronic administration a tolerance develops to the sedative effects.

Therapeutic Uses

1. **Schizophrenia.**
2. **Mania.**
3. **Anxiety neuroses** and **psychosomatic disorders.**
4. **Painful terminal illness.**
5. **Drug-induced psychosis.**
6. **Shock.**
7. **Nausea and vomiting:** Chlopromazine exerts its antiemetic action (in nonsedative doses) by *depressing the chemoreceptor trigger zone* in the medulla. Prochloperazine is used to suppress vestibular function in *Meniere's disease.*
8. **Hiccough.**
9. **Withdrawal symptoms** of addictive drugs (opiods).
10. **Pruritus.**
11. **Mental retardation.**

Adverse Reactions

Antipsychotic drugs are remarkably safe with a **wide margin of safety** and overdoses are seldom fatal in adults.

Disturbances of Central Nervous Function

Extrapyramidal effects: Three of the common reactions are (i) **parkinsonism,** (ii) **akathesia,** marked by aimless motor restlessness, and (iii) **dyskinesia (or dystonia)** characterized by tonic contraction of muscle groups, specially of the face, tongue and neck and sometimes in the pelvis resulting in adoption of awkward postures.

Convulsant action: The phenothiazines may precipitate epileptiform seizures in susceptible individuals.

Endocrine effects: Breast enlargement in men (**gynaecomastia**), and lactation in women (**galactorrhoea**). Weight gain, oedema and fluid retention can occur. ***False positive pregnancy tests have been reported.***

Disturbances of Autonomic Nervous Function

Postural hypotension: It is dose related and more pronounced with parenteral administration.

Anticholinergic effects: These may be manifested as dry mouth, constipation, urinary retention and blurred vision.

Nasal congestion may occur due to alpha-adrenoceptor blockade.

Sexual function: There may be failure of ejaculation, attributable to alpha-adrenoceptor blockade.

Hypothermia is facilitated by peripheral vasodilatation, and reduced muscular activity (anti-shivering effect), and aided by inhibition of sweating.

Miscellaneous Effects

Allergic reactions: Photosensitivity resembling sunburn may occur.

Ocular changes: Pigmented **retinopathy** is probably the most serious phenothiazine induced change.

Skin: Purplish pigmentation of the skin occurs on prolonged therapy.

Hepatotoxicity: Obstructive (cholestatic) jaundice.

Bone marrow toxicity: Agranulocytosis usually occurs during the first 6 to 10 weeks of treatment.

Tolerance and physical dependence: The antipsychotic drugs are not addicting. However, a mild degree of **physical dependence** may occur.

Drug Interactions

Phenothiazines potentiate the actions of analgesics, sedative-hypnotics and anaesthetics. Combination preparations may sometimes be used for treatment of schizophrenia with depression.

Non-phenothiazine Antipsychotics

These drugs are best employed in the following two situations: (i) patients with chronic schizophrenic symptoms which are not controlled by the phenothiazines; and (ii) patients showing hypersensitivity reactions to phenothiazines.

Depot Neuroleptics

Fatty acid esters of phenothiazines are used for the maintenance therapy in schizophrenics. *Single injections may be effective for 2-4 weeks.*

Many depot preparations are available, viz, **fluphenazine decanoate, fluphenazine enanthate, flupenthixol decanoate, perphenazine enanthate** and **fluspirilene.**

ANTIDEPRESSANTS

The two major categories of antidepressant drugs are: (i) the **tricyclic group** of which *imipramine* and *amitriptyline* are the most widely used; and (ii) the **monoamine oxidase inhibitors** (MAOIs) of which *tranylcypromine* and *phenelzine* are the best known.

Classification of Depressions

From the point of view of drug treatment, depression may be classified into: (i) **reactive depression** (exogenous); and (ii) **endogenous depression.**

Reactive depression is characterized by a well-defined precipitating stress, such as the loss of a loved one, adverse effects of drugs, or certain disease states. It is usually **self-limiting.**

Endogenous depression is possibly caused by some **neurochemical imbalance**. The symptoms are usually more severe and often requires life-long therapy.

CLASSIFICATION OF ANTIDEPRESSANTS

1. **Tricyclics**
   Amitriptyline, Clomipramine, Imipramine, Trimipramine.
2. **Selective Serotonin Reuptake Inhibitors (SSRIs)**
   Citalopram, Fluoxetine, Fluvoxamine, Paroxetine, Sertraline.
3. **Monoamine Oxidase Inhibitors (MAOIs)**
   Phenelzine, Tranylcypromine, Selegiline.
4. **Others**
   Maprotiline, Trazodone, Venlafaxine.

Tricyclic Antidepressants

Tricyclic antidepressants are chemically related to the *phenothiazine tranquilizers*. In general these drugs are effective for treating **moderate to severe** depressive illness, associated with loss of appetite and sleep disturbances. ***Improvement in sleep is the first benefit of therapy.***

Pharmacological Actions

The tricyclics act by increasing the availability of **noradrenaline** and **serotonin** as central neurotransmitters by ***blocking their neuronal reuptake,*** which leads to an enhanced neuronal transmission. The tricyclics block the '**amine pump**' which is an active transport system for the re-uptake mechanism.

The **second** major action of the tricyclics is variable ***sedative*** effect.

The **third** action of tricyclics is their potent **central** and **peripheral anticholinergic activity.**

Pharmacokinetics

The tricyclics being lipid-soluble in their non-ionized form are readily absorbed from the gut, but are subjected to considerable **first pass** hepatic metabolism. Protein binding of these drugs is high and *they can interact with other highly protein bound drugs.*

Therapeutic Uses

1. **Depressions:** The tricyclics are mainly used in the treatment of **endogenous depression.**
2. **Enuresis:** For this condition imipramine 25-50 mg orally may have a beneficial effect.
3. **Chronic painful states:** The tricyclics are also used in conditions like **school phobia** in children; **hyperactive child syndrome** and **minimal brain damage.**

Adverse Reactions

i. **Autonomic nervous system:** Dry mouth, blurring of vision, and constipation are commonly reported side effects. Hesitancy in micturition and impotence may occur.

ii. **Central nervous system:** Fine tremor, sedation, insomnia, decreased REM sleep, convulsions and ataxia may occur.

iii. **Cardiovascular system:** Tachycardia and palpitation are often reported.

iv. **Allergic reactions:** Skin reactions, intrahepatic cholestatsis, and agranulocytosis may occur rarely.

v. **Drug interactions:** The tricyclics are likely to interact with the following groups of drug: (i) **Antihypertensives;** (ii) **MAOIs;** and (iii) **Thyroid hormones.**

Dosage: The dosage guide is presented in **Table 2.7.**

Table 2.7: *Dosage guide for antidepressants*

Classification, Generic name	*Dose range mg/day divided in 2-4 doses*
Noradrenaline-Reuptake Inhibitors	
Tricyclics	
Amitriptyline	50-300
Clomipramine	25-250
Doxepin	25-300
Imipramine	30-300
Trimipramine	50-300
Amoxapine	50-600
Desipramine	25-300
Maprotiline (tetracyclic)	50-225
Nortriptyline	30-100
Protriptyline	15-60
Serotonin-Reuptake Inhibitors	
Fluoxetine	20-80
Fluvoxamine	50-300
Paroxetine	10-50
Sertraline	50-200
Venlafaxine	75-225
Atypical Antidepressants	
Bupropion	200-450
Nefazodone	200-600
Trazodone	150-600
Monoamine Oxidase Inhibitors (MAOIs)	
Phenelzine	45-90
Tranylcypromine	30-60
Selegiline (MAO-B inhibitor)	10-40

Newer Antidepressants

Mianserin: This is a tetracyclic compound which ***increases nonadrenaline turnover*** by an unknown mechanism. *Dosage*: 30-120 mg daily in divided doses.

Amoxapine, maprotiline and **trazodone** are claimed to have a more rapid onset of action and a lower incidence of adverse effects. These three are **second generation antidepressants.**

Citalopram

Citalopram *inhibits the re-uptake of serotonin,* and is one of the members of the selective serotonin re-uptake inhibitors (SSRIs). It is used for **depressive illness** and **panic disorders. Side effects** include palpitation, postural hypotension, confusion, impaired concentration, amnesia, migraine and hypersensitivity reaction. **Dose:** 20 mg daily as a single dose (max. dose 40 mg daily). Other member of this group are **fluoxetive, fluvoxamine, paroxetine** and **sertraline.**

Venlafaxine

Venlafaxine promotes neurotransmitter activity in the CNS by *inhibiting the re-uptake of serotonin and nonadrenaline.* **Side effects** include nausea, headache, somnolence, hypotension, asthenia, and nervousness. **Dose:** Initially 75 mg daily in 2 divided doses (max. dose 150 mg daily).

Monoamine Oxidase Inhibitors (MAOIs)

The MAOIs are generally less effective and more toxic than the tricyclics.

The **mode of action** of MAOIs, whereby they elevate the mood, is due to the increased availability of monomine neurotransmitters at synapses in the CNS. The brain levels of **noradrenaline, dopamine** and **serotonin** are increased. The MAOIs produce a feeling of well-being and elation.

Adverse effects: Most often these effects may be minor like dizziness, orthostatic hypotension, oedema, increased intraocular pressure, dry mouth, mydriasis, constipation, difficulty in urination, delayed ejaculation and impotence. **Hepatotoxicity** and other signs of liver damage have been reported.

Selegiline

There are two types of monamine oxidase: MAO-A metabolizes noradrenaline and serotonin; and MAO-B metabolizes dopamine. Selegiline is a *selective irreversible inhibitor of MAO-B,* thereby retards the breakdown of dopamine. It shows marked improvement in patients of *depression.* The **dose** is 5 mg with breakfast and 5 mg with lunch.

Electroconvulsive therapy (ECT): In ECT, a current of 200-150 mA is applied for 0.1-0.6 seconds across the temples. Within a few seconds there is a generalized tonic convulsion; followed by a series of clonic convulsions and then followed by a period of confusion and amnesia lasting 30-90 minutes before full recovery. In practice light anaesthesia is produced by **thiopentone,** and a short-acting muscle relaxant like **suxamethonium** is administered to the patient before applying the shock.

ECT is of benefit in the treatment of ***schizophrenia (Acute episodes)*** and in the treatment of **endogenous depression with marked suicidal tendencies.**

ANTIMANIC DRUGS

Lithium Carbonate

Lithium is an earth metal with an atomic weight of 7. Lithium counteracts mood changes, without producing sedation, and is the only specific antimanic drug for the prophylaxis and treatment of **manic-depressive disorders.** Lithium has a *narrow margin of safety.*

Mode of action: Manic states are brought about by an *excess of noradrenaline* at central adrenergic synapses. Lithium is thought to: (i) **accelerate the presynaptic destruction of catecholamines;** (ii) **inhibit the release of noradrenaline** at the synapse; and (iii) **decrease the sensitivity of the postsynaptic receptor.** These actions tend to correct the presumed overactivity of the catecholaminergic systems in mania.

Pharmacokinetics: Lithium is completely absorbed 6-8 hours after oral administration. It is not bound to the plasma proteins, and is well distributed in the body. Plasma t½ is approximately 7 to 24 hours and lithium is eliminated almost entirely by the kidneys.

Therapeutic uses: Manic-depressive disorder is the best established indication for the use of lithium.

Adverse reactions: Mild to moderate side effects include nausea, malaise, diarrhoea, and fine hand tremors. Thirst, polydipsia, fatigue, muscle weakness, slurred speech and nystagmus may occur. Moderate to severe adverse reactions include persistent nausea and vomiting blurred vision, hyperactive tendon reflexes, hypothyroidism, goiter, epileptiform convulsions, hypokalemia, ECG changes toxic psychosis.

Dosage: Lithium carbonate 0.25-2.0 g orally daily, adjusted by daily blood level tests to achieve a maintenance concentration of 0.5-1.2 mEq/l.

HALLUCINOGENIC DRUGS (PSYCHOTOMIMETICS)

Hallucinogens *produce changes in perception, thought, mood and behaviour.*

Lysergic Acid Diethylamide (Lysergide, LSD-25, LSD)

LSD is the most potent hallucinogenic agent presently available, producing behavioural effects in adult humans after oral doses of 25-50 mcg.

Physiological effects: Within 20-60 minutes of ingestion of LSD, there is a marked sympathetic stimulation, causing *mydriasis, sweating, tachycardia, tremor, gooseflesh, muscular weakness, and hyperthermia.* Fluctuations in mood, *euphoria, dysphoria, hilarity,* followed by extreme anxiety fits of crying and panic are seen.

Psychological effects: Colours, become more intense and kaleidoscopic. Enhanced sensitivity to touch, smell and taste have been noted. The subject believes he is having a **transcendental** experience. Disorientation of **time** and **space** is common. **Depersonalization** is induced.

Mode of action: There is evidence that links LSD action to its effects at the **serotonergic receptor sites** in the CNS. Thus, LSD exhibits **anti-serotonin activity.**

Adverse reactions: Repeated usage of LSD produces tolerance to the psychic effects of the drug within 4 days. **Cross-tolerance** has been demonstrated between LSD, mescaline, psilocybin and psilocyn.

Chronic use of LSD does not produce physical dependence. The adverse reactions include confusion, extreme anxiety, panic and a marked **psychotic state**. LSD causes, **chromosomal damage** probably leading to congenital abnormalities in humans.

Psilocybin and Psilocyn: In 1958, Hofman (of LSD fame) isolated psilocybin and psilocyn from the magic mushroom. These substances have about 1 percent of the potency of LSD.

Mescaline: It is the oldest known drug, with a primary hallucinogenic activity. It was isolated in 1896 from the Mexican cactus, popularly known as the **peyote cactus.** Mescaline is probably the least active of the commonly used psychotomimetic agents.

Trimethoxyamphetamine (TMA) is an alpha-methylated analogue of mescaline and is about 10 times more potent than mescaline.

Amphetamine: This agent also produces a psychosis in which there are visual, auditory, tactile and olfactory hallucinations and excitation.

DOM is about 100 times more potent than mescaline. It is also known as STP (Serenity, tranquility and peace) to the abuser.

MDA is twice as active as mescaline. This compound produces psychotomimetic effects, without perceptual distortions.

Bufotenine is found in Cohaba Snuff, and the skin and parotid gland of the toad (*Bufo marinus*). It causes hallucinations with severe and uncomfortable autonomic effects.

Nutmeg: The nutmeg tree, *Myristica fragrans*, is the source for the spices nutmeg and mace. As a flavouring agent nutmeg is popular and pleasant. Nutmeg causes psychotomimetic effects when large amounts are eaten. Its effects include *euphoria, visual hallucinations , loss of touch with reality, and distortions of time and space.* **Myristicin** is thought to be the active ingredient.

Cannabis (Marihuana, Marijuana)

The plant *Cannabis sativa*, the hemp plant, grows freely in Central Asia and the Himalayas. The psychoactive potency depends on the concentration of the naturally occurring substance **delta-9-tetrahydrocannabinol**, which is abbreviated as THC.

Preparations of Cannabis

There are a number of preparations of the leaves, flowers and the resin. All of them are included in the generic term **cannabis.**

In this country there are three main types of preparations of cannabis: (i) **Bhang** is the preparation of dried leaves and flowering shoots of *Cannabis sativa*. This is roughly equivalent to **marihuana** (usually smoked) as it is known in North America; (ii) **Ganja** is the dried flowering tops of *Cannabis sativa*, usually the female plants. Ganja is usually smoked; and (iii) **Charas** is the resinous exudate collected from the flowering tops and leaves of *C.sativa*. This is the most potent form of Cannabis. Equivalent to **hashish,** as it is known in the United States. Charas or hashish possesses 5 to 10 times the potency of bhang or marihuana. Bhang in this country is incorporated into sweets and drinks (often as a party prank on festive occasions).

Pharmacological Actions

Behavioural Effects

During the **initial phase** the subjects are anxious, restless and experience euphoria, and have enhanced perception of the five senses. In the **sedative phase** the subjects pass into a dream-like state. In high doses, marihuana produces a loss of personal identity. In 'bad trips' panic and psychotic reactions may occur.

Adverse reactions: Cannabis has a low toxicity. The therapeutic index of THC is 40,000. In contrast, the therapeutic indices for alcohol and secobarbital are 10 each.

Regarding the 'abuse potential' of cannabis, there is little **psychological dependence; tolerance** does develop on continuous use; and there is **no physical dependence.**

The possible hazards associated with long-term heavy use of cannabis are: (i) **chromosomal damage;** (ii) **interference with the functioning of the immune system;** (iii) **hormonal changes** which may lead to impotence and temporary sterility and gynaeomastia in males; (iv) **injury to**

the bronchial tract and lungs; (v) **severe personality changes;** and (vi) irreversible brain damage.

The hallucinogenic drugs are drugs of abuse, and are related to problems of drug dependence, dealt with separately in **Chapter 2.10.**

2.9 CENTRAL NERVOUS SYSTEM STIMULANTS

Stimulation of the central nervous system (CNS) can be produced in man and animals by a large heterogenous group of **natural** and **synthetic** substances.

CLASSIFICATION

1. **Cerebral or Psychomotor stimulants**
   Amphetamines
   Atropine
   Cocaine
   Ephedrine
   Xanthines (Caffeine)
   Methylphenidate
   Pemoline
2. **Brainstem stimulants or analeptics**
   Pentylenetetrazol
   Picrotoxin
   Doxapram
3. **Spinal stimulants or convulsants**
   Strychnine

Some therapeutically effective CNS stimulants are:

1. Xanthines (Caffeine).
2. Amphetamines (Dextroamphetamine, Methamphetamine).
3. Methylphenidate.
4. Pemoline.
5. Respiratory stimulants or analeptics (Doxapram).

PSYCHOMOTOR STIMULANTS

Xanthines (Methylxanthines)

The xanthines–**caffeine, theophylline, theobromine**–are closely related plant alkaloids. **Caffeine** is found in coffee bean (*Coffee arabica*), in the leaves of tea (*Thea sinensis*), in the bean of cocoa (*Theobroma cacao*), and in kola nut (*Cola acuminata*).

Pharmacological actions: The methylxanthines have qualitative similarly, but quantitative differences in their effects.

Central nervous system: Caffeine, theophylline and theobromine, in order of decreasing potency, stimulate the CNS. Mental activity, performance, and association of ideas are facilitated. Fatigue and drowsiness are allayed.

The above mentioned effects are produced by 85 to 250 mg of caffeine, the amount contained in 1 to 3 cups of coffee **(Table 2.8).**

Table 2.8: *The caffeine concentration in commonly consumed beverages*

Beverage	*Caffeine content (mg)*
Coffee	
Brewed	100-150/cup
Instant	85-100/cup
Decaffeinated	2-4/cup
Tea	65-75/cup
Cocoa	5-40/cup
Cola drinks	3-5/30 ml

Cardiovascular system: The methylxanthines stimulate the myocardium; increase coronary blood flow, cardiac output, myocardial work and oxygen consumption.

Smooth muscles: The xanthines relax smooth muscles, and their bronchodilator activity has been utilized in the treatment of bronchial asthma.

Skeletal muscles: Caffeine increases muscular work capacity in man by increasing the release of acetylcholine (ACh) at the myoneural junction.

Diuretic action: The methylxanthines, specially theophylline, increase urine production.

Other actions: Caffeine promotes secretion of hydrochloric acid and pepsin in the stomach. The basal metabolic rate (BMR) is increased slightly.

Mode of action: There are two basic cellular actions of the methylxanthines: (i) caffeine augments skeletal muscle twitch response; and (ii) the xanthines increase the accumulation of c-AMP in the cell. They are **competitive inhibitors of phosphodiesterase,** and inhibit the breakdown of c-AMP. An increase in c-AMP in the myocardium produces a positive inotropic effect. Caffeine can stimulate all levels of the CNS.

Pharmacokinetics: The methylxanthines are absorbed on oral, rectal or parenteral administration. Oral absorption of theophylline at times is erratic due to its poor water solubility, and is apt to produce gastric irritation and vomiting. These drugs are metabolized in the liver and excreted largely in the urine.

Therapeutic uses: Caffeine is used to allay fatigue and increase sensory awareness used to treat **mild to moderate respiratory depression. Aminophylline** is used to treat **bronchial asthma** and **status asthmaticus;** and to relieve **acute left ventricular failure**. Caffeine with ergotamine tartrate is used to treat **migraine**.

Adverse reactions: On ingestion of 1 g or more of caffeine insomnia, restlessness, excitement, tachycardia, extrasystoles, quick respiration, and delirium have been observed. An anxiety neurosis like syndrome can occur. High tannin content of tea is likely to cause constipation. Some degree of tolerance and psychic dependence develops to xanthine beverages.

Preparations and Dosage

1. **Aminophylline** (Theophylline ethylenediamine) is the most widely used soluble theophylline salt. It may be administered orally (100-300 mg); by slow IV injection (250-500 mg); or per rectum (360 mg) in suppositories.
2. **Caffeine citrate:** Orally 100 to 200 mg every 4 hours is the usual dose.
3. **Caffeine sodium benzoate** is employed for stimulation of individuals depressed by alcohol or other CNS depressants. It is given in doses upto 500 mg IM or SC.
4. **Dyphylline** has been extensively used in the treatment of bronchial asthma in oral doses of 15 mg/kg, but its efficacy is limited.
5. **Pentoxifylline** is a **haemorheological** agent, a class of drugs that lower blood viscosity and improve erythrocyte flexibility and deformability, i.e., the ability of red cells to change their shape in response to mechanical forces and stresses. It has been used in the treatment of **intermittent claudication, cerebral ischaemia, transient ischaemia attacks** (TIAs), and **chronic occlusive arterial disease of the limbs.** Pentoxifylline is administered in a dose of 400 mg 3 times daily with meals. **Adverse effects** include angina, dyspnoea, hypotension, dizziness, anxiety, and confusion. Rarely cardiac arrhythmias, hepatitis, and bone marrow suppression may occur.

Amphetamines

Amphetamine, Dextroamphetamine, Methamphetamine: The amphetamines are synthetic sympathomimetic amines causing marked CNS stimulation. Amphetamines induce varying degrees of **euphoria** depending on the dose, and the personality of the user. Peripheral effects include elevation of blood pressure, bronchodilation, contraction of urinary sphincter and mydriasis.

The initial effects of amphetamines are generally pleasant, but **tolerance** soon develops to the mood elevating action of these compounds. Prolonged use can lead to **irritability, insomnia, dizziness, jitteriness, easy distractibility,** and **confusion**. In emotionally unstable persons **habituation** and **dependence** occurs.

Mode of action: The net effect is **potentiation of endogenous catecholamine (noradrenaline, dopamine) activity.** The CNS stimulant effect is exerted on the **cerebral cortex** and the **reticular formation.** The **anorexiant** (appetite suppressant) effect is the result of the stimulation of satiety centre in the lateral hypothalamus.

Pharmacokinetics: Oral absorption of amphetamines is complete, and they are widely distributed in the body. They attain high concentrations in the CNS.

Therapeutic Uses

1. As short term (4-8 weeks) adjunct in the treatment of **obesity.**
2. Treatment of **narcolepsy.**
3. Treatment of **attention deficit disorder** (ADD) in children.

Preparations and Dosage

1. **Amphetamine sulphate:** Narcolepsy: 5-60 mg daily in divided doses; ADD: 5 mg one to two times daily, increase by 5 mg/week until optimal response; Obesity: 5 to 30 mg/day in divided doses 30-60 minutes before meals.
2. **Dextroamphetamine sulphate:** Narcolepsy: 5-60 mg/day, in divided doses; ADD: 2.5 to 5 mg/day increase gradually to optimal effect; Obesity: 5-10 mg one to three times daily.
3. **Methamphetamine:** Obesity: 5 mg tid; ADD: 5 mg bid or tid, increase gradually to optimal effect.

Adverse reactions: Side effects with acute amphetamine usage are nervousness, palpitation, tachycardia and insomnia. Other adverse reactions include dizziness, euphoria, headache, chills, tremors, hypertension, cardiac arrhythmias, and anginal pain.

Amphetamines are frequently abused, and **psychological dependence** occurs.

Methylphenidate

Methylphenidate is a CNS stimulant with a pharmacologic profile similar to that of amphetamine.

Therapeutic Uses

1. Adjunctive therapy of ***attention deficit disorder*** (ADD) in children.
2. Narcolepsy.
3. Relief of mild ***depression and withdrawn senile bahaviour.***

Dosage: Methylphenidate is used orally in a dosage of 20 to 30 mg daily in 2 or 3 divided doses.

Adverse reactions: Nervousness and insomnia are the most commonly encountered side effects. Other adverse effects include dizziness, drowsiness, agitation, toxic psychoses, palpitation, anginal attacks, arrhythmias, alopecia and leucopenia.

Pemoline

Pemoline is pharmacologically comparable to amphetamine and methylphenidate. It has a ***lower abuse potential*** than most other CNS stimulants. This drug ***increases dopaminergic function*** in the CNS and its main effects are increased alertness, enhanced motor activity, and mild euphoria.

Pemoline is used as adjunctive therapy of **attention deficit disorder** in children, and in the treatment of **narcolepsy** and **excessive sleepiness.** The recommended starting dose is 37.5 mg/day as a single morning dose.

The most frequent **side effects** of pemoline therapy are **insomnia, anorexia** with **weight loss.**

RESPIRATORY STIMULANTS OR ANALEPTICS

Respiratory stimulants or **analeptics**, are believed to act at the level of the brainstem and peripheral carotid chemoreceptors. **Their use has largely been replaced by ventilatory support.**

Doxapram

Doxapram produces respiratory stimulation by activating the peripheral carotid chemoreceptors, manifested by an *increased tidal volume*, and a slight increase in respiratory rate. A pressor response due to *improved cardiac output* is observed. It effectively *antagonizes opiate-induced respiratory depression*, without affecting the analgesia.

Dosage: Single IV injection of 0.5 to 1 mg/kg not to exceed 1.5 mg/kg, or an infusion of 250 mg doxapram in 250 ml of normal saline may be administered at a rate of 5 mg/min.

Adverse reactions include generalized warmth, sweating, dyspnoea, restlessness, hyperreflexia, laryngospasm, breathholding, tachycardia, and hypertension.

Caffeine sodium benzoate is also employed to treat respiratory depression due to overdosage with CNS depressants (e.g. narcotic analgesics, alcohol).

2.10 DRUG DEPENDENCE

The use of drugs for 'nonmedical' or 'recreational' purposes is becoming increasingly common specially among the youth.

DEFINITIONS

Currently accepted definitions according to the WHO Expert Committee on Drug Dependence are as under:

Drug: A drug is a substance (natural or synthetic) which when taken into the living organism, may modify one or more of its functions.

Drug dependence: It is a state, **psychic** and sometimes also **physical** resulting from the interaction between a living organism and a drug.

i. **Psychologic (psychic) dependence:** It denotes the compulsive need to experience a pleasurable drug reaction, ranging from a mild desire for the drug to an overwhelming need to have the drug at any cost.
ii. **Physical dependence:** It is an altered physiologic state resulting from prolonged use of a drug, and regular usage becomes necessary to avoid the *withdrawal* or *abstinence* syndrome.

In short, drug dependence produced by repeated consumption of a **natural** or **synthetic** drug is characterized by: (i) an overpowering desire or need (compulsion) to continue taking the drug, and to obtain is by any means; (ii) a tendency to increase the dose, tolerance; (iii) a **psychic** or **physical** dependence on the effects of the drug; (iv) appearance of a characteristic **withdrawal syndrome** on withholding the drug; and (v) a general **detrimental effect** on the patient and society.

DRUGS OF ABUSE

Classification

The drugs of abuse may be classified as under:

1. **CNS depressants**
   a. Alcohol
   b. Barbiturates
   c. Antianxiety drugs
2. **CNS stimulants**
   a. Amphetamines
   b. Anorectics
   c. Cocaine
3. **Narcotics**
   a. Heroin
   b. Morphine
   c. Codeine
4. **Psychotomimetics**
   a. LSD, DOM, DMT
   b. Psilocybin
   c. Mescaline

Table 2.9 : *Abuse characteristics of drug groups*

Drug group	Psychic dependence	Physical dependence	Tolerance
CNS depressants	++	+++	++
Amphetamines	+++	+	+++
Cocaine	++	++	+
Narcotic analgesics	+++	+++	+++
Psychotomimetics			
LSD	0	0	++
Marihuana	0	+	+

Key : +++ = marked; ++ = moderate; + = slight; 0 = absent

5. **Volatile inhalants**
   Acetone, benzene, trichloroethylene, toluene, paint thinner, amyl nitrite, nail polish remover, and petrol
6. **Marihuana (Cannabis)**
7. **Nicotine.**

The abuse characteristics of the main drug groups are listed in **Table 2.9.**

CNS Depressants

Alcohol

Alcohol abuse is a major drug problem in terms of damaged health, accidents, family discord and socially unacceptable behaviour.

The characteristics of **acute alcohol intoxication** depend on the blood level, ranging from euphoria to profound cardiorespiratory depression and coma. **Chronic alcohol abuse** is marked by GI disturbances, liver damage, pancreatitis, malnutrition, cardiac impairment, and psychotic disturbances.

Chronic alcohol ingestion results in development of **tolerance** and ultimately **physical dependence.** Withdrawal of alcohol after several weeks of consumption may result in **tremors, anxiety, confusion, GI disturbances, weakness, insomnia,** and **delusions.**

Treatment of acute alcohol withdrawal is largely symptomatic and involves use of sedatives or anticonvulsants e.g., diazepam. Chronic alcoholism management requires *psychiatric counselling* and supportive social interaction (Alcoholics Anonymous).

Barbiturates

The shorter acting barbiturates like **amobarbital, pentobarbital, secobarbital** are most sought after agents because they produce **euphoria.**

Withdrawal reactions on abrupt termination of barbiturate use range from **anxiety, confusion, weakness, anorexia, insomnia** due to rebound REM sleep, and **tremors** to **delirium, disorientation, hallucinations** and **convulsions.**

Management of the withdrawal state is symptomatic.

Antianxiety Agents

Chronic use of a number of other sedativehypnotics and antianxiety drugs can result in dependence and an abstinence syndrome. *Methaqualone* has been withdrawn from the market, but remains one of the 'street drugs of choice' and is widely abused. A combination of the antihistamine *diphenhydramine* and *methaqualone* (Mandrax) is more dangerous than methaqualone alone.

The **benzodiazepines** are the most widely used antianxiety drugs. Benzodiazepines are frequently misused by patients of anxiety neuroses or other psychosomatic disorders.

Prolonged use of benzodiazepines has resulted both in **psychologic** and **physical dependence.** Abrupt discontinuation of usage result in cramps, sweating, agitation, aggressivity, disorientation, confusion, tremors, depression, auditory and visual hallucinations, and paranoia. Diazepam withdrawal has been reported to result in coma and death.

CNS Stimulants

Amphetamines

They are widely abused drugs for their CNS stimulant effects by students, truck drivers, executives, athletes, doctors, nurses and pharmacists. **Methamphetamine** (Speed) by IV injection elicits an almost instantaneous euphoria or orgasm-like reaction. **Tolerance** to this effect develops rapidly and larger doses have to be taken.

Amphetamines induce **physical dependence** and abrupt withdrawal results in fatigue, muscle pain, lethargy and depression. Withdrawal symptoms are treated symptomatically.

Diazepam may be used if sedation is required.

Anorectics

A number of amphetamine-related anorectics are employed as adjuncts in the short-term treatment of **obesity.** They are frequently misused chronically as appetite suppressants and produce symptoms of chronic amphetamine use, like insomnia, elevated blood pressure, tachycardia and anxiety. These drugs on chronic usage result in **tolerance** and **physical dependence.**

Cocaine

Cocaine is a natural product extracted from the leaves of *Erythroxylon coca* (coca plant). Its legitimate use in medicine is as a local anaesthetic for the nasal and oral cavity. In high doses cocaine induces **euphoric excitement** and **hallucinations.** This property ranks it highest among the drugs causing **psychic dependence.** No physical dependence develops.

The powdered drug is commonly administered by inhalation or **'snorting'** and is rapidly absorbed from the nasal mucosa. On IV administration a brief rapturous sensation follows. **Crack,** a new hardened form of cocaine, is heated in a glass pipe and smoked; it produces intense euphoria within minutes.

Treatment of abuse is difficult. Regular supportive therapy, along with tranquilizers and antidepressant drugs is employed.

Narcotics

Opioid addiction is one of the oldest afflictions of mankind. The **narcotic analgesics** including **heroin, morphine, codeine** and other **synthetic** and **semisynthetic** derivatives have similar abuse characteristics. **Heroin** is the opioid with the widest illicit use. **Morphine** and **pethidine** are sometimes abused by persons (doctors, nurses and pharmacists) who have ready access to these drugs. A crude form of heroin called **'brown sugar'** has lately found wide illicit use and is smoked.

The **characteristics of dependence** of the morphine type are strong **psychic dependence,** and early development of **physical dependence** which increase in intensity, parallel to the development of **tolerance.**

Heroin or **opium** may be smoked , but most heroin addicts resort to IV injection of heroin and other potent narcotics as it promptly results in a sensation of exquisite pleasure (orgasmic effect, 'rush') and a feeling of extreme contentment.

Diagnosis of opiate addiction: The best evidence of narcotic additiction is provided by the injection of a narcotic antagonist like **naloxone** or **nalorphine** which precipitates a sudden withdrawal syndrome.

Treatment of abuse: Withdrawal symptoms can be suppressed by substitution of another narcotic for an opiate. Frequently oral *methadone* initially 20 mg once or twice daily is given, then the dose is gradually reduced.

Psychotomimetics

Psychotomimetic drugs also termed **hallucinogens** are a group of naturally occurring compounds (like psilocybin, mescaline) and synthetic compounds (like LSD, DOM) capable of producing profound distortion of reality.

The term **psychedelic** means 'mind expanding', i.e., these drugs can increase creativity of the mind. These drugs are capable of producing changes in (i) *perception,* (ii) *thought,* (iii) *mood,* and (iv) *behaviour.*

Lysergic acid diethylamine (LSD): It is the most potent hallucinogen available and effects usually last for 8-12 hours.

Mescaline (Peyote): Peyote buttons are chewed or swallowed. Oral doses of 250-500 mg produce LSD like hallucinations for 6-12 hours.

DOM: Structural analogue of mescaline also known as STP, an acronym for 'serenity, tranquility and peace'. DOM is a psychotomimetic producing intense, prolonged psychic alteration at a dose of 5 mg lasting for several days.

Drugs of the LSD type induce a state of excitation of the CNS, and central autonomic hyperactivity manifested by changes in mood (usually euphoria, sometimes depression).

Abuse syndrome: Daily use of hallucinogens produces **tolerance**, although it dissipates rapidly and ends after 3 days. **Psychic dependence** to the LSD type of drugs varies greatly but is usually not intense. There is no evidence of the development of physical dependence.

Treatment of abuse: Rest, reassurance, sympathy and support in a quiet environment are most successful in treating the anxiety and panic reactions. Benzodiazepines like **diazepam** can be safely used.

Volatile Inhalants

Volatile hydrocarbons such as **acetone**, **benzene, carbon tetrachloride, trichloethane, trichloroethylene** and **toluene** are present in many household products like **glue, paint, lighter fluid, nail polish remover** and **varnish thinner.** These volatile liquids are commonly placed on a handkerchief and inhaled. The initial effects are CNS **excitation**, sense of **exhilaration**, **dizziness** and occasionally auditory or visual **hallucinations**. Lately, **amyl nitrite** inhalation has been abused as a sexual stimulant.

Marihuana (Cannabis)

Cannabis, obtained from the leaves and flowering tops of hemp plants (**Cannabis sativa**, **Cannabis indica**) is a very ancient drug. Other names for cannabis and its products are **hashish**, **charas**, **bhang**, **ganja** and **marijuana** or **marihuana**. **Delta–9–tetrahydrocannabinol** (THC) is the major psychoactive ingredient. Marihuana is also nicknamed as '**pot**', '**weed**' and '**grass**'.

The most commonly reported effects that smokers report within 15 minutes of inhaling an adequate dose is a feeling of **floating** and **drowsiness** and they find it **pleasurably relaxing**. Colour seems brighter and richer. Perception of time and distance is distorted . Psychic symptoms include impaired concentrations, expression and recall.

Chronic use of marihuana may result in **psychologic** dependence but **physical dependence** is rare.

Nicotine

Nicotine is an alkaloid found in tobacco in a concentration between 1 to 2 percent. It is rapidly absorbed by the lungs and causes mild CNS stimulation. **Tolerance** develops to these effects but is variable in nature and duration. Withdrawal from nicotine may result in **nausea, diarrhoea, increased appetite, headache, drowsiness, insomnia, irritability,** and **poor concentration.** For management of the psychic dependence, gradual reduction of nicotine consumption is usually less effective over the long-term than abrupt cessation.

MECHANISMS OF TOLERANCE AND DEPENDENCE

Tolerance to, and dependence on drugs are very closely linked. Without tolerance to a drug physical dependence is most unlikely.

Tolerance: Several mechanisms of tolerance to a drug may be delineated: (i) **behavioural tolerance** may be developed as in the case of chronic alcoholics; (ii) **metabolic tolerance** may occur due to continued exposure to the drug; (iii) **immune tolerance** may develop through the formation of antibodies to the drug; and (iv) **pharmacodynamic tolerance,** i.e., tolerance based on a lessened degree of drug effect.

Dependence: Two types of dependence are recognized: Psychological and physical. **Psychological dependence** is manifested by a strong craving for the drug, but not necessarily with the appearance of physical signs on abrupt withdrawal of the drug. In **physical dependence** psychologic and physical symptoms of withdrawal develop, as exemplified by the withdrawal reactions that occur in heavy users of alcohol, and opiates. *As a rule psychological dependence is seen in all who develop physical dependence although the converse is not true.*

2.11 ANTIPARKINSONIAN DRUGS

Parkinson's disease or *paralysis agitans* is a chronic progressive disorder of the central nervous system (CNS) which is the result of damage to cells located in the basal ganglia of the brain. The *three* main manifestations of Parkinson's disease are:

1. **Akinesia (Bradykinesia):** This is a lack or difficulty in initiating voluntary muscle

movement resulting in a mask-like facies; impaired postural reflexes; and inability to care for oneself.
2. **Rigidity:** This is usually of the plastic or cogwheel type, i.e., it gives way in a series of jerks.
3. **Tremor:** Coarse (3-6 cycles/sec), repetitive muscle activity usually worse when the patient is at rest, is commonly manifested as a 'pill-rolling' motion of the hands and bobbing of the head.

Parkinson's disease affects either sex usually over the age of 50 years. As the disease progresses common functions like *walking*, *eating*, and *writing* become difficult.

NEUROCHEMICAL BASIS OF PARKINSONISM

The normal function of the extrapyramidal system depends on **a balanced action** of the excitatory and inhibitory components. The excitatory transmitter is **acetylcholine,** while the inhibitory transmitter is **dopamine.** In parkinsonism the inhibitory component is deficient, and the concentration of dopamine in the basal ganglia is low. The pathological lesion in parkinsonism lies in the **corpus striatum** and **basal ganglia.**

ANTIPARKINSONIAN DRUGS

1. **Dopaminergic agents**
   a. Dopamine precursor (e.g. *levodopa*)
   b. Dopamine releasing agent (e.g. *amantadine*)
   c. Dopamine receptor agonists (e.g. *bromocriptine*)
   d. Inhibition of dopamine inactivation (e.g. *selegiline*).
2. **Anticholinergic/antihistaminic agents**
   a. Anticholinergics (e.g. *benztropine, biperiden, ethopropazine, orphenadrine, procyclidine, trihexyphenidyl*)
   b. Antihistaminic (e.g. *diphenhydramine*).

Adjunctive therapy for parkinsonism includes **physical therapy** to delay disability, and **emotional support** to lessen feelings of helplessness.

Dopaminergic Agents

Levodopa , Carbidopa/Levodopa, Benserazide/Levodopa

Dopamine (DA) itself fails to cross the blood-brain barrier in adequate amounts and is not effective in treating the disease. **Levodopa** (L-DOPA, 1-dihydroxyphenylalanine), the metabolic precursor of dopamine, penetrates the blood-brain barrier and is converted to dopamine in the brain, thereby replenishing the deficient neurotransmitter. The enzyme **dopa decarboxylase** which converts dopa to dopamine is not only present in the brain, but also in the plasma. As such a significant fraction of an oral dose of L-DOPA is converted to DA in the plasma and cannot penetrate the blood brain barrier. Thus, very large amounts of L-DOPA are required to provide clinically effective levels.

To overcome this problem fixed-dose combinations (1:4, 1:10) of **carbidopa** and **levodopa** are available.

Carbidopa is a peripheral dopa decarboxylase inhibitor, retarding the peripheral breakdown of L-DOPA. This allows a greater fraction of the L-DOPA dose to cross the blood-brain barrier, producing higher DA levels in the central motor regulatory areas. Carbidopa itself does not cross the blood-brain barrier. *Levodopa dosage requirements are reduced by about 75 percent by combination with carbidopa.*

Benserazide is another peripheral dopa decarboxylase inhibitor which is used in combination with levodopa in a ratio 1:4.

Mode of action: Levodopa is a precursor of DA that readily passes the blood-brain barrier, where it is decarboxylated to DA. This restores depleted DA level and improves the symptoms of parkinsonism.

Therapeutic Uses

1. Levodopa is widely used for the treatment of ***all types of parkinsonism*** (idiopathic, postencephalitic, or arteriosclerotic) *except* those associated with antipsychotic drug therapy.

Preparations and dosage: Carbidopa/Levodopa tablets are available in a fixed ratio of either 10 mg carbidopa/250 mg levodopa, 25 mg carbidopa/100 mg levodopa, or 25 mg carbidopa/250 mg levodopa. Initially 1 tablet daily until 6 tablets per day.

Adverse reactions: Common side effects are nausea, vomiting, anorexia, orthostatic, hypotension, salivation, dysphagia, ataxia, headache, confusion, dizziness, weakness, hand tremor, insomnia, anxiety, euphoria, choreiform and other involuntary movements, nightmares and agitation.

Drug Interactions

1. Effects of L-dopa are **decreased** by antipsychotics, papaverine, pyridoxine, and benzodiazepines.
2. Effects of L-dopa may be **potentiated** by propranolol, methyldopa, and anticholinergics.

Amantadine

Amantadine is a synthetic antiviral agent. It effectively relieves symptoms or parkinsonism specially **akinesia** and **rigidity.** It is effective in about 40 percent of patients, but its *efficacy diminishes within 1 to 2 years.*

The **mode of action** of amantadine is incompletely understood. It causes release of DA from presynaptic nerve endings, and blocks its presynaptic reuptake.

Amantadine is used for the symptomatic treatment of parkinsonism in doses of 100 mg once or twice daily (maximum 400 mg/daily).

Side effects seen with amantadine are irritability, anxiety, nausea, dizziness, ataxia, confusion, depression, constipation, urinary retention, oedema and livedo reticularis (skin mottling).

Bromocriptine

It is a dopamine agonist acting directly on the postsynaptic dopamine receptors. It is primarily used orally as adjunctive therapy to provide additional therapeutic control. Such cases are referred to as '*late L-DOPA failures*'.

Bromocriptine mesylate is available in 2.5 mg tablets and 5 mg capsules. For Parkinson's disease the dosage varies from 30 to 50 mg/day. **Adverse reactions** include nausea, vomiting, dizziness, ankle oedema, skin mottling, skin rashes, muscle cramps, and Raynaud's syndrome.

Selegiline

Physiologically the enzyme MAO-B catalyzes the metabolism of dopamine in the brain. Selegiline *irreversibly inhibits MAO-B enzyme in the nerve endings in the brain* thereby increasing the intraneuronal levels of dopamine.

The usual **dosage** is 5 mg a day, at breakfast and lunch. **Adverse reactions** include confusion, vivid dreams, headache, anxiety, insomnia, hallucinations, palpitation, and urinary retention.

Anticholinergic/Antihistaminic Agents

Since the introduction of levodopa these agents have played a **secondary** role in the management of parkinsonism. They are used in ***combination with levodopa*** to obtain a better control on the disease.

Mode of action: These agents exhibit a *post-synaptic blocking effect on central cholinergic excitatory pathways.*

Therapeutic uses: The central anticholinergics are used as adjunctive agents in the treatment of parkinsonian symptoms, specially rigidity. They are also used for the prevention and relief of extrapyramidal reactions resulting from antipsychotic drug therapy. Their usual dosage range is detailed in **Table 2.10.**

Adverse reactions: Common side effects are dryness of mouth, blurred vision, dizziness, nausea, nervousness and urinary hesitancy. Severe adverse effects include confusion, agitation, delirium, hallucinations, depression, memory loss, constipation, mydriasis, diplopia and increased intraocular pressure.

DRUG MANAGEMENT OF PARKINSONISM

Patients with **mild,** early parkinsonism are good candidates for **anticholinergic** drug therapy. Treatment is started with small doses of **trihexyphenidyl.** Later the patient may be switched on to a more potent agent like **benztropine.**

Table 2.10 : *The central anticholinergic drugs used for parkinsonism*

Drug	Dosage range	Comments
Benztropine	0.5-6 mg	Used orally and parenterally for parkinsonism and extrapyramidal system reactions induced by antipsychotic drugs.
Biperiden	2-20 mg	Most effective against akinesia and rigidity.
Diphenhydramine	75-200 mg	Effective in mild parkinsonism and extrapyramidal reactions
Ethopropazine	50-500 mg	Controls most symptoms including tremor.
Orphenadrine	150-250 mg	Relieves rigidity; controls autonomic manifestations.
Procyclidine	10-20 mg	Anticholinergic and antispasmodic; most effective against rigidity; controls excessive salivation.

The combination of **carbidopa with levodopa** (Sinemet) is considered to be the most effective current drug treatment for most advanced cases of parkinsonism.

ALZHEIMER'S DISEASE

Alzheimer's disease (AD) is characterized by progressive impairment of memory and cognitive functions, leading to a complete vegetative state. It is a disease of the ageing population. Impairment of short-term memory (STM) is usually the first symptom of the disease, while long-term memory (LTM) remains preserved.

In AD there is marked atrophy of the cerebral cortical and subcortical neurones, i.e., a senile dementia of Alzheimer type. The presence of **senile plaques** which are aggregates of **beta amyloid** are pathognomic of the disease. The **'cholinergic hypothesis'** proposes that a **deficiency of acetylcholine** (ACh) is critical in the genesis of the confusional state in the disease. There is evidence of a marked *decrease in choline acetyltransferase* in cholinergic neurones.

Treatment: Patients of AD are very uncooperative, and at times are helped by **neuroleptics** like promazine or haloperidol.

Anticholinesterases: The reversible AChE inhibitor **physostigmine** has shown some efficacy in improving cognitive function in Alzheimer type dementia.

Tacrine is an acridine derivative approved by the FDA for the treatment of AD. It **inhibits** both AChE and butyrylcholinesterase. It also increases the release of ACh from cholinergic nerve endings. Studies bear evidence that oral tacrine in combination with lecithin is effective in improving memory in patients of AD. **Adverse effects** of tacrine like abdominal cramps, nausea, vomiting, diarrhoea and hepatotoxicity are a limiting factor. **Dosage:** Initial dose is 10 mg qid daily for 6 weeks. Later, increase the dose to 20 mg qid/day.

Donepezil (5-10 mg OD), **Rivastigmine** (3-12 mg/day in 2 divided doses) , and **Galantamine** (8-32 mg/day in 2 divided doses) are three newer *cholinesterase inhibitors* approved for control of moderate Alzheimer's disease. However, they are unable to reverse the degenerative changes occurring in AD.

Memantine has been tried in the treatment of moderate-to-severe cases of Alzheimer's disease.

Drugs Acting on the Peripheral Nervous System

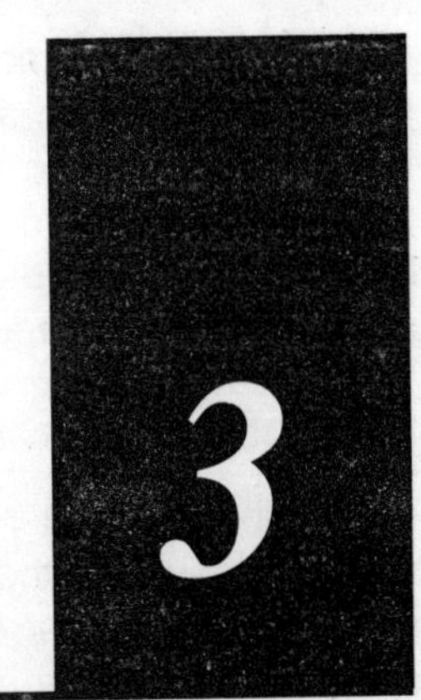

3.1 GENERAL CONSIDERATION

ANATOMY OF THE AUTONOMIC NERVOUS SYSTEM

The ANS regulates the vital functions in the body including **blood pressure, body temperature, water balance, urination, digestion** and many others.

The ANS comprises two major subdivisions, **sympathetic** and **parasympathetic.** The main nerve centres for these autonomic reflex arcs are located in the **hypothalamus, medulla oblongata** and **spinal cord.** Both these divisions have ***opposing effects*** on the innervated viscera and most of the viscera have a ***dual*** nerve supply. The general arrangement of the ANS is shown in **Fig. 3.1.**

Parasympathetic Nervous System

The parasympathetic outflow comprises both **cranial** and **sacral** components. Cranial outflow is carried in cranial nerves III (oculomotor), VII (facial), IX (glossopharyngeal) and X (vagus). Sacral outflow is carried in the spinal nerves of sacral segments 2,3 and 4 of the spinal cord. ***Acetylcholine*** (ACh) is the chemical transmitter between the postganglionic parasympathetic neurones and the effector cells.

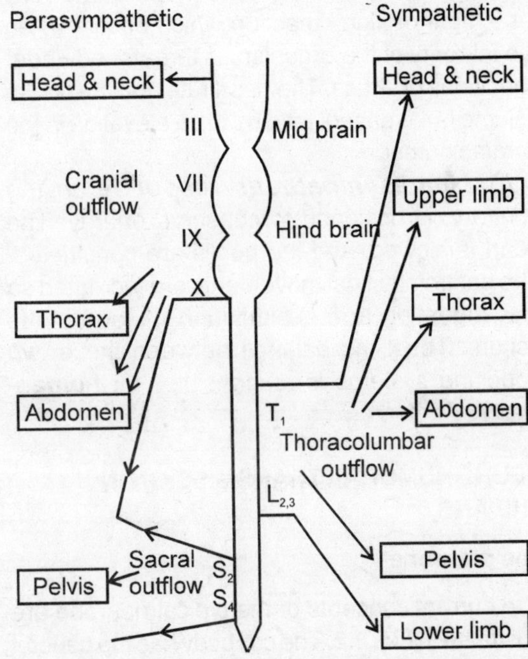

Fig. 3.1: *The efferent outflow of the autonomic nervous system. The parasympathetic pathways (left) are bilaterally paired. Most of the sympathetic pathways (right) are paired except the prevertebral ganglia (coeliac, superior and inferior mesenteric ganglia).*

Sympathetic Nervous System

The sympathetic outflow is described as **thoracolumbar** since the preganglionic neurones emerge from the CNS in the ventral roots of the spinal nerves of the first thoracic to second or third lumbar segments. **Noradrenaline** (NA) is the chemical transmitter between the postganglionic sympathetic neurones and the effector cells, except to the **sweat glands** which are supplied by sympathetic cholinergic fibres.

PHYSIOLOGICAL FUNCTIONS OF THE ANS

The sympathetic system, working with the adrenal medulla regulates the expenditure of energy, specially in times of **stress.** The parasympathetic system on the contrary helps the body to store and save energy.

The ***sympathetic response*** prepares the body for a 'fight or flight' reaction which occurs when the integrity of the organism is threatened under conditions of stress. The heart rate and the stroke volume is increased, leading to an elevation in the cardiac output.

The ***parasympathetic response*** on the contrary, is designed to conserve energy. The heart is slowed, and the pupils are constricted. The gastrointestinal movements are facilitated so that digestion and assimilation of food stuffs occurs. Thus, the balance between these two opposing systems is responsible for **homeostasis.**

NEUROHUMORAL TRANSMISSION IN THE ANS

The Neurone

The current concepts of the typical neurone are illustrated in **Fig. 3.2.** The cell body has the general function of maintaining neuronal integrity. The nucleus contains DNA, in which is encoded information for all the enzymes needed for normal cell function. Amongst the enzymes are those needed for the synthesis and degradation of the particular *neurotransmitter.* The cell bodies possess the appropriate mechanism to take up the specific neurotransmitter precursor from the surroundings, i.e., the cholinergic neurone takes up **choline,** the adrenergic neurone takes up **tyrosine,** and the tryptaminergic neurone takes up **tryptophan.**

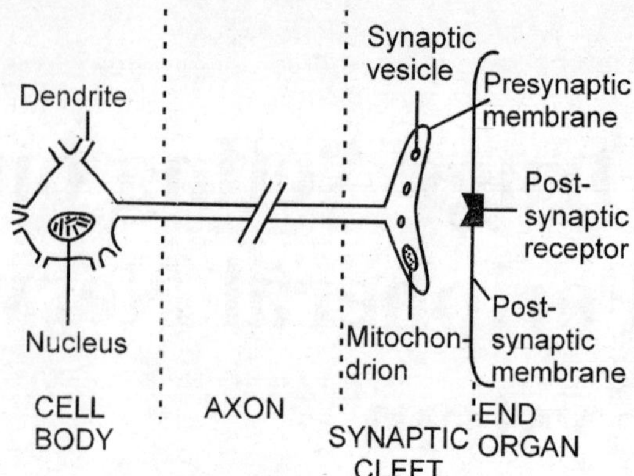

Fig.3.2 : *Schematic diagram of a typical neurone.*

The synaptic vesicles are aggregated in neuronal terminations, and store the neurotransmitter. During nervous activity the vesicles release the neurotransmitter into the **synaptic cleft** by a process of **exocytosis.** The released transmitter diffuses across the synaptic cleft, and combines with the specific receptors on the **postsynaptic membrane** in the end organ and produces the response. Drugs which activate receptors are termed **'agonists'**, and those which block the effect of agonists are termed **'antagonists'.**

Cholinergic Transmission

Autonomic and somatic nerves that synthesize, store and release acetylcholine (ACh) are called **cholinergic.** ACh molecules are stored in a bound, or inactive form in tiny storage sac, called **synaptic vesicles.** On the arrival of the action potential at the nerve ending, free ACh molecules are discharged into the synaptic cleft by a process of **exocytosis.** This active ACh combines with the cholinergic receptors. The cholinergic receptors are of two types, **muscarinic** and **nicotinic.**

Adrenergic Transmission

Sympathetic postganglionic nerve fibres that synthesize store and release noradrenaline (NA) are called **adrenergic.** NA is stored in a bound, or inactive form, in the granules (**synaptic vesicles**) of adrenergic neurones. On the arrival of the action potential at the nerve ending, free NA is liberated in the synaptic cleft by a process of **exocytosis.** This free NA then combines with the adrenergic receptors located on the postsynaptic membrane, and produce the response. The adrenergic receptors are of two types, **alpha** and **beta.** The **alpha-receptors** are mainly excitatory in nature, except in the intestines where their stimulation produces relaxation. The **beta-receptors** are mainly inhibitory, except in the heart where their stimulation produces cardioacceleration and increased myocardial contractility **(positive inotropism).**

STEPS IN NEUROHUMORAL TRANSMISSION

Irrespective of the type of neurone, the fundamental steps in chemical transmission are as under:

1. Biosynthesis of the neurotransmitter.
2. Storage of the neurotransmitter.
3. Release of the neurotransmitter.
4. Interaction with the postsynaptic membrane.
5. Inactivation of the neurotransmitter.
6. Recovery of the postsynaptic membrane (Repolarization).

To summarize, the **parasympathetic** system is mainly concerned with the sedentary activities like digestion, emptying of the bowels and urinary bladder. Whereas, the **sympathetic** system is concerned with functions involving increased activity of tissues, e.g., stimulation of the heart during exercise and stress. Generally the viscera have a nerve supply from each of the two divisions of the ANS, e.g., the heart, pupil and intestines. The **two** divisions of the ANS balance each other and are responsible for the maintenance of **homeostasis.**

3.2 CHOLINERGIC AGENTS (PARASYMPATHOMIMETICS)

The cholinergic drugs are chemicals that act at the same sites as the neurotransmitter acetylcholine (ACh), and mimic the actions of acetylcholine. Thus, these drugs are also called **parasympathomimetics.**

THE CHOLINERGIC RECEPTORS

The cholinergic receptors are of two types: (i) **muscarinic** which are located in tissue innervated by the postganglionic parasympathetic nerves, sweat glands and blood vessels; and (ii) **nicotinic** which are located in the autonomic ganglia (both parasympathetic and sympathetic), the neuromuscular junction, the adrenal medulla and in the CNS. ACh is the physiological stimulant of both muscarinic and nicotinic receptors.

The distinction between the two types of receptors has practical importance, because the response of organ systems to stimulants (agonists) and blockers (antagonists) differs **(Table 3.1).**

CLASSIFICATION OF CHOLINERGIC DRUGS

The cholinergic drugs may be grouped as under :

Direct-acting cholinergics

Group I **Acetylcholine and related choline esters**
Acetylcholine, Methacholine, Carbamylcholine, Bethanechol.

Group II **Cholinomimetic alkaloids**
Pilocarpine, Muscarine, Arecholine,

Indirect-acting cholingerics

Group III **The anticholinesterase agents**

a. **Reversible anticholinesterases**
Physostigmine, Neostigmine, Pyridostigmine, Ambenonium, Edrophonium, Distigmine, Demecarium.

b. **Irreversible anticholinesterases**
Di-Isopropylfluorophosphonate (DFP), Ecothiopate, Malathion, Parathion

Choline Esters

Acetylcholine (ACh)

Choline, the parent substance produces ACh-like effects but the activity is very feeble. Its activity is

Table 3.1 : *The cholinergic receptors and drug response*

	Muscarinic receptors	Nicotinic receptors	
Agonists	Acetylcholine Carbachol Muscarine Methacholine Pilocarpine	Acetylcholine Carbachol Nicotine	
Antagonists	Atropine Hyoscine Homatropine etc.	Hexamethomium Mecamylamine Pempidine etc.	at autonomic ganglia
		Tubocurarine Gallamine etc.	at skeletal neuromuscular junction

increased several thousand times by *esterification*.

ACh is the acetic acid ester of choline and is the physiological stimulant of both muscarinic and nicotinic receptors.

Muscarinic Actions

The muscarinic actions of ACh correspond to those produced by the alkaloid, **muscarine.** They are exerted on the **cardiovascular system, smooth muscles and exocrine glands.** A few sympathetic postganglionic nerves are also cholinergic and produce muscarinic actions like **secretion of sweat,** and **vasodilatation in skeletal muscle.** The muscarinic actions are:

1. Slowing of the heart, arteriolar vasodilatation, and a fall in blood pressure.
2. Stimulation of smooth muscles of the bronchi, gastrointestinal tract, gall bladder and bile duct, urinary bladder and ureters.
3. Relaxation of the sphincters in the gastrointestinal, biliary and urinary tracts.
4. Stimulation of the salivary, sweat, nasopharyngeal, and lacrimal glands, and stimulation of the secretory activity of the stomach, intestines and pancreas.
5. Constriction of the pupil (miosis) and accommodation of the lens for near vision.

The muscarinic actions of ACh are blocked or inhibited by **atropine,** and other anticholinergic drugs.

Nicotinic Actions

These are so called because they resemble the pharmacological actions of small quantities of the alkaloid, **nicotine**. They are exerted at the **skeletal neuromuscular junction, autonomic ganglia, adrenal medulla** and the **CNS.** The nicotinic actions are:

1. Stimulation of the skeletal muscle.
2. Stimulation of sympathetic and parasympathetic ganglia, and stimulation of the adrenal medulla.

The nicotinic actions of ACh are blocked or inhibited by **curare (d-tubocurarine)** at the neuromuscular junction, and by **ganglion blocking agents (pentolinium)** at the autonomic ganglia.

Mechanism of Action

The result of ACh action is either **hyperpolarization** (as in myocardial pacemaker cells), or **depolarization** (as in smooth muscles). Because of such a **dual action** ACh relaxes the smooth muscles in many peripheral blood vessels (**hyperpolarization**), and stimulates the smooth muscle of the gut (**depolarization**).

Table 3.2 : *Cholinergic receptor activation profile of choline esters*

Drug	Muscarinic Receptor Activation			Nicotinic Receptor Activation	Inactivation by Cholinesterase
	GI/Urinary	Cardiovascular	Ocular		
Acetylcholine	++	++	+	++	Yes
Methacholine	++	++	+	None	Slow hydrolysis
Carbamylcholine	+++	+	++	+++	No
Bethanechol	+++	+	++	None	No

Key : Strong +++; Moderate ++; Weak +

Therapeutic uses: ACh has no safe therapeutic use.

Methacholine (Acetyl Beta-methylcholine)

Methacholine has a longer duration of action than ACh, and is specific for muscarinic receptors.

Therapeutic Uses

Paroxysmal atrial tachycardia: Methacholine in a dose of 10 to 40 mg subcutaneously may be administered.

Carbamylcholine (Carbachol)

It is the **most potent** choline ester. It is not readily hydrolysed by cholinesterase, and has **both** muscarinic and nicotinic actions, but the muscarinic actions predominate **(Table 3.2).**

Therapeutic uses: Carbachol may be used to treat postoperative **intestinal atony** and **retention of urine.** Occasionally, it is used to treat **paroxysmal atrial tachycardia,** and **glaucoma.** Administered subcutaneously in doses of 0.25 to 0.5 mg, or orally 1 to 4 mg daily.

Bethanechol

Bethanechol has structural features common to both methacholine and carbachol. It is not hydrolysed by cholinesterase. It is devoid of nicotinic actions of ACh, and is principally a muscarine agent.

Therapeutic uses: It is used to treat *abdominal distention,* **paralytic ileus** and for **post-operative urinary retention.** Bethanechol is active by mouth (dose 30-120 mg daily).

Cholinomimetic Alkaloids

Pilocarpine

Pilocarpine is an alkaloid obtained from the leaflets of *Pilocarpus microphylus.* It stimulates the muscarinic receptors at the postganglionic neuroeffector junction **directly.**

Pilocarpine has a marked **diaphoretic** effect, and produces profuse sweating. It acts as a **sialogogue**, and increases salivary secretion.

Pilocarpine when injected subcutaneously or instilled in the eye causes a **constriction of the pupil (miosis),** and **spasm of accommodation** which lasts for 2 to 3 days.

Pilocarpine is mainly employed in the treatment of **chronic glaucoma** as a 0.5 to 4 percent solution. Pilocarpine ocular therapeutic system (Ocusert Pilo) is a continuous release form of pilocarpine (20 mcg/hour or 40 mcg/hour) placed into the lower conjunctional cul-de-sac. It provides for effective concentrations of pilocarpine in **open-angle glaucoma** for a week.

Muscarine

Muscarine is an alkaloid obtained from the poisonous mushroom *Amanita muscaria.* It is a choline derivative, and like ACh stimulates the effector cells in organs innervated by cholinergic nerves. Muscarine has ***no therapeutic uses.***

Arecholine

Arecholine is obtained from the betel nut *Areca catechu*. It has a ***muscarinic*** and ***weak nicotinic activity*** somewhat like pilocarpine. Betel nuts as such and preparations containing powered betel nuts are popularly chewed in India to promote salivary secretion and to aid digestion.

ANTICHOLINESTERASES

Anticholinesterases or **cholinesterase inhibitors** inhibit the enzyme acetylcholinesterase so that it is unable to hydrolyse ACh, and thus they preserve ACh at the nerve ending. Their action is **indirect.** Anticholinesterase agents are classified as **reversible** or **irreversible** inhibitors of acetylcholinesterase (AChE).

Mechanisms of Action

Physostigmine and neostigmine can delay hydrolysis of ACh from 1 to 8 hours.

The **irreversible cholinesterase inhibitors** are mostly *organophosphate* compounds. They are widely used as ingredients of many **insecticides** (malathion, parathion) and **war gases** (sarin, tabun). The organophosphates produce almost a permanent inactivation of the enzyme AChE, and their therapeutic usefulness is limited.

REVERSIBLE ANTICHOLINESTERASES

Physostigmine (Eserine)

Physostigmine salicylate and ***sulphate*** are the salts of an alkaloid obtained from the dried ripe seeds of *Physostigma venenosum*. It is well absorbed from the gastrointestinal tract and enters the CNS. It is equally active against true cholinesterase (AChE) and pseudocholinesterase.

Therapeutic uses and dosage: Physostigmine salicylate is administered orally in doses of 0.5 to 1.0 mg with a maximum dose of 3 mg in 24 hours, or by IM route in a dose of 0.5mg. ***Physostigmine sulphate*** is preferred to salicylate in eye-drop preparations which contain 0.25 or 0.5 percent physostigmine sulphate.

The main use of physostigmine in the form of eye-drops is as a miotic to treat **glaucoma.** Its systemic use is in the **treatment of atropine poisoning.** Physostigmine may be used in the early stages of **Alzheimer's disease.**

Neostigmine

Neostigmine is a synthetic quaternary ammonium compound with a rapid onset of action and similar reversible anticholinesterase activity to physostigmine. It differs from physostigmine in that it is a **quaternary nitrogen** compound, and is irregularly absorbed from the gastrointestinal tract, and it **does not cross the blood-brain barrier. This minimizes CNS toxicity.** It produces the contraction of the skeletal muscle by two ways: **firstly,** by a direct action on the skeletal muscle, and **secondly** by inactivation of cholinesterase. It has **anticurare** action.

Therapeutic uses: Neostigmine is used in the treatment of **myasthenia gravis**. The unwanted side effects may be abolished by atropine. It may be given by injection or more conveniently orally (dose 15 to 30 mg tid or qid daily). It is also used as an **antidote for curare poisoning.**

Dosage: Orally, neostigmine bromide 15 mg thrice daily; neostigmine methylsulphate 0.25 to 1.0 mg SC or IM.

Pyridostigmine

Pyridostigmine is chemically and pharmacologically closely related to neostigmine. It is slow in onset, weaker in action (½ to ¼ th) than neostigmine, but has a **longer duration of action.** Pyridostigmine is used in the treatment of **myasthenia gravis.** The dosage of pyridostigmine bromide is 60 to 240 mg orally, or 1 to 5 mg IM or SC.

Ambenonium

Ambenonium is a bis-quaternary reversible anticholinesterase agent with about **six times greater activity than neostigmine.** It is given orally in a dose of 5 to 25 mg to patients of **myasthenia gravis.**

Edrophonium

Edrophonium is a **short-acting cholinesterase inhibitor.** It is a weak anticholinesterase agent. Its use in **myasthenia gravis** is limited to the **differential diagnosis** of the disease, and in emergency treatment of a **myasthenic crisis.**

Distigmine

Distigmine has a **longer duration of action** than neostigmine and its action lasts for 24 hours. It is used to treat **atony** of the bladder and intestines, and may be repeated every second or third day. The usual dose is 5 mg orally or 0.5 mg by IM injection.

Demecarium

It is more potent than neostigmine. Its main use is in the management of **glaucoma.** The dosage in glaucoma is from 2 drops of a 0.25 percent solution instilled twice weekly to 1 to 2 drops twice daily.

Irreversible Anticholinesterases

Organophosphate cholinesterase inhibitors like DFP, phospholine, parathion and malathion are highly toxic compounds as they produce an **irreversible *inhibition of both acetylcholinesterase and pseudocholinesterase.*** These agents were developed for potential **chemical warfare,** mainly in Germany. Later they were developed as **insecticides** and **pesticides** for use in agriculture. Only the following two agents are used in ophthalmic practice.

DI-isopropylflourophosphonate (DFP)

DFP is a clear liquid and forms unstable solutions in water. For clinical use it is dissolved in arachis oil. ***Its duration of action is about 10 days.***

DFP is used topically as an instillation of a 0.1 percent solution into the conjunctival sac for the treatment of **glaucoma.** It is employed only when other miotics have failed.

Ecothiopate

Ecothiopate has the advantage over DFP that it forms a **stable** solution in water, and avoids the need for oily drops. When instilled into the eye, ecothiopate produces a miotic effect within 45 minutes which may **persist for one to four weeks.**

Ecothiopate iodide is available as a 0.06, 0.0125 and 0.25 percent aqueous solution. The usual dose in the treatment of **glaucoma** is 1 drop once or twice daily.

Organophosphate Anticholinesterase Poisoning

Most pronounced effects are profuse sweating and salivation; mental confusion and marked ataxia; severe dehydration; bronchoconstriction and increased bronchial secretions; ***respiratory paralysis*** and ***death.***

TREATMENT OF ANTICHOLINESTERASE POISONING

1. **Atropine:** it is a specific and effective antidote. It is given in a dose of 1mg IM or subcutaneously, repeated frequently.
2. **Supportive measures** include artificial respiration and fluid/electrolyte therapy.
3. **Pralidoxime (Pyridine-2-aldoxime methiodide, PAM):** It is an antidote of a different kind and is a **cholinesterase reactivator.** ***The enzyme is freed and reactivated to hydrolyse the excess of ACh*** at the receptors sites.

In severe poisoning **pralidoxime** is given in an **initial** dose of 1 to 2 g infused intravenously with 1 to 2 mg of **atropine.**

PHARMACOTHERAPY OF MYASTHENIA GRAVIS

Myasthenia gravis is a chronic disease characterized by *progressive weakness and rapid fatiguability* of the skeletal muscles due to impaired neuromuscular transmission. **Dysphagia** and **dysarthria** may be the first symptoms. This disease is more common in women. The drugs employed are:

a. **Reversible anticholinesterases:** The drugs used are neostigmine, pyridostigmine, ambenonium and edrophonium (diagnosis only). Parasympathetic side effects are an indication for atropine. The usual dosage is as under:
Neostigmine–15-30 mg tid or qid orally.
Pyridostigmine 60-120 mg 3 to 4 hourly orally
Ambenonium–5-25 mg tid or qid orally.
b. **Adrenal glucocorticoids:** Long-term ***alternate day treatment*** with prednisone produces good results. **Plasmapheresis** may be useful to prepare patients for **thymectomy.**
c. **Ephedrine sulphate:** This sympathomimetic amine has appreciable **anticurare action** in a dose of 12 mg with each dose of neostigmine.

PHARMACOTHERAPY OF GLAUCOMA

The glaucomas constitute a group of ocular diseases in which an elevated intraocular pressure (IOP) damages the optic nerve head, causing visual loss. There are **two** types of primary glaucoma: (i) open or wide angle (chronic, simple) and (ii) narrow angle (acute, congestive). The drugs employed are:

a. **The miotics:** When applied topically to the eye these drugs cause **constriction of the pupil, contraction of the ciliary muscle, and a fall in IOP due to the decreased resistance to the outflow of the aqueous humour.**
   i. **Parasympathomimetics:** Pilocarpine, Carbachol.
   ii. **Short-acting anticholinesterase:** Physostigmine.
   iii. **Long-acting anticholinesterases:** Demecarium, DFP, Ecothiopate.
b. **Adrenergic agents: Dipivalyladrenaline** is a new adrenaline analogue. It is a 'prodrug' that undergoes biotransformation to become active adrenaline, and can be used in far smaller amounts without sacrificing its IOP reducing effects. Topical adrenaline lowers IOP apparently both by ***increasing aqueous outflow, and by decreasing aqueous humour formation.***
c. **Beta-adrenoceptor blockers:** *Timolol* is the agent used to lower IOP in patients with primary open-angle glaucoma and secondary glaucomas. It ***decreases the production*** of aqueous humour.
d. **Carbonic anhydrase inhibitors:** *Acetazolamide, dichlorphenamide, ethoxzolamide and methazolamide* may be used. These agents are given systemically to reduce IOP.
e. **Osmotic agents:** Hypertonic solutions of *glycerine, isosorbide* and *mannitol* are used for the short-term reduction of IOP.

3.3 CHOLINERGIC BLOCKING AGENTS (PARASYMPATHOLYTICS)

Cholinergic blocking agents **block** or **interfere** with the actions of acetylcholine (ACh) at the postganglionic parasympathetic nerve endings. These agents have been variously named as **parasympatholytics, spasmolytics** and **anticholinergics.**

THE BELLADONNA FAMILY

The **three** noteworthy plants are **Atropa belladonna, Hyoscyamus niger** and **Datura stramonium.**

Atropine

The principal alkaloids of belladonna are **atropine, hyoscyamine** and **scopolamine** (hyoscine). The most important alkaloid is **atropine.**

Mode of action: Atropine, hyoscine and the synthetic anticholinergics cause a prolonged blockade of **muscarine cholinergic receptors** which prevents the ACh or choline esters to reach receptor sites. This antagonism is **competitive** in nature.

Pharmacological Actions of Atropine

Central Nervous System

Atropine *stimulates* the cerebral cortex and the

medulla. The action is dose-dependent.

Cardiovascular System

The primary action of atropine is to **alter the heart rate.** In small doses (0.5 to 0.6 mg) it stimulates the vagus centrally and the pulse rate is *slightly slowed.* Larger doses (1 to 2 mg) block the cardiac vagus peripherally, and the central action is masked, resulting in an *increase in heart rate.*

Gastrointestinal System

The cholinergic supply is **secretomotor** to the stomach, and **motor** to the intestines. In small doses atropine **diminishes gastric secretion in peptic ulcer.** Atropine relaxes the gall bladder and the bile duct.

Other Smooth Muscles

Atropine relaxes the bronchi and bronchioles, resulting in a widening of the airway. The bronchial secretions are dried up and may lead to 'mucus plug' formation and obstruction. The tone and contractions of the ureter are decreased. The detrusor muscle of the bladder is relaxed.

Effect on Secretions

The secretion of mucous glands lining the respiratory tract, mouth, nose, pharynx and bronchi is diminished. Sweating (which involves sympathetic cholinergic nerves) is suppressed, and the skin becomes hot and dry, and the body temperature rises.

Effect on the Eye

The intrinsic muscles of the eye have a dual (parasympathetic and sympathetic) nerve supply (**Fig. 3.3**). The parasympathetic supply is carried via the oculomotor nerve, and innervates the **constrictor pupillae,** the stimulation of which causes **miosis.** The sympathetic supply is via the superior cervical ganglion, and innervates the **dilator pupillae,** the stimulation of which causes **mydriasis.** When atropine is administered orally, parenterally or a dilute solution (0.5 to 1.0%) is instilled into the conjunctional sac, a dilatation of the pupil (**mydriasis**), and paralysis of accommodation (**cycloplegia**) occurs. The lens becomes less convex, and the eye is **fixed for distant vision.**

Mydriatics (Pupillary dilators)	*Miotics (Pupillary constrictors)*
A. <u>Sympathomimetics</u> (stimulate radial muscles) e.g. ephedrine, phenylephrine	A. <u>Parasympathomimetics</u> (stimulate circular muscles) e.g. eserine, pilocarpine
B. <u>Parasympatholytics</u> (Inhibit/paralyse circular muscles) e.g. atropine, homatropine	B. <u>Sympatholytics</u> (Inhibit/paralyse radial muscles)e.g. guanethidine tolazoline

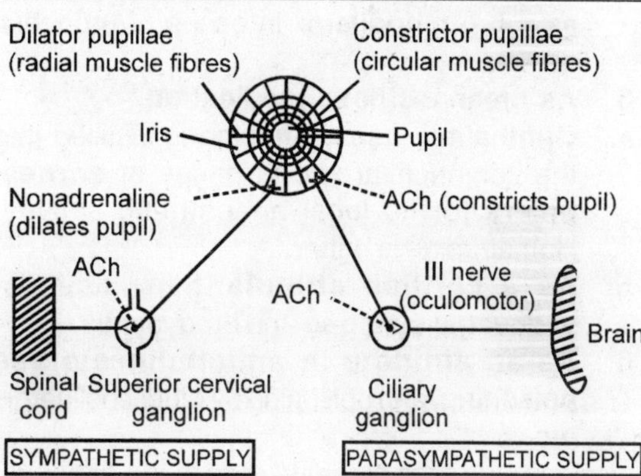

Fig. 3.3: *Innervation of the intrinsic muscles of the eye (diagrammatic mode of action of mydriatics and miotics.*

The mydriasis produced by atropine pushes the mass of the iris muscle against the cornea, blocking the cornea-iris angle. This reduces the drainage of ciliary fluid, and the ***intraocular pressure (IOP) has a tendency to rise.*** Atropine is **contraindicated in glaucoma.**

Other Actions

Atropine in large doses has a ***weak* local anesthetic** action, and exerts a **weak antihistaminic** activity. Large doses of atropine increase body temperature as a result of diminished sweat secretion and a reduced heat loss.

Pharmacokinetics

Atropine is readily absorbed from the intestines. In the blood it is appreciably bound to the plasma proteins, and elimination by the kidney is almost complete (85 to 90%) within 24 hours. A ***drop of the suspected urine, when instilled into the conjunctival sac of a cat, produces mydriasis.*** Atropine is hydrolysed in the liver by atropine esterase.

Therapeutic Uses

1. **CNS disorders:** Scopolamine and antihistamines are effective in the treatment of nausea and vomiting of **motion sickness.**
2. **As antispasmodics:** They relax the spasm of smooth muscles (colic) of the **intestinal**, **urinary** and **biliary tracts.** Atropine is used as a **bronchodilator** in cases of bronchial asthma.
3. **As preanaesthetic medication.**
4. **Ophthalmic uses:** Atropine is instilled into the conjunctival sac in cases of **corneal ulcers** for its local anaesthetic activity. Homatropine is better.
5. **As a cardiac stimulant** in cases of **vasovagal syncope** and bradycardia.
6. **As an antidote in anticholinesterase poisoning,** and poisoning by other cholinergic drugs.

Dose: Atropine sulphate (oral, subcutaneous) 0.5 to 1.0 mg . For instillation into the eye a 1-2 percent solution is used.

Contraindications

Atropine is contraindicated in patients with **glaucoma** and **prostatic hypertrophy.**

Adverse Reactions

1. **Dryness of the mouth and throat** (xerostomia) due to reduced salivation, leading to dysphagia.
2. **The skin is dry**, hot and red, specially in the region of the face and neck (atropine flush).
3. **Blurred vision** due to paralysis of accommodation. The intraocular pressure may rise leading to **glaucoma.**
4. **Urinary retention.**
5. **Palpitation and tachycardia.**
6. **Constipation**.

Atropine/Belladonna Poisoning

The symptoms of intoxication are severe dryness of the mouth and throat, wide pupillary dilatation, dsyphagia and thirst, tachycardia, redness of the skin specially in the blush area, muscle incoordination, rise in body temperature, delirium, hallucinations, mania, apathy, stertorous breathing, stupor, coma and finally respiratory collapse.

Treatment of Poisoning

1. The antidote of choice is **physostigmine salicylate** (it readily crosses the blood-brain barrier). A slow IV injection of 1-4 mg of physostigmine readily controls the delirium and coma. It may be repeated within 1 to 2 hours.
2. Hyperpyrexia and delirium may be treated by an ice cap, and **cold sponging.**
3. Respiratory stimulants like caffeine with sodium benzoate or oxygen-carbon dioxide mixtures may be used.
4. **Artificial respiration** instituted, if necessary.
5. Diazepam may be used if mental symptoms are disturbing.

Scopolamine (Hyoscine)

The main difference in the action of atropine and scopolamine is on the CNS. Atropine in therapeutic doses has little effect on the CNS, but in higher doses it produces a mild stimulation. With still **higher does atropine is a strong stimulant of the CNS.** Scopolamine on the contrary is a **primary depressant** of the CNS, and in therapeutic doses causes drowsiness, amnesia, euphoria, fatigue and sleep.

Therapeutic Uses

1. **Scopolamine** is used with **morphine** in obstetrics to produce amnesia or **'twilight sleep'.** The drug combination produces a

blurred consciousness. For producing amnesia morphine 15 mg and scopolamine 0.5mg is injected subcutaneously.

2. Scopolamine may be used for **preanaesthetic medication** to reduce salivary and bronchial secretions.
3. Used in some cases of **motion sickness.**

Dose: Scopolamine hydrobromide 0.3 to 0.6 mg orally or subcutaneously. **Transdermal hyoscine** is also available for prevention of motion sickness.

SYNTHETIC ANTIMUSCARINICS (ATROPINE SUBSTITUTES)

Numerous synthetic compounds, as well as derivatives of the natural alkaloids have been prepared to: (i) obtain a greater **selectivity** of action than atropine; and (ii) to **lessen the side effects** produced. These **atropine-like drugs** may be classified into the following **three** groups:

Group I — **Atropine-like Mydriatics**
- Homatropine hydrobromide
- Eucatropine hydrochloride
- Cyclopentolate hydrochloride
- Tropicamide

Group II — **Antisecretory-Antispasmodics (Peptic ulcer)**
- Propantheline bromide
- Oxyphenonium bromide
- Dicyclomine

Group III — **Antiparkinsonian Drugs**
- Benzhexol
- Benztropine
- Orphenadrin

To summarize, atropine is a typical competitive antagonist for the muscarinic effects of ACh in the body. Major clinical uses of atropine are based on its muscarinic blocking action in the **heart, eye, gastrointestinal tract** and the **brain.**

3.4 ADRENOCEPTOR STIMULANTS (SYMPATHOMIMETICS)

Sympathomimetic drugs mimic the effects of sympathetic nervous stimulation of organs, and structures that contain the adrenergic receptors.

THE ADRENERGIC RECEPTORS

Ahlquist in 1948 suggested that the effects of adrenaline at peripheral sites could be divided in to **two** groups, which depended on two types of postsynaptic receptors: **alpha** and **beta type**. Stimulation of ***alpha-receptors*** produces ***excitation*** in most adrenergically innervated organs and tissues, except in the *gastrointestinal tract*. In contrast, stimulation of ***beta-receptors*** produces ***inhibition*** in most adrenergically innervated organs and tissue, except in the *heart*.

There are **two** distinct types of alpha-receptors (**alpha$_1$**, **alpha$_2$**), and two types of beta-receptors (**beta$_1$**, **beta$_2$**). The difference is based primarily on their location. Thus, **alpha$_1$** receptors are found **postsynaptically** on vascular smooth muscle, gastrointestinal, and urinary sphincters, eye, pancreas, spleen and certain glands. **Alpha$_2$** receptors are located **presynaptically** where they control the release of noradrenaline by a **negative feedback** mechanism. **Beta$_1$** receptors are located primarily in the heart, and adipose tissue, while **beta$_2$** receptors are located in the bronchial, gastrointestinal, uterine and urinary smooth muscle, skeletal muscle blood vessels, and in the liver and kidney.

Adrenaline has a mixed action; **noradrenaline** is a predominant alpha-agonist; and **isoprenaline** is a beta-agonist.

In addition to adrenergic alpha and beta receptors there are specific **dopaminergic** receptors located on the renal and visceral blood vessels. Their activation by **dopamine** results in vasodilation and reduced vascular resistance in the renal and visceral blood vessels. **Isoprenaline** is an example of a mixed beta$_1$/beta$_2$ adrenoceptor agonist, whereas **salbutamol** and **terbutaline** act selectively on beta$_2$ adrenoceptors.

Biosynthesis, Storage and Release of Catecholamines

The noradrenergic neurones (conventionally called adrenergic neurones) synthesize, store and release noradrenaline as their neurotransmitter. The synthesis of NA is the first step in the process of noradrenergic transmission **(Fig. 3.4).**

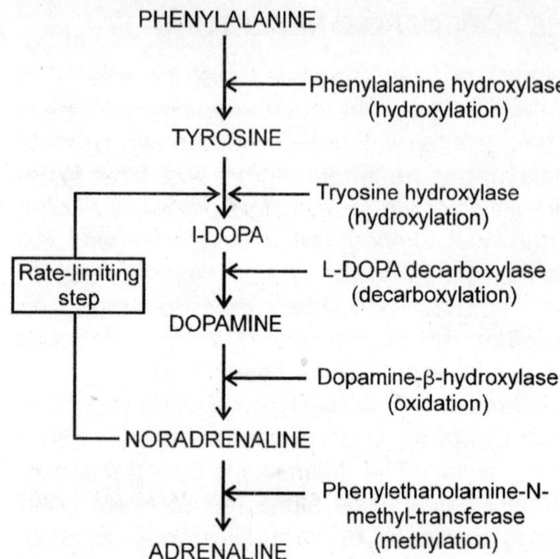

Fig. 3.4 : *Biosynthesis of catecholamines. Phenylalanine is converted in the circulation (extraneuronally) into tyrosine. Tyrosine is taken up from the blood stream by noradrenergic neurones and chromaffin cells of the adrenal medulla. In the cytoplasm of the neurones tyrosine is converted to l-DOPA, and l-DOPA to dopamine. Dopamine is taken up into noradrenaline storage vesicles, and converted to noradrenaline. The conversion of noradrenaline to adrenaline does not occur in the noradrenergic neurones, but takes place in the chromaffin cells of the adrenal medulla which store adrenaline.*

FATE OF CATECHOLAMINES

The two major enzyme systems involved in the metabolism of catecholamines are **monoamine oxidase (MAO),** and **catechol-O-methyl-transferase (COMT).** A major mode of termination of the action of noradrenaline is by re-uptake (80-90 percent) into the adrenergic neurone to be re-used as transmitter. The end products, **vanillyl-mandelic acid** (VMA) and **metanephrines** are excreted in the urine.

CLASSIFICATION OF SYMPATHOMIMETIC AMINES

Group I **Directly-acting amines:** Adrenaline, Noradrenaline, Isoprenaline, Dopamine, Dobutamine.

Group II **Indirectly-acting amines:** Amphetamine, Tyramine.

Group III **Mixed action amines:** Ephedrine, Metaraminol, Methoxamine

Chemically speaking, the sympathomimetic amines can be classified under *two* heads:

i. *Catecholamines* (Group I), and
ii. *Noncatecholamines* (Groups II and III).

Catecholamines

Adrenaline (Epinephrine)

Adrenaline is found in ***nervous tissue, adrenal medulla,*** and in the ***chromaffin cells*** scattered throughout the body. Adrenaline is a **prototype** sympathomimetic agent, and exerts both alpha and beta effects.

Pharmacological Actions

Cardiovascular System

The cardiovascular effects produced in man by an intravenous infusion of adrenaline are shown in **Fig. 3.5.** The *systolic blood pressure is raised,*

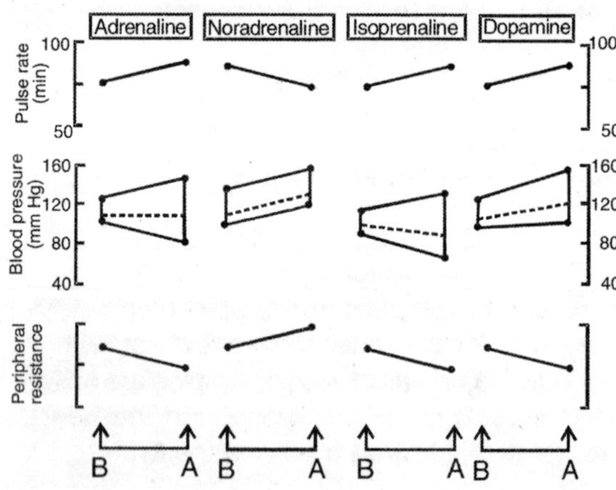

Fig. 3.5 : *Comparison of the circulatory effects of adrenaline, noradrenaline, isoprenaline and dopamine (diagrammatic). The middle panel depicts the drug effect on arterial blood pressure as : upperline for systolic, lower line for diastolic, and dashed line for mean (diastolic + 1/3 pulse pressure) blood pressure B = before drug; A = after drug.*

while the *diastolic pressure is lowered* and the *mean blood pressure registers little change*. Heart rate is increased and the **overall peripheral resistance is reduced. The cardiac output is elevated by adrenaline.**

Respiratory System

The bronchial muscle is *relaxed* (beta-effect) and the microcirculation in the bronchial mucosa is constricted (alpha-effect). These changes lead to a ***decreased bronchial resistance.***

Metabolic Effects

The metabolic actions of adrenaline lead to: (i) a marked **increase in oxygen consumption** by tissues; (ii) an **increased glycogenolysis** in liver; (iii) **decreased glucose utilization** by tissues; (iv) **release of lactic acid** from muscle; and (v) an **elevation of free fatty acid (FFA)** levels in blood. These actions are largely caused by the promotion of the formation of cyclic AMP (c-AMP). The glycogenolytic action of adrenaline on the liver and skeletal muscle leads to **hyperglycaemia.**

Eyes: On intravenous administration adrenaline contracts the radial muscles of the iris inducing **active mydriasis** (alpha-effect), but no cycloplegia. Adrenaline ***lowers intraocular pressure*** in normal subjects and in glaucoma.

Skeletal muscle: Adrenaline facilitates neuromuscular transmission by a presynaptic action which increases the amount of acetylcholine liberated at the myoneural junction. It has an **antifatigue action.**

Gastrointestinal tract: The tone, frequency and amplitude of peristalsis are reduced (alpha- and beta-effects). The sphincters are constricted (alpha-effect).

Glandular secretions: The *salivary secretion* becomes thick and mucoid. *Adrenaline-induced sweating provides indirect evidence for an adrenergic sweating mechanism in man.*

Urogenital tract: The detrusor muscle of the bladder is relaxed (beta-effect). The trigone and the sphincters are constricted (alpha-effect). The human gravid uterus contracts.

Central nervous system: In certain individuals it may induce a feeling of **anxiety, apprehension, restlessness,** and sometime **tremors** and **weakness.**

Absorption, Fate and Excretion

Adrenaline is poorly absorbed and rapidly destroyed in the gastrointestinal tract. Hence it has to be given parenterally by the **intramuscular** or **subcutaneous** route, or by **inhalation.**

Therapeutic Uses

1. **Bronchial asthma.**
2. **Hypersensitivity reactions:** In allergic emergencies the first drug to use is adrenaline.
3. **Heart block and cardiac arrest:** For the treatment of heart block with syncope **(Stokes Adams attacks)** 0.3 to 0.6 ml of adrenaline (1 in 1000) may be given subcutaneously. For the treatment of **cardiac arrest** about 0.3 to 0.5 ml of adrenaline (1 in 1000) may be injected directly into the right atrium.
4. **Control of bleeding:** Adrenaline is frequently used as a topical haemostatic agent to produce vasoconstriction, which stops epistaxis (nose bleed).
5. Adrenaline is **added to local anesthetics like lignocaine** to limit the absorption from the site of infiltration, and prolong the duration of action.

Contraindications

Adrenaline is contraindicated in ***thyrotoxicosis*** and cardiovascular diseases like ***hypertension***, ***arteriosclerosis***, and ***coronary insufficiency***.

Adverse Reactions

The most common ill effects of adrenaline are *anxiety, fear, pallor, tachycardia, palpitation, tremors, restlessness* and *throbbing headache*. Extreme hypertension may occur and precipitate cerebral haemorrhage, and there may be convulsive episodes. *Cardiac arrhythmias* and fatal *ventricular fibrillation* may develop.

Dosage: Adrenaline hydrochloride in a 1:1000 aqueous solution is available for subcutaneous or intramuscular injection. The usual dose ranges between 0.1 to 0.5 ml subcutaneously.

Noradrenaline (Norepinephrine, Levarterenol)

Noradrenaline chemically differs from adrenaline in that the 'nitrogen is without' methyl substitution.

Pharmacological Actions

Noradrenaline predominantly acts on the alpha-adrenoceptors, i.e., **it is an alpha-agonist,** and it has only minimal effects on cardiac beta-receptors.

Cardiovascular System

Noradrenaline raises both **systolic** and **diastolic** blood pressures; mainly due to an increase in the total peripheral resistance (**Fig. 3.5**). The cardiac output is only slightly affected.

Cardiac oxygen consumption is increased, but to a lesser extent compared to adrenaline. The **coronary arteries are dilated** and the coronary flow is increased. Noradrenaline also possesses a **positive inotropic effect** on the heart.

Therapeutic Uses

Noradrenaline is used as a vasopressor agent in the treatment of **hypotensive states** like **surgical** or **myocardial infarction.**

Adverse Reactions and Contraindications

Rapid administration may cause dangerous cardiac arrhythmias. Caution is to be observed in patients of **hypertension** and **cardiovascular diseases.**

Dosage: Noradrenaline bitartrate injection is available in 2 ml ampoules containing 1mg/ml noradrenaline base (1 in 1000) solution of noradrenaline base). It should not be used if the solution is brown in colour or contains a precipitate. The solution is diluted to contain 4 mcg/ml of noradrenaline base which is obtained by diluting 4 ml of official injection (2 ampoules) in 1000 ml of 5 percent dextrose injection. The rate of infusion (0.5 to 1.0 ml/min) is adjusted to maintain the desired level of blood pressure. Blood pressure is taken every 5 minutes till it is stabilized.

Isoprenaline (Isoproterenol, Isopropyl-noradrenaline)

Isoprenaline is a synthetic catecholamine derived from noradrenaline. Isoprenaline acts almost exclusively on the beta-adrenoceptors.

Pharmacological Actions

Cardiovascular System

As a result of stimulation of the cardiac beta-adrenoceptors, isoprenaline exerts a *positive* **inotropic** and **chronotropic** effect on the heart, causing an increase in the cardiac output. It *lowers peripheral vascular resistance*, mainly in the skeletal muscle, and also in the renal and mesenteric vessels. The mean pressure is ***slightly reduced*** (**Fig. 3.5**).

Bronchial Muscles

Isoprenaline relaxes all smooth muscles in the body. This **spasmolytic action** is most marked on the **bronchial** and **gastrointestinal** musculature.

Therapeutic Uses

1. **Bronchial asthma:** Isoprenaline may be administered as a sublingual tablet or by inhalation.
2. **Heart block:** It is useful for the immediate treatment of heart block.
3. Isoprenaline may be employed in **cardiogenic shock** and in **septicaemic shock.**

Adverse Reactions and Contraindications

Isoprenaline may cause ***palpitation***, ***tachycardia***, ***headache*** and ***flushing of the skin***. Serious arrhythmias, anginal pain, tremors, dizziness and sweating occasionally occur. It is ***contraindicated*** in patients of cardiac arrhythmias, coronary insufficiency, hyperthyroidism, and diabetes mellitus.

Dosage: Isoprenaline hydrochloride inhalation solutions are available in strengths of 1 : 100, 1 : 200 and 1 : 400 solution of isoprenaline base. ***Sublingual tablets*** of 10 and 15 mg, and sustained release tablets of 30 mg are available.

Dopamine

Dopamine is the naturally occurring catecholamine, which is the immediate precursor of noradrenaline in the body. Although dopamine has specific dopaminergic receptors in the CNS, injected dopamine has no central effects as it does not cross the blood-brain barrier.

Pharmacological Actions

The haemodynamic response in man to an infusion of dopamine is that the *cardiac output is increased, peripheral resistance is decreased, and there is little change in the mean arterial pressure and the heart rate* (**Fig. 3.5**).

Therapeutic Uses

Dopamine is used for the treatment of shock resulting from **trauma, surgery**, and **myocardial infarction**. Also used in the treatment of **congestive heart failure**, **renal** and **liver failure**.

Adverse Reactions and Contraindications

Toxic effects include nausea, vomiting, tachycardia, and ectopic beats. Precordial pain and occasionally hypertension may develop. Dopamine is contraindicated in patients of *tachyarrhythmias* and *pheochromocytoma*.

Dosage: Dopamine hydrochloride is available as a sterile solution containing 40 mg/ml of the drug in 5 ml ampoules. The contents of the ampule are diluted in 250 or 500 ml of 0.9% sodium chloride, or 5% dextrose solution to give a final concentration of 800 or 400 mcg/ml. This is given as a drip infusion at a rate between 5 to 20 mcg/kg body weight. The blood pressure, heart rate and urine flow must be continuously monitored.

Dobutamine

Dobutamine is a synthetic catecholamine related to dopamine.

Pharmacological Actions

Dobutamine acts directly on beta$_1$-adrenoceptors in the heart. It has little or no action at beta$_2$- or alpha-receptors. ***It increases the contractile force of the heart raising the stroke volume and cardiac output***. Like dopamine, it produces ***vasodilation of the renal and mesenteric vessels***. Dobutamine has a very short duration of action (plasma t½ is 2 minutes), as it is rapidly metabolized and excreted.

Therapeutic Uses

Dobutamine is used in the short-term management of **acute cardiac decompensation**. Dobutamine is more useful than dopamine in the treatment of **cardiogenic shock**.

Adverse Reactions and Contraindications

Premature ventricular beats occur in patients. Less frequently headache, palpitation, nausea, anginal pain and dyspnoea may occur.

Dosage: Dobutamine is available as a powder for injection (250 mg/vial). It is administered by IV infusion, diluted in 5 percent dextrose injection. The usual dosage range is 2.5 to 10 mcg/kg/min of either 250, 500 or 1000 mcg/ml solution.

Noncatecholamines

A number of sympathomimetics lack the catechol nucleus and are used clinically. Their effects depend partly upon **release** of stored noradrenaline from the noradrenergic nerve terminals, and partly upon a **direct** action on the effector cells. The indirectly-acting compounds (**amphetamine, tyramine**) predominantly act by releasing noradrenaline, which stimulates the adrenoceptors, whereas **ephedrine, metaraminol** and **methoxamine** have a mixed action. **Amphetamine** and **ephedrine** are prototypes.

In contrast to catecholamines most of the non-catecholamines are ***effective orally,*** and have a much ***longer duration of action.***

Amphetamine

Amphetamine has powerful CNS stimulant activity. The name **amphetamine** (Benzedrine) refers to the racemic form of the drug, and ***dextro-amphetamine*** (Dexedrine) to the d-isomer. Both are synthetic in origin.

Pharmacological Actions

Cardiovascular System

Amphetamine given orally **raises both systolic and diastolic blood pressures.** The pulse pressure is usually increased as it has an effect on both alpha- and beta-receptors. The heart rate is reflexly slowed.

Central Nervous System

Amphetamines have a powerful **psychostimulant action** on the CNS. **Dextroamphetamine** is most active in this respect, and is 3 to 4 times as potent as the l-isomer.

In man the effects of an oral dose (10 to 30 mg) of amphetamine are: alertness, wakefulness, decreased fatigue, elevation of mood, increased motor and speech activity. Performance of simple mental tasks may be improved. The effect on memory is undecided. Physical performance is improved. Prolonged use leads to mental depression and fatigue.

Amphetamine leads to a suppression of appetite, i.e., it has an **anorexigenic** or **anorexiant** effect. The site of anorexiant action is the feeding centre, whereby the hunger drive is diminished.

Therapeutic Uses

Amphetamine is employed in the treatment of : **narcolepsy, hyperkinetic behaviour disorders** in children, **depressive states, enuresis, epilepsy, motion sickness, postencephalitic parkinsonism, orthostatic hypotension** and **obesity.**

Adverse Reactions and Precautions

Amphetamine may induce dryness of mouth, difficulty in micturition, agitation, restlessness, insomnia and anorexia. With higher doses there may be hypertension, tachycardia, anginal pain and cardiac arrhythmias. On prolonged use **tolerance** and **dependence** on amphetamine may develop.

Dosage: Amphetamine sulphate, amphetamine phosphate and dextroamphetamine sulphate are available usually in 5 or 10 mg tablet forms. The usual initial oral dose is 2.5 to 5.0 mg.

Ephedrine

In olden days ephedrine was isolated from plants like *Ephedra equisetina* or *E.sinica*. It is now obtained entirely by chemical synthesis. Its central actions are less pronounced than those of the amphetamines. Ephedrine partly owes its peripheral action to **release** of noradrenaline from neuronal storage sites, and has **direct** action also on the adrenoceptors, i.e., it has a **mixed action.** Ephedrine stimulates both alpha- and beta-receptors.

Pharmacological Actions

Cardiovascular system: Ephedrine in many ways has ***similar cardiovascular effects as adrenaline,*** but the effects persist ***seven to ten times longer***.

Smooth muscles: The **bronchodilator** effect of ephedrine is weaker, slower in onset, but more persistent than that of adrenaline. Consequently, ephedrine is of value only in the ***prevention of acute attacks of bronchial asthma.***

Central nervous system: The central *stimulant effects* of ephedrine are similar to those of amphetamine, but are less marked.

Therapeutic uses: Ephedrine is used in mild or moderate cases of **bronchial asthma**. It may be used as a **nasal decongestant**. Other uses include **Stokes-Adams syndrome, hypotension during spinal anaesthesia, and narcolepsy.**

Adverse Reactions and Precautions

In therapeutic doses ephedrine stimulates the CNS, manifested as insomnia, restlessness, tremors, anxiety and agitation. Tolerance is developed after several weeks of continued use, but disappears on discontinuing the therapy.

Dosage: Ephedrine sulphate and **ephedrine hydrochloride** are preparations available as nose drops, sprays or tablets. The oral dose varies from 15 to 50 mg. In **hypotensive states** ephedrine sulphate 15 to 50 mg may be given subcutaneously.

OTHER SYMPATHOMIMETIC AMINES

A large number of sympathomimetic amines, some of them not included in the text so far, are usefully employed clinically. Their details are beyond the scope of this text.

3.5 ADRENOCEPTOR BLOCKING AGENTS (SYMPATHOLYTICS)

Adrenoceptor blocking drugs **inhibit** or **prevent** the response of effector cells to both sympathetic nerve activity, or sympathomimetic amines by their blocking action on the adrenoceptors.

ADRENOCEPTORS

Noradrenaline is the neurotransmitter released at the noradrenergic nerve terminals. Two types of adrenoceptors have been recognized and designated as α (Alpha) and β (beta) adrenoceptors. Subsequently they were further classified into α_1 and α_2 and β_1, β_2 and β_3 receptor subtypes.

The α_1- adrenoceptors are located at **post-synaptic** sites on tissues innervated by adrenergic neurones. The α_2 adrenoceptors have **presynaptic location,** and are involved in the **feedback inhibition** of noradrenaline release from nerve terminals. The β_1 adrenoceptors are found chiefly in the **heart**, while β_2 adrenoceptors are located in a number of sites including bronchial muscle and skeletal muscle blood vessels. The β_3-adrenoceptor are located in the *adipose tissue.*

ALPHA-ADRENOCEPTOR BLOCKING AGENTS

Classification of Alpha-Blockers

1. *Haloalkylamine:* Phenoxybenzamine.
2. *Imidazolines:* Tolazoline, Phentolamine.
3. *Ergot alkaloids:* Ergotamine and dihydroergotamine, ergotoxine and dihydroergotoxine, ergometrine.
4. *Other compounds:* Thymoxamine, Prazosin, Chlorpromazine, Yohimbine

Mode of Action

1. **Competitive short-acting antagonists:** The *ergot alkaloids*, *tolazoline* and *phentolamine* belong to this group. Their duration of action is short. These agents are also called **reversible** alpha-blockers.
2. **Noncompetitive, long-acting antagonist:** *Phenoxybenzamine* belongs to this group and produces a non-competitive antagonism which cannot be overcome by increasing the concentration of the alpha-agonist noradrenaline.

Haloalkylamine

Phenoxybenzamine

Phenoxybenzamine is the only haloalkylamine in clinical use. It is a potent alpha-adrenoceptor blocker.

In the early stages the alpha-blockade induced by phenoxybenzamine is **competitive,** but once the blockade is fully developed it becomes **non-competitive** in nature.

In hypertensive patients phenoxybenzamine produces a marked reduction in blood pressure. Phenoxybenzamine increases the cardiac output and decreases the total peripheral resistance which leads to a **better tissue perfusion.**

Therapeutic uses: Phenoxybenzamine is used to treat peripheral vasospastic conditions like **Raynaud's disease,** and **intermittent claudication.** It has been successfully used in the treatment of **inoperable pheochromocytoma**. It is used in the treatment of **shock-syndromes** marked by hypotension and extreme vasoconstriction.

Adverse reactions: Side effects include nasal congestion, bronchoconstriction and miosis. Serous effects of overdosage are postural hypotension, reflex tachycardia, congestive heart failure, cerebral stroke or kidney failure.

Dosage: Phenoxybenzamine hydrochloride is started at a dose level of 10 mg daily orally. The daily dose is adjusted usually between 20 and 60 mg.

Imidazolines

Tolazoline

Tolazoline is a **weak** alpha-blocker and causes peripheral vasodilatation mainly by its direct relaxant effect on the vascular smooth muscle. It causes a weak **competitive blockade** of alpha-receptors in man. Tolazoline decreases peripheral resistance, increases venous capacity with little change in the arterial pressure as the cardiac output is increased.

Tolazoline is used to increase blood flow in peripheral vasospastic conditions like **Raynaud's syndrome, chilblains, causalgia, frostbite, acrocyanosis** and **intermittent claudication.**

Adverse effects include pilomotor stimulation (goose flesh), tachycardia, increased gastrointestinal motility, and hyperchlorhydria.

Dosage: Tolazoline hydrochloride 25 to 50 mg three times a day. An injection solution (25 mg/ml) is also available.

Phentolamine

Phentolamine is a more potent alpha-blocker compared to tolazoline. This alpha-blocker is almost exclusively used for the **diagnosis of pheochromocytoma,** and for the prevention of hypertension during operative removal of this adrenal medullary tumour.

Adverse reactions to phentolamine include orthostatic hypotension, tachycardia and nasal stuffiness.

Dosage: Phentolamine hydrochloride 50 mg four to six times a day orally prior to surgery on patients of pheochromocytoma. Phentolamine mesylate is injectable intravenously, and 5 mg ampules are available.

Ergot Alkaloids

Ergot is a parasitic fungus (***Claviceps purpura***) which grows on rye and certain other grains. It contains twelve alkaloids (six isomeric pairs) of complex chemical structure. Two major actions of ergot alkaloids are: (i) to stimulate smooth muscles, and (ii) to block alpha-adrenoceptors.

Ergotamine

Ergotamine possesses both vasoconstrictor and alpha-blocking activity. Dihydrogenation of ergotamine (dihydroergotamine) increases the alpha-blocking potency and reduces the smooth muscle stimulant activity. Both ergotamine and dihydroergotamine are used to treat **migraine.**

Ergotamine tartrate for the *prevention of migraine* may be given orally as 2 or 3 tablets (1 mg / tablet) repeated for 2 to 3 doses. It may be injected in a dose of 0.25 mg SC. Combination of ergotamine tartrate 1 mg, and caffeine 100 mg (Cafergot) in tablet from is available for use, and 2 tablets may be administered at onset of attack.

Other Ergot Alkaloids

Ergometrine has weak alpha-blocking activity, but is a powerful stimulant of the uterus (oxytocic action), and is mainly used in obstetrics to reduce *post-partum haemorrhage.*

Ergotoxine is a mixture of three different alkaloids **ergocornine, ergocristine** and **ergocryptine.** The dihydrogenated derivatives of this mixture (dihydroergotoxine) have increased alpha-blocking potency, and very little smooth muscle stimulant activity.

Dihydroergotoxine has been used in vasospastic disorders like **Raynaud's syndrome.** It has been used to **improve the mental status of elderly patients** with signs of inadequate cerebral blood flow.

Dihydroergotoxine may be administered sublingually in doses upto 4.5 mg per day in tablet form. It may be injected IM or intra-arterially in doses of 150 to 600 mcg to relieve vasospasm.

Side effects include **nausea, vomiting, blurred vision, nasal stuffiness, skin rashes and chronic effects like convulsions, abortion, peripheral vascular stasis and gangrene.**

Bromocriptine

Bromocriptine (2-bromo-alpha-ergocryptine) is a compound related to the ergot alkaloid **ergocryptine.** It **suppresses prolactin secretion** by a direct action on the anterior pituitary possibly by a **specific dopamine receptor agonistic action.**

Bromocriptine has been employed in the treatment of **hypogonadism** in both men and women. It has been shown to restore fertility in women with or without **hyperprolactinaemia.** It is also used for the **suppression of puerperal lactation.**

Side effects include nausea, vomiting, postural hypotension and micturition syncope. On prolonged therapy mild constipation, muzziness, nasal congestion, night cramps in legs and dystonic reaction may occur.

Dosage: Bromocriptine mesylate for suppression of lactation is given orally in a dose equivalent to 2.5 mg bromocriptine base for 2 to 3 days, and later 2.5 mg twice daily for 14 days.

Other Compounds

Prazosin

Prazosin is of value in the treatment of hypertension (**Chap. 4.2**), and congestive heart failure (**Chap. 4.3**). It has potent ***alpha$_1$-adrenoceptor blocking activity.***

Chlorpromazine

Chlorpromazine amongst its many actions possesses alpha-adrenoceptor blocking activity. However it is not used clinically as an alpha-blocker.

Yohimbine

Yohimbine is a plant alkaloid related to reserpine. It produces a short-acting competitive blockade of **alpha-receptors,** and also **blocks the 5-hydroxytryptamine** receptors. In addition, it is a **strong stimulant of the brain,** and is reputed to possess **aphrodisiac** properties, which presumably are attributable to stimulation of the CNS, and vasodilatation in the genitalia. Convincing evidence for its aphrodisiac action is lacking.

BETA-ADRENOCEPTOR BLOCKING AGENTS

Beta-blockers are **competitive inhibitors** of the effects of catecholamines at beta-adrenergic receptor sites. The main effect is to **reduce cardiac activity by diminishing beta$_1$- receptor stimulation in the heart.** The response of the heart to stress and exercise is reduced. These properties qualify them to be used in the treatment of **angina pectoris** to reduce the oxygen consumption, and increase exercise tolerance of the patient. They are used to control **cardiac arrhythmias** as they block adrenergic stimulation of the cardiac pacemaker. Beta-blockers are also beneficial in the ***long-term treatment of hypertension.***

Classification

I. **Non-selective beta-blockers:** Propranolol, pindolol, sotalol, timolol, penbutolol.
II. **Cardioselective beta-blockers:** Metroprolol, atenolol, acebutolol, bevantolol, betaxolol, tolamolol.
III. **Beta-plus alpha-blocker:** Labetalolol.

Mode of Action

Propranolol is the *prototype* beta-blocker. Blockade of cardiac ($beta_1$) receptors ***reduces heart rate, myocardial contractility, and cardiac output. The atrioventricular conduction time is slowed, and the automaticity is suppressed.*** Consequent upon this the blood pressure falls. *Renin release is reduced* by about 60 percent.

Pharmacokinetics

Propranolol is almost completely absorbed from the gut, but is metabolized by the liver during its **first-pass** through the portal circulation, and only one-third reaches the systemic circulation. Propranolol is almost completely metabolized before excretion in urine.

Therapeutic Uses

1. **Hypertension:** All beta-blockers are equally effective antihypertensives.
2. **Angina pectoris:** Propranolol may be used for the long-term management of patients with angina pectoris.
3. **Cardiac arrhythmias:** Beneficial effects have been observed in patients of **supraventricular arrhythimias, tachyarrhythimias due to thyrotoxicosis, persistent atrial extrasystoles** refractory to conventional treatment, **atrial flutter** and **fibrillation.**
4. **Myocardial infarction:** Propranolol and timolol are indicated in clinically stable patients who have survived the acute phase of MI.
5. **Pheochromocytoma:** After primary treatment with an alpha-blocker, propranolol may be useful as *adjunctive therapy* if the control of tachycardia becomes necessary before or during surgery.
6. **Idiopathic hypertrophic subaortic stenosis.**
7. **Migraine.**
8. **Hyperthyroidism:** Propranolol rapidly controls tachycardia, tremors and anxiety in patients of thyrotoxicosis.
9. **Parkinson's disease and essential tremor:** Propranolol combined with levodopa may benefit a patient of Parkinson's disease.
10. **Glaucoma:** Beta-blockers lower intraocular hypertension by decreasing the production of aqueous humour. **Timolol** is the best topical ophthalmic preparation available. Topically one drop of a 0.25 percent solution is instilled into the conjunctival sac twice daily.
11. **Anxiety:** Propranolol and other beta-blockers suppress objective signs of anxiety like ***diarrhoea, palpitation, tachycardia*** and ***tremor.*** There is increasing interest in the use of beta-blockers for **acute situational anxiety.** The lay press popularizes these drugs by using the term 'confidence drugs'.

Contraindications

Beta-blockers are contraindicated in *sinus bradycardia; congestive heart failure: cardiogenic shock; and hypersensitivity* to beta-blockers. Propranolol, timolol and pindolol are contraindicated in patients with **bronchial asthma.**

Adverse Reactions and Precautions

Gastrointestinal: Vomiting, diarrhoea and flatulence.

Cardiovascular: Marked bradycardia and hypotension specially on intravenous administration. Propranolol may precipitate **heart failure** in patients with inadequate cardiac reserve.

Propranolol may cause **cold extremities** and precipitate or aggravate **Raynaud's phenomenon** or **intermittent claudication.**

Respiratory: Propranolol induces bronchoconstriction and may provoke asthmatic attacks.

Metabolic: Propranolol may mask some hypoglycaemic symptoms like tachycardia in patients on insulin therapy.

Neurologic: Fatigue and lethargy are common central side effects. **Vivid dream** or **nightmares,** with or without insomnia occur frequently. **Depression** and **memory loss** are not uncommon.

INDIVIDUAL BETA-BLOCKERS

1. **Propranolol:** It is the most commonly used non-selective blocker. Its indications include *hypertension, cardiac arrhythimias; myocardial infarction, hypertrophic subaortic stenosis, pheochromocytoma, migraine, and angina pectoris*. Propranolol is given in doses of 40 mg bid upto 480 mg/day.
2. **Timolol:** It is useful for *chronic wide angle glaucoma and aphakic glaucoma*. It can be used as an antihypertensive agent in a dose of 10-40 mg/day in 2 divided doses.
3. **Metoprolol:** It is a ***selective beta$_1$-receptor*** blocker devoid of ISA. Because of its relative **cardioselectivity,** metoprolol may be preferred to a nonselective agent in asthmatics. It is given in a dose of 50-200 mg twice daily.
4. **Atenolol:** The antianginal effect of this long-acting (half-life 6 hours) beta-blocker appears to be comparable to that of propranolol. It is a selective *beta$_1$- antagonist*. It is given in a dose of 50-200 mg once daily.
5. **Labetalol:** This agent combines selective postsynaptic alpha$_1$-adrenergic blocking, and non-selective beta-adrenergic blocking activity. ***Both alpha- and beta-blocking action of labetalol contribute to a decrease in blood pressure in hypertensives.*** It is given in a dose of 100 mg bid.

Propranolol is the most extensively used beta-blocker. It is used in **angina pectoris, essential hypertension, cardiac arrhythmias, thyrotoxicosis** and **anxiety.**

3.6 GANGLION BLOCKING AGENTS

Drugs which *inhibit* or *block* the nerve impulse transmission across the synapses in autonomic ganglia are known as **ganglion blocking agents.** These agents block transmission across both **sympathetic** and **parasympathetic ganglia,** i.e., they are ***non-selective*** in their action.

Mode of Action

Transmission across the ganglia is **cholinergic** in nature, and the **nicotinic receptors** are involved. Suppression or blockade of ganglionic transmission by drugs may be induced: (i) by the **occupation of nicotinic cholinoceptors on the postsynaptic membrane** which does not permit the released ACh to occupy these receptors and cause a depolarization, i.e., such drugs act by *competition* with ACh and are called **non-depolarizing ganglion blockers,** and (ii) by causing **persistent depolarization** of the post-synaptic membrane, and thereby rendering it inexcitable. Such drugs are called **depolarizing ganglion blockers** and they cause an initial facilitation of transmission followed by paralysis.

CLASSIFICATION

I. **Non-depolarizing blocking agents**
   - Trimetaphan.
   - Mecamylamine.

II. **Persistent depolarizing blocking agents**
   - Nicotine.

NON-DEPOLARIZING BLOCKING AGENTS

The autonomic ganglion blockers today are of ***historical interest*** and have a small but not insignificant place in therapeutics.

All ganglion blocking agents essentially produce the same qualitative effects, since they block both sympathetic and parasympathetic ganglia.

Trimetaphan Camsylate

Trimetaphan is a very short-acting ganglion blocker. It is used to produce **'controlled hypotension'** during surgical procedures specially in vascular and neurosurgery to provide a **'bloodless field'** for the operation.

Trimetaphan is administered in a dose of 50 mg to 1 g as an intravenous infusion (1 mg/ml). The infusion may continue upto 2 hours, and on stoppage the blood pressure returns to normal in about 5 minutes.

Mecamylamine Hydrocholoride

Mecamylamine was the first **non-quaternary** ganglion blocker to be used clinically in the treatment of **moderate to severe hypertension. Tolerance** to the drug develops on prolonged use.

PERSISTENT DEPOLARIZING BLOCKING AGENTS

Autonomic Ganglion Stimulants

Nicotine

Nicotine is the colourless, volatile and highly toxic **liquid alkaloid** obtained from the leaves of the tobacco plant ***Nicotiana tabacum,*** and acquires a brown colour on standing. It has no therapeutic use, but is of considerable interest because of its wide use in **tobacco smoking** and **tobacco chewing.**

Mode of Action

Nicotine is a **persistent depolarizing ganglion blocker,** as initially it behaves like a **partial agonist** at the ganglia producing depolarization, and later due to **prolonged depolarization** it blocks the ganglia. Thus it has a 'dual action'. Nicotine first stimulates and then depresses the autonomic ganglia, adrenal medulla, neuromuscular junction, and the central nervous system.

Pharmacological Actions

Central nervous system: Small doses of nicotine have a stimulating effect on the CNS, and larger doses depress it. The **conditioned reflexes** are first inhibited, and later completely lost. **Tremors** are a characteristic effect in man, which are due to both central and direct stimulation of the skeletal muscle.

Cardiovascular system: The action on circulation is the result of divergent actions of the drug on the ***vasomotor*** and ***vagal centres*** in the medulla, the **sympathetic** and **parasympathetic** ganglia, the **adrenal medulla** and the **chemoreceptors of the carotid sinus,** and aortic body. The electrocardiogram (ECG) may show a **depression or inversion of the T wave.**

Smooth muscles: On the gastrointestinal tract nicotine induces **powerful contractions of the stomach, which extend to the intestinal tract exhibiting a marked increase in the tone and peristalsis.**

Fate of Nicotine

Nicotine ingested or inhaled by man is partially degraded in the body mainly in the liver. The remainder is excreted in the urine unchanged.

Tolerance to Nicotine

Tolerance to nicotine develops fairly rapidly. The excitation, salivation, nausea and the burning sensation of the buccal mucosa in the uninitiated individual (non-smoker) diminish on repeated use of tobacco. ***Non-smokers*** are nauseated by 1 to 2 mg of nicotine administered orally, whereas smokers may tolerate upto 8 mg of the alkaloid. **Smokers** usually absorb about 0.3 to 0.6 mg of nicotine per cigarette.

NICOTINE AND TOBACCO SMOKING

Tobacco through the ages has been **snuffed, chewed** and **placed under the lips,** but the most popular route of intake is by **smoking.** The pleasureable qualities of tobacco consumption are usually ascribed to the soothing effect exerted by nicotine on the CNS. This leads to the tobacco habit. **Physical dependence does not develop.** About 90 percent nicotine is absorbed from the smoke inhaled into the lungs, whereas, only 10 to 25 percent is absorbed if the smoke is merely taken in the mouth and expelled. Numerous other compounds have also been isolated from tobacco smoke. Some of these are polycyclic hydrocarbons known as **'tars'** and are responsible for the greater incidence of **lung cancer** among smokers. In addition to **lung cancer, respiratory, cardiovascular** and **gastrointestinal diseases** have been related to cigarette smoking.

The use of tobacco may lead to **palpitation, extrasystoles,** and **paroxysmal auricular tachycardia**. It induces peripheral vasoconstriction evidenced by an **increase** in the **systolic** and **diastolic blood pressures. Emphysema and bronchitis** are six times more prevalent in smokers than in non-smokers. ***Anginal attacks*** may be provoked by tobacco. **Complete blindness** in one or both eyes (**tobacco amblyopia**) may develop.

Cigarette smoking is **contraindicated** in hypertension, angina pectoris, postcoronary conditions, Raynaud's disease, Buerger's disease, intermittent claudication, and other vasospastic conditions, atherosclerosis, peptic ulcer, bronchial coughs, emphysema and lung cancer.

Tobacco Smoking

According to WHO estimates India has nearly 12 crore smokers. Out of them 70% desire to quit smoking, but only 30% actually try each year, and only 3% to 5% succeed in quitting.

Nicotine Replacement Therapy (NRT) combined with **motivational therapy** is employed for quitting the cigarette smoking habit. Two agents have been developed for this purpose: (i) **Bupropion HCl** which is an antidepressant. It is used for nicotine replacement therapy in a dose of 150 mg OD orally for 6 days, then 150 mg bid for 7- 9 weeks, and (ii) **Varenincline** which activates the *nicotine receptor*, fooling the smoker whose craving is satisfied. With the pills the quit rate is around 50%, and it is 7% to 10% with the "patch" or"gum".

3.7 SKELETAL MUSCLE RELAXANTS

There are **three** varieties of clinically useful skeletal muscle relaxants: (i) those that act peripherally at the neuromuscular junction termed as **neuromuscular blocking agents;** (ii) those that act in the brain and spinal cord termed as **centrally acting muscle relaxants;** and (iii) the **directly acting muscle relaxant** dantrolene sodium.

NEUROMUSCULAR TRANSMISSION

Transmission of impulses at the neuromuscular junction is mediated by **acetylcholine (ACh),** which is released from the nerve terminals where it is stored in the presynaptic vesicles (**Fig. 3.6**).

The ***sequence of events*** during neuromuscular transmission may be summarized as under:

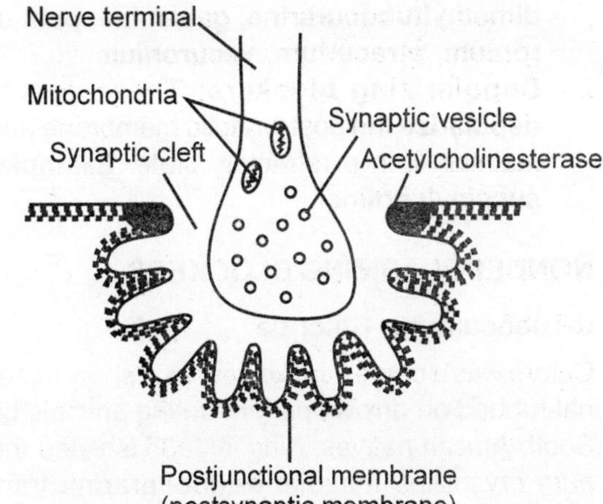

Fig. 3.6 : *The skeletal neuromuscular junction (diagrammatic).*

1. Arrival of nerve action potential in the nerve terminal.
2. Release of ACh into the synaptic cleft, from the synaptic vesicles by **exocytosis.**
3. Diffusion of ACh across the synaptic cleft, and its association with the **nicotinic cholinoceptors.**
4. Depolarization of the motor end plate to give the **end plate potential** (epp).
5. The epp crosses the **threshold potential** and the **action potential** is triggered to the muscle cell (propagated muscle potential).
6. Ca^{++} release from the intracellular sites causes shortening of myofibrils and development of muscle tension.
7. Dissociation of ACh: Receptor complex, followed by hydrolysis of ACh by AChE.
8. Transport of choline back into the nerve terminal.
9. Resynthesis of ACh.
10. Storage of ACh in synaptic vesicles.

CLASSIFICATION OF NEUROMUSCULAR BLOCKING AGENTS

1. **Nondepolarizing blockers:** These agents competitively block the receptor sites, and ACh fails to reach the nicotinic cholinoceptor. **Examples** include **d-tubocurarine,**

dimethyltubocurarine, gallamine, pancuronium, atracurium, vecuronium.

2. **Depolarizing blockers:** These agents **depolarize** the postsynaptic membrane and maintain it in a refractory state. **Example: succinylcholine.**

NONDEPOLARIZING BLOCKERS

d-Tubocurarine Chloride

Curare was a crude, tar-like, resinous sticky material rubbed on arrow tips for hunting animals by South African natives. King in 1935 isolated the pure crystalline material **d-tubocurarine** from ***Chondrodendron tomentosum***. Synthetic tubocurarine is also available.

Mode of Action

When d-tubocurarine is injected intravenously it is distributed throughout the extracellular body fluid, but does not cross the blood-brain barrier. A small part combines locally and **reversibly** with the **nicotinic cholinoceptors** on the surface of the skeletal muscle fibres in the region of the end plate.

The **tubocurarine: receptor complex** formed, keeps ACh away from the nicotinic cholinoceptors, and the end plate potential fails to develop.

Actions of d-tubocurarine: In man, tubocurarine, causes a **flaccid paralysis** of all skeletal muscles. The extraocular muscles are affected **first**, followed by those of the face, limbs, and trunk then the intercostal muscles and **finally** the diaphragm is paralysed. **The use of tubocurarine therefore almost always requires some ventilatory assistance.**

Therapeutic uses: Tubocurarine is used with **general anaesthesia** to produce muscle relaxation during surgical procedures; to reduce the severity of muscle spasm in severe **tetanus**; and to facilitate **controlled ventilation.**

Toxicity: A **fall in blood pressure** with a slight increase in heart rate may occur. Rarely it may induce **bronchospasm** due to histamine release. Overdosage causes **respiratory failure** by paralyzing the intercostal muscles and the diaphragm. Occasionally **postoperative apnoea** resistant to neostigmine may occur.

Dose: Average dose is 6 to 9 mg intravenously.

Dimethyltubocurarine Iodide

This is a **semisynthetic** derivative of tubocurarine and is about **twice as potent** as tubocurarine, but has a **shorter duration of action.** Its ***average dose*** is 2 mg intravenously.

Gallamine Triethiodide

Gallamine is a **synthetic** agent. Its mode of action is similar to tubocurarine. Gallamine has a shorter duration of action and lesser potency than tubocurarine. Its ***average dose*** is 80 mg intravenously.

Pancuronium Bromide

Pancuronium is approximately **5 times as potent** as tubocurarine, although the mechanism of neuromuscular blockade is the same. **Dose** is 4 to 6 mg intravenously.

Atracurium

Atracurium functions as a **competitive antagonist** with ACh at the cholinergic receptor sites on the motor end plate. Haemodynamic changes seldom occur.

An initial dose of 0.4 mg/kg produces neuromuscular blockade within 2 to 5 minutes. **Adverse reactions** include skin rash, dyspnoea, bronchospasm, laryngospasm, hypotension, and prolonged muscle relaxation.

Vecuronium

Vecuronium is another nondepolarzing neuromuscular blocker. An initial dose of 0.08 to 0.1 mg/kg given as an IV bolus produces neuromuscular blockade within 3 to 5 minutes. **Adverse reactions** include excessive muscle weakness, decreased respiratory reserve and apnoea.

Antagonists of Nondepolarizing Blockers

The **anticholinesterases** are useful in combating

the toxic effects of nondepolarzing blockers. They exert a **decurarizing effect** mainly by inhibiting the enzyme acetylcholinesterase at the motor end plate. The compounds which may be used (SC or IM or IV) are **neostigmine methylsulphate** 1 to 3 mg or **pyridostigmine** 5 to 15 mg with *atropine* 1 mg to antagonize the muscarinic action. **Artificial respiration,** preferably with oxygen under pressure should be carried out.

DEPOLARIZING BLOCKERS

These drugs cause a **persistent depolarization** of the neuromuscular junction, i.e., they have the same effect as the natural neurotransmitter ACh but of a longer duration. **This type of neuromuscular block is not antagonized by anticholinesterases.**

Succinylcholine Chloride

Succinylcholine has a rapid onset (1 minute) and short duration of action (5 minutes), because it is rapidly hydrolysed by the **plasma cholinesterase** (pseudocholinesterase). Prolonged paralysis (**succinylcholine apnoea**) does not occur unless the plasma cholinesterase level is low or the individual has an *atypical plasma cholinesterase.*

Therapeutic uses: Succinylcholine is used primarily as an **ultrashort-acting** muscle relaxant. It is used for brief procedures like **endotracheal intubation**, relief of **laryngospasm, endoscopy**, **orthopaedic manipulations** and **electroconvulsive therapy.**

Toxicity: The initial stimulation of muscle fibres leads to **muscle fasciculations,** which may cause considerable **soreness of the muscles**. Severe **ventricular arrhythmias** and **cardiac arrest** have followed succinylcholine administration. Succinylcholine may precipitate **malignant hyperthermia** in genetically predisposed patients.

Dose: Average initial dose is 30 mg intravenously. For continuous infusion the average rate is 2.5 mg/minute.

Antagonists of Depolarizing Blockers

There are no clinically effective antagonists for the depolarizers. The safest treatment is **controlled ventilation** until the block reverses spontaneously.

CENTRALLY ACTING MUSCLE RELAXANTS

These centrally acting muscle relaxants act on higher centres, and are commonly employed as **antianxiety agents.**

Muscle spasm often results from injury to peripheral musculoskeletal system structures, usually associated with pain. **Muscle spasticity** is the result of damage to the neurones in the CNS rather than in the peripheral structures. The resulting hypertonicity is permanent and can lead to crippling **contractures.**

Therapeutic Uses

The dosage and therapeutic uses of some commonly employed centrally acting muscle relaxants are summarized in **Table 3.3.**

Table 3.3: *Some commonly used centrally acting muscle relaxants*

Compound	*Usual single oral dose (mg)*
Diazepam	2-10
Methocarbamol	500-2000
Carisoprodol	250-350
Chlordiazepoxide	25-50
Chlorzoxazone	250-750
Baclofen	5-20

The available neurospasmolytic agents are used in two clinical conditions: (i) **Musculo-skeletal disorders,** e.g., muscle strains and sprains, whiplash injuries of the cervical spine processes, herniated disc, low backache, dislocations and fractures, arthritis, fibrositis, bursitis and neuritis; and (ii) **Neurological disorders,** e.g., cerebral palsy, multiple sclerosis, poliomyelitis, hemiplegia, quadriplegia, Parkinson's disease, and strychnine poisoning.

DIRECTLY ACTING MUSCLE RELAXANT

Dantrolene Sodium

Dantrolene is a hydantoin derivative that acts **directly** on the contractile mechanism of the voluntary muscle. It acts by ***interfering with the release of calcium***. Dantrolene facilitates the effects of GABA, which results in reduced efferent spinal motor neurone activity, and depressed brainstem reticular function.

Therapeutic uses: Dantrolene has been used in patients with strokes, multiple sclerosis, cerebral palsy, spinal cord injury, postencephalitic athetosis and dystonia.

Toxicity: The common adverse effects are weakness and diarrhoea. Hepatic dysfunction and phototoxicity may also occur. Rarely insomnia, nervousness, skin rashes, visual disturbances, and psychotic reactions may occur.

Dose: Dantrolene sodium is initially administered in a dose of 25 mg twice daily by mouth. Prolonged therapy is not desirable.

To conclude, the use of neuromuscular blocking agents is largely limited to anaesthesia. The centrally acting muscle relaxants have clinical usefulness in some musculeskeletal, and neurological spastic disorders. The directly acting agent *Dantrolene*, offers a new approach to the treatment of spasticity.

3.8 LOCAL ANAESTHETICS

Local anaesthetics may be **defined** as drugs which reversibly block nerve conduction beyond the point of application when applied locally in an appropriate concentration.

CLASSIFICATION

According to their **clinical usage**, the local anaesthetics are classified into the following types:

1. **Topical anaesthetics:** benzocaine, butacaine, butyl aminobenzoate, cocaine, benoxinate. *Others* are dibucaine, lidocaine and tetracaine.
2. **Infiltration and block anaesthetics:** procaine, chloroprocaine, hexylcaine, lidocaine. *Others* are bupivacaine, mepivacaine, piperocaine, prilocaine and tetracaine.
3. **Spinal anaesthetics:** tetracaine. *Others* are procaine, dibucaine, lidocaine, mepivacaine and piperocaine.
4. **Epidural and caudal anaesthetics:** lidocaine, prilocaine, and mepivacaine.

CLINICAL USES AND TECHNIQUES OF ADMINISTRATION

1. **Topical anaesthesia:** In this the local anaesthetic is applied in the form of a ***solution***, ***ointment***, ***cream*** or ***powder*** directly to the site which is to be anaesthetized.
2. **Infiltration and block anaesthesia:** It is produced by injecting the agent throughout the area to be rendered insensitive. This form of anaesthesia is used for minor operations, e.g., *drainage of a carbuncle or the excision of a small superficial cyst.*
   Two types of block anaesthesia are usually applied:
   (i) **Field block:** In this the anaesthetic agent is not injected in the area to be dissected, but into the surrounding area. Field blocks are applied to the **scalp** and **anterior abdominal wall,** and (ii) **Nerve block** in which the local anaesthetic is deposited close to the mixed nerve, e.g., radial, ulnar, pudendal, or a cord of the brachial plexus and many others.
3. **Spinal anaesthesia:** In spinal anaesthesia the solution is injected into the **subarachnoid space,** so that it reaches the roots of the spinal nerves and dorsal root ganglia (**Fig. 3.7**). The site of injection is chosen to block the roots of those nerves which supply the site of operation.
4. **Epidural and caudal anaesthesia:** The point of the needle rests in the epidural space (**Fig. 3.7**) which is not fluid filled, and extends from the foramen magnum to the sacral hiatus.

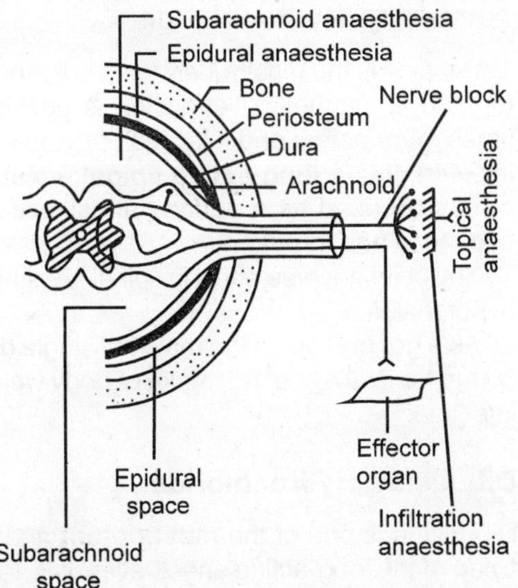

Fig. 3.7 : *Sites of application of local anaesthetics*

Caudal anaesthesia is a simple variation of epidural anaesthesia. Anaesthesia of the most caudal segments only can be achieved, making the method **suitable for obstetric analgesia.** Optimal caudal anaesthesia almost completely **relieves labour pains.**

ABSORPTION AND METABOLISM

The rate of absorption from the sites of injection depends upon the **vascularity** and blood flow of the region. Metabolism of the local anaesthetics does not take place at the site of application but in the **plasma** or **liver.**

MODE OF ACTION

The local anesthetics in current use consist of an aromatic **lipophilic** group, connected by an intermediate carbon chain to the **hydrophilic** amino group. The linkage between the intermediate group and the aromatic group may be an amide (lignocaine) or an ester (procaine).

The principal site of action of the local anaesthetics is the outer part of cell membrane. They reduce the membrane permeability changes to Na^+ and K^+, which occur in response to an excitatory stimulus, as they have a **membrane stabilizing effect.**

PHARMACOLOGICAL ACTIONS

Local anaesthetics largely exert their effect on a restricted area. These local effects are **loss of pain, temperature, and touch, vasodilatation, and loss of motor power.** In addition, they exert effects on the CNS, and the cardiovascular system.

Central Nervous System

All local anaesthetics, under certain conditions have CNS stimulating effects. High doses may cause convulsions and respiratory depression.

Cardiovascular System

During the phase of CNS stimulation the blood pressure may be elevated. But later during the phase of CNS depression profound and dangerous hypotension may occur. They have a **direct depressant action** on the heart, and also cause a **direct peripheral vasodilatation.**

TOXICITY OF LOCAL ANAESTHETICS

Transient or persistent CNS stimulation followed by CNS and cardiovascular depression may occur. Very profound CNS stimulation may lead to ***convulsions***, which may be treated with **diazepam** intravenously. Rarely systemic allergic reactions may occur, and **topical sensitization** may lead to dermatitis on the fingers of dentists who repeatedly come in contact with the drug.

The sequelae of spinal anaesthesia are **hypotension** due to blockade of sympathetic vasoconstrictor fibres. Trauma of lumbar puncture may cause a **transient headache.**

COMMON LOCAL ANAESTHETIC AGENTS

Cocaine Hydrochloride

This alkaloid obtained from the coca shrub was the first clinically important local anesthetic. The use of cocaine is restricted to **topical anesthesia** of the eye, nose and throat, and in bronchoscopy. Onset of action is rapid (1 minute), and the duration upto 2 hours. Dropped into the eye it produces prompt surface anesthesia, vasoconstriction and mydriasis.

Adverse effects are mydriasis, dryness and damage to the cornea. On systemic absorption it can lead to hypertension, tachycardia, tremors and convulsive seizures. It causes **psychological** and possibly **physical dependence** on repeated use. For topical application it is used as a 5 to 10 percent solution.

Procaine Hydrochloride

Procaine is rapidly effective when injected, but is not effective as a topical anesthetic. Its duration of action is relatively short (1 hour), but it can be lengthened by adding adrenaline to the solution. It is used for **peripheral** and central **nerve blocks.** It was the preferred local anesthetic for injection for many years, but now it has been replaced by lidocaine for *infiltration, nerve block,* and *subarachnoid anesthesia.* It is rapidly hydrolysed by plasma cholinesterase and also by the liver.

Solutions of 1 to 2 percent are employed for central block procedures. The total dose for spinal anaesthesia is 50 to 200 mg intrathecally.

Lidocaine Hydrochloride

This amide is one of the most widely used local anesthetics for **infiltration, regional, nerve block, epidural and subarachnoid anaesthesia**. It also is commonly used for topical anesthesia. It is more potent than procaine.

Adverse reactions include stimulation or depression of the CNS. There may be a bradycardia and hypotension. Allergic reactions may occur.

Usually a 1 to 2 percent solution is employed for nerve blocks. For **spinal anesthesia** a 5 percent hyperbaric solution is used. It may be applied topically as a 2 percent ointment. Also available as suppositories (100 mg) for use prior to proctoscopic and sigmoidoscopic examination.

Tetracaine Hydrochloride

Tetracaine is the most widely used subarachnoid (spinal) anaesthetic. Tetracaine is possibly 10 times more potent and toxic than procaine when injected. It is a **long-acting spinal anesthetic.** It may be used as a surface anesthetic in the eye, nose and throat.

The chief adverse effect in spinal anesthesia is hypotension.

As a general guide the maximal single dose is 50 mg topically, and 1.5 mg/kg of body weight by injection.

Dibucaine Hydrochloride

Dibucaine is one of the **most potent** and **most toxic** of the long-acting anesthetics. It is 15 to 20 times more potent, and 15 times more toxic than procaine when injected. The onset of action is slow (upto 15 minutes) and the duration of spinal anesthesia is 3 to 4 hours and can be prolonged upto 6 hours by the addition of **adrenaline.**

Mepivacaine Hydrochloride

This agent is chemically and pharmacologically related to lidocaine and is indicated for **infiltration, nerve block** and **epidural anesthesia**. The maximal single dose is 7 mg/kg of body weight, or 400 mg total, whichever is less.

Bupivacaine Hydrochloride

This agent is chemically related to mepivacaine and is used for **infiltration, nerve block and epidural anaesthesia**. It is particularly useful when administered by continuous epidural technique to **relieve pain of labour**. The maximal single dose should not exceed 200mg without adrenaline, and 250 mg with adrenaline.

CLINICAL PROPERTIES OF LOCAL ANESTHETICS

The **latency** of a local anesthetic is defined as the time required for the onset of analgesia/anaesthesia after its administration. They fall into the following categories:

Fast-acting: lidocaine, mepivacaine
Intermediate-acting: procaine, bupivacaine
Slow-acting: tetracaine, dibucaine

Another factor to be considered while choosing a local anaesthetic agent is its **duration of anaesthetic action**, for which they are categorized as under:

Short duration (about 1 hour): procaine, chloroprocaine.

Intermediate duration (1-2 hour): lidocaine.

Long duration (2-3 hours): mepivacaine.

Very long duration (over 3 hours): Tetracaine, dibucaine, bupivacaine.

Oxygen, and vasopressor drugs with apparatus for resuscitation should be available at hand.

Drugs Acting on the Cardiovascular System

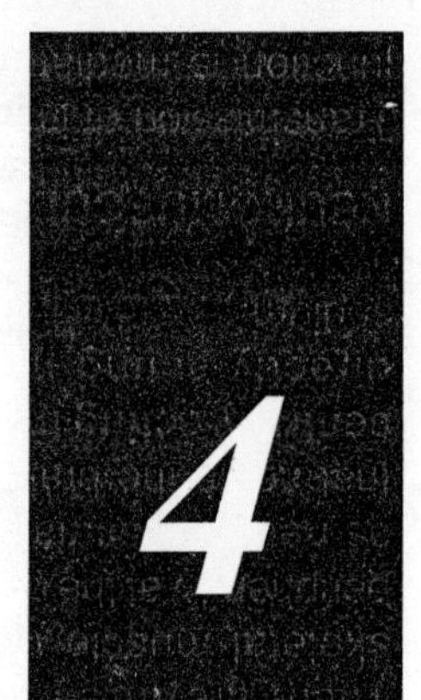

4.1 GENERAL CONSIDERATION

The human heart is a four-chambered muscular organ, which by means of its rhythmic contractions pumps blood through two circuits–a shorter **pulmonary** circulation, and a longer **systemic** circulation. A unidirectional flow of blood is ensured by valves within the heart, and in some of the veins.

THE CONDUCTING SYSTEM

The system for initiating and conducting the impulses is made up of: (i) the **sinoatrial**, or SA node, which sends impulses over certain atrial pathways to (ii) the **atrioventricular** or AV node, from which they are passed onto (iii) the AV bundle or **bundle of His**. This divides into (iv) **two bundle branches**, the right and left, which break up into a network of fine fibres, the **Purkinje fibres**, which make contact with the muscle fibres of the ventricles. This conduction system is responsible for the normal heart beat rhythm.

BLOOD SUPPLY TO THE HEART

The heart is supplied by two **coronary arteries**, which are the first branches of the aorta and arise just above the aortic valves. Coronary venous blood is collected into the **coronary sinus**, which opens into the right atrium.

NERVE SUPPLY TO THE HEART

The heart receives fibres from both the **parasympathetic** and **sympathetic** divisions of the autonomic nervous system. The parasympathetic fibres are carried in the **vagus** nerves and mainly supply the atria, the SA node, and the AV node. The sympathetic fibres are located in the **upper thoracic** and **inferior cervical ganglia**, and these fibres supply all parts of the heart.

AUTOMATICITY

The heart exhibits an **intrinsic rhythmicity** which is independent of external nervous or hormonal activity. The beat is initiated by the **pacemaker**. The cells exhibit a **spontaneous depolarization**. The action potentials are conducted across the atria via the internodal tracts to the AV node. The conduction at the AV node is slower to provide time for the atria to empty into the ventricles, before the ventricles contract.

There is another variety of automatic cells known as the **"latent pacemakers",** located in the AV node and Purkinje system. The rate of phase 4 **spontaneous depolarization** of latent pacemaker cells is much slower than the pacemaker cells.

CONDUCTIVITY

The SA node, or **pacemaker,** triggers the passive firing of the rest of the conducting system by means of its excitatory action potentials.

REFRACTORY PERIOD

The inability of the myocardium to be re-excited immediately after an action potential is called **refractoriness**, and the period during which the excitability is reduced is called the **refractory period**. The Effective Refractory Period (ERP) is followed by the **relative refractory period** (RRP), in which only an abnormally strong stimulus can initiate a propagated muscle potential. The RRP is followed by the **supernormal period** (SNP), in which even stimuli slightly smaller than the threshold stimuli elicit a propagated response. The interval between depolarization and complete recovery to normal resting excitability is the **full recovery time** (FRT).

REGULATION OF HEART RATE

Under resting conditions, the normal heart rate of an adult man is about 70 beats per minute. In well trained athletes the heart rate is about 50 beats per minute, which indicates a higher efficiency of the heart. Strenuous exercise, fever and emotional stress increase the heart rate. Basically the heart rate is maintained by means of nervous control mechanisms.

Cardiac arrhythmias arise as a result of abnormalities in either or both of the fundamental electrophysiological properties of the heart, i.e., **automaticity** and **conductivity.**

THE ELECTROCARDIOGRAM (ECG)

The electrocardiograph records the patterns of electrical activity generated in the heart. These patterns of electrical activity are shown by the electrocardiogram (ECG) recorded on a moving strip (25 mm/sec) of calibrated paper. Electrocardiography is an important **diagnostic** and **prognostic** tool for the detection and management of cardiac arrhythmias.

In the normal ECG three main components are seen. The P wave corresponds to **atrial depolarization**, the QRS complex indicates **ventricular depolarization,** and the T wave records **ventricular repolarization.** A small U wave of uncertain origin follows the T wave in some leads **(Fig. 4.1).**

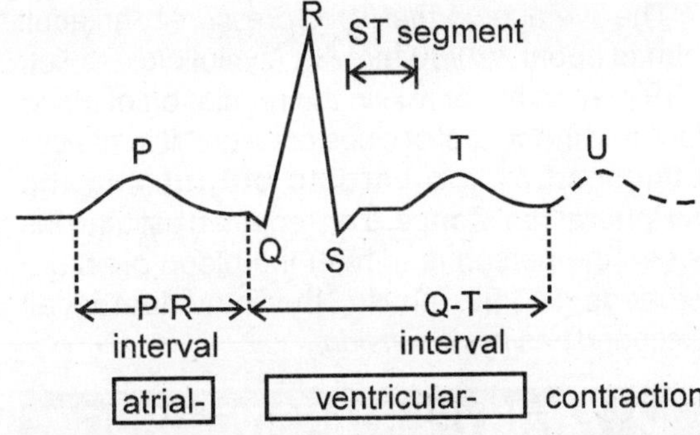

Fig. 4.1: *The normal electrocardiogram, its waves, complexes and intervals. The boxes at the bottom roughly indicate the timing of the atrial and ventricular muscle contraction.*

CARDIAC OUTPUT

The volume of blood pumped by the heart per minute is termed as the **cardiac output.** It depends upon the amount of blood expelled by each contraction or stroke of the left ventricle (stroke volume) and the heart rate.

Cardiac output = Stroke volume × Heart rate
(ml/min) (ml/contraction) (beats/min)

The normal cardiac output in man is 5.5 litres of blood per minute.

BLOOD PRESSURE

The **arterial blood pressure** fluctuates with each contraction of the heart. The maximum arterial pressure resulting from ventricular contraction or systole, is termed as **systolic blood pressure**. During the relaxation or diastolic phase of the cardiac cycle, the pressure falls, and a steep fall is avoided by the elastic recoil of the arteries. This lower blood pressure is called the **diastolic blood pressure.** The **pulse pressure** is the difference between the systolic and diastolic blood pressures. The **mean blood pressure** is not the arithmetic mean of the systolic and diastolic blood pressures. The value of mean blood pressure is given by the formula:

$$\text{Mean BP} = \text{diastolic pressure} + \frac{\text{pulse pressure}}{3}$$

The average *normal blood pressure* in an adult man is about 120/80 mm Hg (systolic/diastolic). ANS plays a major role in the regulation of blood flow, and the control of blood pressure. It is directly influenced by the **cardiac output** and the **peripheral resistance.** If on repeated estimations (when the person is at rest) the blood pressure exceeds 140/90 mmHg, the individual in all likelihood has *hypertension.*

4.2 ANTIHYPERTENSIVE DRUGS

The term 'hypertension' literally means an abnormally raised arterial blood pressure. There are many conditions which elevate arterial pressure, including primary renal disease, pheochromocytoma, hyperthyroidism, hyperaldosteronism, and coarctation of aorta, leading to **secondary** hypertension. In about 80 to 85 percent of patients of hypertension, no specific cause is evident, and such a condition is labelled as **primary** or **essential** hypertension.

It is agreed that if the values of systolic/diastolic BP on repeated determinations exceed 140/90 mm Hg, it is likely that the person is suffering from hypertension.

REGULATION OF BLOOD PRESSURE

In order to understand how antihypertensive drugs act, it would be useful to review the factors which regulate blood pressure (**Fig. 4.2**).

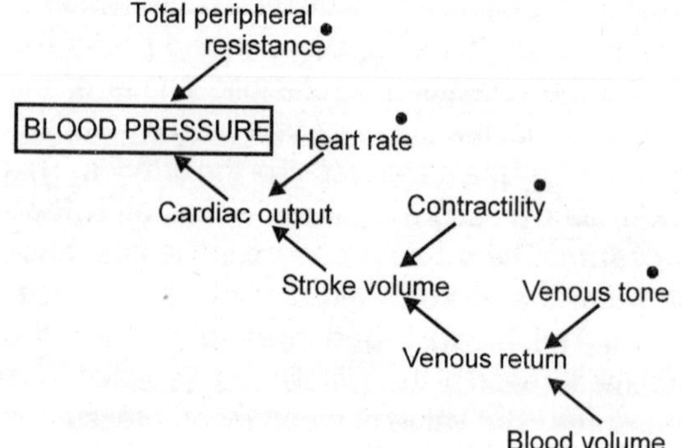

Fig. 4.2 : *Scheme for physiological maintenance of blood pressure (see text).*

Essential hypertension is a 'disease of regulation'. The four factors, namely **total peripheral resistance (TPR), heart rate, myocardial contractility,** and **venous return** are directly under the control of the sympathetic nervous system which is supposed to be defective in a hypertensive patient. There is strong evidence that in hypertensives, the **Renin: Angiotensin: Aldosterone system** is also faulty.

THE RENIN: ANGIOTENSIN: ALDOSTERONE SYSTEM

The demonstration that renal ischaemia leads to hypertension led to the discovery of a kidney enzyme, **renin**, which is derived from the granules of the juxtaglomerular apparatus. On renal ischaemia renin is released which acts on a substrate in the blood, called **angiotensinogen** which is converted into **angiotensin I**, a decapeptide. This is converted into **angiotensin II** or **angiotensin**, an octapeptide, by the converting enzymes located in the lungs. Angiotensin stimulates the adrenal cortex to release **aldosterone.**

Angiotensin is a **very potent vasopressor** agent, and is 40 times more potent than noradrenaline. It causes strong arteriolar constriction, and a rise in both **diastolic** and **systolic** blood pressures.

ANTIHYPERTENSIVE DRUGS

Hypertension according to the level of blood pressure may be categorized as under:

Pressure (mm Hg)	Category
Diastolic	
Less than 85	Normal
85-90	High normal
91-105	Mild
106-115	Moderate
Greater than 115	Severe
Systolic (with diastolic less than 90)	
Less than 140	Normal
140-160	Borderline systolic
Greater than 160	Isolated systolic

Borderline hypertension can be controlled by **weight reduction, salt restriction, cessation of smoking, and change in life style.** Now **isolated systolic hypertension** is also recognized as a disease entity and drug therapy must be seriously considered.

Classification

Drugs influence arterial blood pressure at **four** effector sites: **arterioles**, **veins**, **heart**, and the **kidneys.**

I. Diuretics
   i. **Thiazides** and related agents (hydrochlorothiazide, chlorthalidone etc.).
   ii. **Loop diuretics** (frusemide, bumetanide, ethacrynic acid).
   iii. **Potassium-sparing diuretics** (spironolactone, triamterene, amiloride).

II. Sympatholytic drugs
   i. **Centrally acting agents** (methyldopa, clonidine).
   ii. **Ganglion blocking agent** (trimethaphan).
   iii. **Adrenergic neurone blocking agent** (guanethidine).
   iv. **Beta-adrenoceptor blockers** (propranolol, metoprolol, atenolol etc.).
   v. **Alpha-adrenoceptor blockers** (prazosin, phenoxybenzamine).
   vi. **Alpha + beta blocker** (labetalol).

III. Vasodilators
   i. **Arterial** (hydralazine, minoxidil, diazoxide).
   ii. **Arterial and venous** (nitroprusside).

IV. Calcium channel blockers
Verapamil, nifedipine, nicardipine, felodipine, amlodipine.

V. Angiotensin converting enzyme inhibitors
Captopril, enalparil, lisinopril.

VI. Angiotensin II receptor blockers
Losartan, valsartan, telmisartan.

VII. Potassium channel opener
Pinacidil.

The **stepped-care approach** of treating hypertension consists of **sequential** prescribing steps, beginning with a **single** agent in increasing dosage, then adding or substituting other agents.

I. DIURETICS

Thiazide Diuretics

Chlorothiazide was the first potent orally effective diuretic. The hydrogenated compounds have a more favourable Na^+/K^+ excretion ratio. A few thiazides are listed in **Table 4.1.**

Table 4.1 : *The dosage and duration of action of some thiazides*

Thiazide	*Dose*	*Duration of action (hrs)*
Chlorothiazide	1000	6-12
Hydrochlorothiazide	25	6-12
Hydroflumethiazide	25	6-12
Bendroflumethiazide	2.5	24
Polythiazide	4	36
Chlorthalidone*	25	72

* Pthalimidine derivative

Mode of action: The thiazides initially induce a Na^+ and water loss, leading to a fall in plasma volume and extracellular fluid (ECF), which in turn **lowers** the cardiac output and BP. On prolonged thiazide treatment the plasma volume and ECF return to normal, but their hypotensive effect continues. This is due to the **reduced sensitivity** of the vascular bed to circulating **catecholamines** (CA) and **angiotensin.**

Adverse reactions: Certain degree of **hypokalemia** can occur, which can be avoided by combining K^+-sparing diuretics like **spironolactone** or **triamterene.** Other side effects are ***hyperglacaemia***, and ***hyperuricaemia.*** Rarely cholestatic jaundice, bone marrow depression, and postural hypotension may occur.

Loop Diuretics

The drugs in this class are **frusemide, bumetanide,** and the less used **ethacrynic acid**. Loop diuretics inhibit active tubular reabsorption of Na^+ and Cl^- in the thick ascending loop of Henle, and segments of the proximal and distal tubules. They have a strong **natriuretic** activity. Magnesium and calcium excretion is increased secondarily, and their chronic use can result in **hypomagnesaemia** and **hypocalcaemia**. Loop diuretics can cause **dangerous hypokalaemia.** In the treatment of hypertension usually frusemide is used in a dose of 40 mg once or twice daily.

Potassium-Sparing Diuretics

Spironolactone, triamterene and **amiloride** produce modest diuresis in comparison to the thiazides and loop diuretics. The important feature is that the loss of Na^+ is not accompanied by loss of K^+, and they exert a **potassium-sparing** effect. Potassium-sparing diuretics are employed with other potent diuretics to minimize K^+ loss.

II. SYMPATHOLYTIC DRUGS

Centrally Acting Agents

Methyldopa

Methyldopa (alpha-methyldopa) is recommended for the treatment of most types of hypertension.

Mode of action: In the central neurones it is converted to **alpha-methylnoradrenaline** by the enzyme dopa decarboxylase. Alpha-methylnoradrenaline is a potent **alpha$_2$-receptor agonist** located presynaptically. This leads to a **decreased sympathetic outflow** from the brain, which in turn causes peripheral vasodilation and reduction of TPR.

Adverse reactions: Marked drowsiness, depression, nightmares, fluid retention, enlargement of breast, drug fever, hepatic dysfunction, and ***haemolytic anaemia*** may occur.

Dose: Methyldopa initially 250 mg bid or tid can be increased upto 500 mg qid.

Clonidine

Clonidine is used primarily in the treatment of moderate hypertension.

Mode of action: Clonidine, is a central **alpha$_2$-adrenoceptor agonist** and inhibits the **outflow of sympathetic vasoconstrictor and cardioaccelerator** impulses from the brainstem.

Adverse reactions: Dry mouth and drowsiness are the most frequent side effects. Other adverse reactions observed are: **GI**–anorexia, nausea, vomiting, parotid pain, liver dysfunction, **CNS**–insomnia, nervousness, anxiety, depression, vivid dreams or nightmares; **Cardiovascular**–Raynaud's phenomenon, flushing, congestive heart failure; **Others**–weight gain, hyperglycaemia, gynaecomastia, impotence, muscle aches.

Dose: Clonidine HCl is available as 0.1 and 0.2 mg tablets. The usual oral dose initially is 0.1 mg bid. If necessary it may be increased to 0.6 mg tid or qid. **Clonidine transdermal patch** is available in three strengths. The patch is applied to the skin at 7-day intervals.

Ganglion Blocking Agents

The ganglion blockers have largely been replaced by the **adrenergic neurone blockers.**

Trimethaphan

Trimethaphan is a short-acting ganglion blocking agent. The blocking action is exerted at the postsynaptic cholinergic receptor in autonomic ganglia. This **competitive antagonism** is short-lived. It also has a direct relaxant effect on the vascular smooth muscle.

Trimethaphan is used to produce **controlled hypotension** during surgery to reduce bleeding. It is also used to control **hypertensive emergencies**, and for the treatment of **pulmonary oedema secondary to pulmonary hypertension.**

Trimethaphan is available as an injection solution (50 mg/ml) and is administered by IV infusion. A 1 mg/ml infusion solution is prepared by diluting 10 ml (500 mg) to 500 ml of 5 percent dextrose injection.

Adrenergic Neurone Blocking Agents

Guanethidine

Guanethidine is a potent drug for the relief of **severe hypertension** and has relatively lower incidence of side effects.

Mode of action: Guanethidine is taken up into the adrenergic neurone by the Na^+ transport mechanism. It depletes the NA stores exhibiting a **reserpine-like** effect; and finally it blocks the membrane amine pump impairing the re-uptake of NA.

Guanethidine sensitizes the adrenergic receptor, and thus is **absolutely contraindicated in pheochromocytoma.**

Adverse reactions: Diarrhoea, nasal congestion, postural hypotension, and parotid pain occur. In the male it may prevent ejaculation, without affecting erection. Due to sympathetic inhibition and hot environment the BP is likely to markedly fall usually after exercise.

Dose: 10 mg per day initially. Can be increased by 10 mg increments every 7 days. Maintenance dose 25-300 mg daily.

Beta-Blockers

Propranolol

All beta-blockers share the common property of being **competitive inhibitors** of catecholamines.

Mode of action: Beta-blockers exhibit an effect on the CNS, an **adrenergic neurone blocking effect**, **antirenin effect**, and the **resetting of the baroreceptors.** The cardiac output falls, and on prolonged use an initial rise in TPR is followed by a fall.

Side effects: Depression, lethargy, impotence, headache and vertigo have been observed. Propranolol may precipitate bronchial asthma. Left ventricular insufficiency, congestive heart failure, hypotension, hypoglycaemia, cardiomyopathy and thrombocytopenic purpura may occur.

Dose: Propranolol 10 mg tid or qid orally. Beta-blockers like **acebutolol**, **atenolol** and **metoprolol** are **relatively cardioselective** in therapeutic doses.

Alpha-Blockers

Prazosin

Prazosin acts by a **competitive postsynaptic alpha$_1$-adrenoceptor blockade.** It dilates both ***resistance*** (arterioles) and ***capacitance*** (veins) vessels. It is employed in the management of **essential hypertension**, and chronic **congestive heart failure.**

Adverse reactions: Severe postural hypotension can occur. Paroxysmal tachycardia and vivid dreams can also occur.

Dose: 2 mg tid for 4 to 6 weeks. Later, graded increments, but total dose not to exceed 20 mg.

Phenoxybenzamine

It is used for the control of **episodes of hypertension associated with pheochromocytoma.** It literally produces a '**chemical sympathectomy**'. The initial dose is 10 mg/day, increased by 10 mg every 4 days till the desired response is attained. **Adverse reactions** like orthostatic hypotension, nasal congestion, miosis, tachycardia and impaired ejaculation can occur.

Alpha + Beta Blocker

Labetalol

Labetalol has an alpha$_1$ blocking action, with a nonspecific beta$_1$ and beta$_2$ adrenoceptor blocking action. It lowers BP primarily by blocking alpha-receptors in the peripheral arterioles, reducing the TPR. *Labetalol lowers both systolic and diastolic pressures, without postural or exercise induced hypotension.*

Side effects: Nasal stuffiness, vivid dreams and epigastric pain may occur.

Dose: Labetalol 100 mg tid orally increasing upto 200 mg tid or qid after 1 or 2 weeks.

Vasodilators

Hydralazine

Hydralazine is a potent direct relaxant of vascular smooth muscle. It **reduces both systolic and diastolic BP**. It increases renal blood flow and is useful in hypertension with renal dysfunction. It is employed in cases of **mild to moderate hypertension**, and **toxaemia of pregnancy.**

Adverse reactions: Headache, palpitation nasal congestion, peripheral neuropathy and bone marrow suppression can occur.

Dose: Hydralazine 20 mg tid raising to 50-75 mg orally. In malignant hypertension upto 20 mg may be given slowly intravenously.

Minoxidil

Minoxidil dilates arteriolar resistance vessels with minimal effects on venous capacitance vessels. It **reduces calcium uptake** through the cell membrane thereby reducing arteriolar tone, and **lowering peripheral vascular resistance**. Reflex tachycardia, increased renin secretion, and salt and water retention occur.

Minoxidil is reserved for the treatment of **severe hypertension**, usually given with a diuretic and beta-blocker to minimize fluid retention and reflex tachycardia respectively. It is also used to treat **alopecia areata,** and **androgenic alopecia** (male pattern baldness) as a topical lotion or ointment.

Adverse reactions: The most commonly seen side effect is *hypertrichosis* (elongation and thickening of fine body hair). This begins in the facial region and later spreads to the back, arms, legs and scalp.

Dose: Minoxidil is available as 2.5 and 10 mg tablets. Initially 5 mg/day as a single dose increased step-wise upto 40 mg/day in divided doses (Maximum is 100 mg/day).

Diazoxide

It is a *non-diuretic thiazide*. On prolonged use it leads to diabetes mellitus. Although not permanent in nature. It is employed for **emergency reduction of BP** as a short-term therapy, not exceeding 2 to 3 days.

Mode of action: It acts directly on the arterioles, lowering the TPR. The heart rate and cardiac output is increased.

Adverse reactions: Salt and water retention, hypogammaglobulinaemia, hypotension, dizziness, hyperglacaemia and transient diabetes mellitus may occur.

Dose: Diazoxide 300 mg by rapid intravenous injection over 30 seconds with the patient in the supine position.

Sodium Nitroprusside

Sodium nitroprusside is a short-term hypotensive agent. It reduces TPR by a direct action on blood vessels and may be used in the treatment of **hypertensive crisis**. It may also be used for **controlled hypotension** during general anaesthesia.

Side effects: It may produce anorexia, nausea, vomiting, abdominal pain, apprehension, dizziness, disorientation, palpitation, retrosternal pain and muscle weakness. **Methaemoglobinaemia** and **hypothyroidism** may occur rarely.

Dose: Stock solution is prepared by dissolving 60 mg in 25 ml of isotonic saline. This 25 ml of the stock solution is added to 1000 ml of isotonic saline or 5 percent glucose solution. The infusion is started at a rate of 5 to 10 drops per minute, the BP being checked every 10 minutes or less.

Calcium Channel Blockers

Verapamil

Verapamil is a calcium channel blocker used in the chronic management of **angina pectoris**, and in the control of **supraventricular arrhythmias**. Verapamil is also useful in the control of **mild to moderate hypertension**. Verapamil relaxes vascular smooth muscle, thereby decreases peripheral vascular resistance.

Adverse reactions: Constipation occurs frequently, and other side effects include dizziness, nausea and oedema.

Dose: Verapamil is available as 40 and 80 mg tablets, and also as 240 mg **sustained release tablets** which are administered once daily.

Nifedipine 10 to 20 mg sublingually or orally has been recommended in **hypertensive emergencies** when close monitoring is not possible. The hypotensive effect is seen within 10 minutes, with a maximal effect in 30-40 minutes.

Amlodipine is a prototype second generation calcium channel blocker. *Amlodipine* and *felodipine* do not reduce myocardial contractility.

Amlodipine is used in the treatment of ***mild to moderate hypertension; chronic stable angina pectoris; or vasospastic angina (Prinzmetal's or variant).***

Dose: In hypertension or angina, initially 5 mg once daily, and adjusted to a maximum dose of 10 mg once daily. *Adverse reactions* include headache, oedema, fatigue, dizziness, nausea, flushing, palpitation, pruritus, muscle cramps, and gum hyperplasia.

Angiotensin Converting Enzyme Inhibitors

Captopril, Enalapril, Lisinopril

Angiotensin converting enzyme inhibitors are orally effective antihypertensives. Captopril is used for controlling severe and resistant forms of hypertension.

Mode of action: These drugs inhibit the angiotensin converting enzyme (ACE), which hydrolyses the inactive angiotensin I to the active angiotensin II. Thus, inhibition of ACE reduces the formation of angiotensin II, and decreases the angiotensin mediated secretion of aldosterone from the adrenal cortex. As a result ***peripheral vascular resistance is lowered*** and salt and water retention is reduced.

Adverse reactions: Common side effects with captopril are loss of taste sensation, rash, and pruritus. Side effects with enalapril are headache, dizziness and fatigue, with lisinopril are GI upset, lightheadedness and fatigue.

Other adverse reactions noted occasionally with all the three drugs include: CNS–insomnia, paresthesias; GI-nausea, vomiting, diarrhoea, altered taste sensation (dysgeusia): CVS – chest pain, palpitation, hypotension. Others–cough, rash, angioedema, bone marrow depression, impotence, and muscle cramps.

Therapeutic uses: The ACE inhibitors can be used to treat **all degrees of hypertension** either alone or in combination with other antihypertensives. These agents are also used as adjuncts in the treatment of **refractory congestive heart failure** with digoxin and a diuretic.

Dose: Captopril–The initial dosage for mild to moderate hypertension is 12.5 to 25 mg bid or tid.

Enalapril–The initial dose is 5 mg once daily. The usual dose range is 10 to 40 mg once or twice daily.

Lisinopril–Initially, 10-20 mg once daily. Usual dosage range is 20-40 mg daily.

Angiotensin II Receptor Blockers

Angiotensin (AT) receptor subtypes–There are two AT receptor subtypes, the AT_1 receptor subtype is located predominantly in the vascular and myocardial tissue, brain, kidney and the adrenal glomerulosa which secretes aldosterone, and the AT_2 receptors are located in the adrenal medulla and possibly in the brain. In the management of hypertension AT_1 subtype selectivity is desirable.

Losartan is a blocker of the AT_1 receptor. Two of the adverse effects of ACE inhibitors (angioedema and cough) are not associated with angiotensin II receptor antagonists.

Dose: Initially 50 mg/day with the usual dose range of 25-100 mg/day.

Newer agents, **Valsartan** (80-160 mg/day) and **Telmisartan** (20-80 mg/day) are used in the treatment of *moderate hypertension, diabetic nephropathy,* and *heart failure.*

Potassium Channel Opener

Pinacidil

Pinacidil is a potent vasodilator and is the first antihypertensive drug classified as a *potassium channel opener.* Pinacidil acts at the level of the arteriolar (resistance) vessels, directly causing relaxation of the vascular smooth muscle.

Pinacidil appears to be a promising alternative agent for the treatment of ***moderate to severe hypertension.*** **Dose:** Adults, 12.5 to 25 mg bid. *Adverse reactions* are related to vasodilation, specially oedema, tachycardia, palpitation, T-wave abnormalities, headache, and flushing.

Miscellaneous Antihypertensive Agents

Phentolamine

Phentolamine is a nonselective alpha-adrenoceptor blocker, used by injection to control hypertensive episodes that occur in patients with **phenochromocytoma** during surgery for removal of the tumour.

Mecamylamine

Mecamylamine is a potent, orally effective ganglion-blocker which exhibits a considerable **orthostatic hypotensive effect**. Due to its many side effects, it is used only for control of **severe hypertension** in patients not responding to other antihypertensive drug combinations.

Indapamide

Indapamide decreases peripheral resistance in hypertensive subjects, and *reduces vascular reactivity to pressor agents like adrenaline, noradrenaline and angiotensin.* It is effective in a single daily dose of 2.5 mg in mild to moderate hypertension. As indapamide is an indoline thiazide derivative, in large doses it exerts diuretic activity. **Side effects** like epigastric pain and nausea have been reported. It is **contraindicated** in severe hepatic and renal insufficiency.

PHARMACOTHERAPY OF HYPERTENSION

The ultimate goal of therapy is to reduce BP to normotensive levels. Periodic blood urea nitrogen (BUN) estimations are a practical guide to therapy. The moment there is a tendency of the BUN to rise, therapy should be titrated afresh.

Mild hypertension may often be treated with one antihypertensive (monotherapy), but more severe hypertension usually requires two or more agents.

4.3 CARDIAC GLYCOSIDES

The term 'Cardiac glycosides' is used to describe a group of compounds of common basic chemical structure, which increase the work performance of the heart. They have a **cardiotonic action**, and this is most marked on the 'failing heart'.

Historically, the English physician and botanist, William Withering (1741-1799) brought this old vegetable drug into modern medicine.

CONGESTIVE HEART FAILURE (CHF)

Congestive heart failure is a gradually developing inability of the heart to pump sufficient blood to satisfy the needs of the body, i.e., it fails to function as an efficient pump. This results in an ***inadequate cardiac output*** causing ***breathlessness on exertion*** or ***even at rest, chronic venous congestion, salt and water retention (dependent oedema), fatigue, confusion*** and ***renal failure*** (underperfusion of tissues).

In the early stages of heart failure, the compensatory mechanisms are activated to maintain cardiac output. Ultimately in advanced congestive heart failure, the heart has no functional reserve, and the heart becomes ***decompensated*** and ***dilated.***

ACUTE PULMONARY OEDEMA

Acute pulmonary oedema occurs in the presence of underlying cardiovascular disease like ***acute myocardial infarction, cardiac arrhythmias, malignant hypertension, aortic valvular diseases, pulmonary embolism*** or ***acute fluid*** or ***salt overload.*** It is precipitated by an acute decrease in left ventricular output. The gas exchange in the lungs suffers, leading to ***marked breathlessness*** (orthopnoea).

AIMS OF THERAPY

There are *three* main aims of therapy:

i. **To reduce cardiac work:** The measures include rest from physical activity; if obese, restrict caloric intake; and restrict salt intake.
ii. **To decrease pulmonary congestion and peripheral oedema:** For urgent reduction in pulmonary congestion, the patient should be *propped up* in bed; administered 60 percent *oxygen* (6 litres/minute); and given IV *aminophylline* for its bronchodilator, vasodilator and positive inotropic effect; and given a *loop diuretic* like *frusemide* for its potent and prompt action.
iii. **To increase cardiac output:** The **cardiac glycosides** are employed to improve the efficiency of the failing heart. **Digoxin** is the prototype.

CARDIAC GLYCOSIDES

Source and Chemistry

Official digitalis is the dried leaf of the **purple foxglove plant** or ***Digitalis purpurea.*** Other plant sources of cardiac glycosides are the white foxglove or ***Digitalis lanata***, and ***Strophanthus kombe.***

Each glycoside represents the combination of an **aglycone** with one to four molecules of sugar. The pharmacological property resides in the aglycone. The aglycones can be released from the cardiac glycosides by ***hydrolysis***.

Pharmacological Actions

The main actions of all glycosides are similar and exerted on the heart. The differences are only in the *potency, onset* and *duration* of action. The primary action may be divided into *three* components: (i) **a positive inotropic effect** on the heart; (ii) **partial blockade of AV conduction;** and (iii) **reduction in the heart rate.** These glycosides cause these effects by their **direct** and **indirect** actions on the cardiac cells.

Effect on myocardial contraction: Digitalis by its direct actions increases the contractility of the myocardium (**positive inotropic effect**), and as a result the cardiac output in the failing heart is increased. The ***diastolic size of the heart is decreased.***

Effect on other myocardial properties: The effects of digitalis on myocardial *automaticity* and *excitability* depend on the dose, and the different parts of heart react differently.

i. **Decreased SA nodal rate:** The spontaneous discharge rate of the SA node is decreased (pulse rate slowed) by a **direct** and **indirect** action of the glycosides which is dose-dependent.
ii. **Slowed AV conduction:** Digitalis slows conduction through the AV node and the bundle of His. **The effective refractory period of the AV node Is prolonged, and the rate of conduction in the atrioventricular bundle is reduced**.
iii. **Increased ventricular contractility:** Digitalis exerts a definite direct effect. The **refractory period is shortened**, and the Purkinje cells show enhanced automaticity.

The effects of digitalis on the ECG are: There is a ***sagging of the ST-segment*** below the isoelectric line, the ***T-wave becomes smaller, disappears or may be inverted***, the ***P-R interval is prolonged*** (delayed atrioventricular conduction), and the **Q-T interval is shortened.**

Effects secondary to relief of CHF: When congestive heart failure is relieved certain secondary changes follow: (i) **diuresis** occurs due to the improved renal circulation; (ii) the **blood pressure returns towards normal**; (iii) the **tachycardia accompanying CHF declines**; (iv) the **venous pressure is reduced**; and (v) the **heart size decreases.**

Effect on Other Systems

Blood and vascular system: Digitalis has a direct constrictor action on the vascular smooth muscle.

Gastrointestinal system: Nausea and vomiting induced by digitalis are both central and reflex in origin. The emetic action is due to the **stimulation of the chemoreceptor trigger zone** in the medulla.

To **summarize,** the action of cardiac glycosides on the failing heart are: (i) direct stimulation of the myocardium and **increased contractility**, with a resultant **increase in cardiac output, reduction in heart size, improved cardiac efficiency,** and more work per ml of oxygen consumed; (ii) **depression of conduction;** (iii) **increased vagal activity** which decreases the auricular refractory period with conversion of flutter to fibrillation, and (iv) the **increased cardiac excitability** makes the heart more vulnerable to arrhythmias.

Pharmacokinetics

The clinically used preparations are (i) **Digoxin,** (ii) **Digitoxin,** (iii) **Lanatoside C** (Cedilanid), (iv) **Deslanoside** (Cedilanid-D), and (v) **Ouabain** (Strophanthin-G) obtained from *S. gratus*, the quickest acting IV glycoside.

Table 4.2 : *Comparison of the pharmacokinetics of digoxin and digitoxin*

Parameter	Digoxin	Digitoxin
Lipid solubility	Less	Greater
Intestinal absorption	40-80%	80-100%
Single dose	0.25 mg	0.10 mg
Plasma albumin binding	20-30%	More than 90%
Biotransformation	Limited	Hydroxylated in the liver
Kidney excretion	Glomerular filtration and tubular secretion	Filtration of unbound digitoxin, and passive tubular reabsorption
Drug in urine	90% as uncharged digoxin	10% as unchanged digitoxin
Half-life (t½)	1-2 days	5-9 days

Digoxin and **digitoxin** are the two preparations, generally satisfactory for all purposes. The pharmacokinetics of digoxin and digitoxin is detailed in **Table 4.2**.

Mode of Action

The evidence for the **inhibition of NA^+/K^+ ATPase enzyme** by cardiac glycosides is so strong that it has been postulated that this enzyme acts as a **receptor** for digitalis. Although not firmly established, the intracellular rise in Na^+ concentration allows more calcium (Ca^{++}) to enter the cell with each action potential. More of Ca^{++} available to the myofilaments is responsible for a more powerful muscle contraction.

Digitalis enhances excitation, contraction, and coupling by which chemical energy is converted to mechanical work on the depolarization of the membrane.

Therapeutic Uses

1. **Heart failure (left sided, right sided or combined) with sinus rhythm or atrial fibrillation.**
2. **Atrial fibrillation.**
3. **Atrial flutter.**
4. **Paroxysmal atrial tachycardia (PAT).**
5. **Prevention of paroxysmal atrial arrhythmias.**

Contraindications and Precautions

1. **Recent myocardial infarction.**
2. **Ventricular tachycardia.**
3. **Partial heart block.**
4. **Acute myocardial insufficiency.**
5. **Previous digitalis therapy.**
6. **Calcium administration.**
7. **Potassium depletion.**

Toxicity

1. **Gastrointestinal effects:** Anorexia, nausea and vomiting are usually the early signs.
2. **Neurological effects:** Headache, fatigue, insomnia and mental symptoms like confusion, delirium and convulsions may occur.
3. **Visual disturbances:** Yellow or green vision, white halos around objects, snow covered appearance of objects is reported by patients.
4. **Cardiac arrhythmias:** Digitalis overdose can simulate every pathological arrhythmia. The most common being ventricular ectopic beats.

Treatment of Digitalis Toxicity

1. **Withdrawal of the drug or reduction in the dose.**
2. **Administration of potassium:** To correct

hypokalaemia, potassium chloride about 2 g every 4 hourly to a total of 4 to 6 g daily may be given.

3. **Antiarrhythmic drugs: Phenytoin** and **lignocaine** are the preferred agents.
4. **Digoxin immune Fab-Ovine** (Digibind) contains antigen-binding fragments derived from antidigoxin antibodies produced in immunized sheep. Digoxin immune Fab is used to treat life-threatening digoxin toxicity.

Preparations, Dosage and Digitalization

The initial saturating process by larger doses of digitalis is designated as **'digitalization'.** After adequate digitalization the **'maintenance dose'** of the glycoside is administered daily, and the attempt is to maintain the patient in a **'compensated'** state with optimal cardiac efficiency. The available preparations and dosages are detailed in **Table 4.3.**

Methods of Digitalization

No fixed routine for either *rapid or slow* digitalization guarantees freedom from toxicity. Depending on the severity of CHF *slow* or *rapid* digitilization may be done.

Drug Interactions

Digitalis is a dangerous drug with a low therapeutic index. During its use it is likely to interact with certain drugs partially listed in **Table 4.4.**

To **summarize** the drug treatment of congestive heart failure consists of administration of **cardiac glycosides, diuretics** and **potassium supplementation** with other measures like dietary salt restriction and rest. **Oxygen inhalations** for hypoxaemic patients, and **intermittent positive pressure breathing** is beneficial. **Loop diuretics** are administered to relieve pulmonary congestion. **Rapid intravenous digitalization** of the patient is carried out cautiously.

Table 4.4: *Drug interactions with digitalis*

Drug (a)	*Drug (b)*	*Effect of (b) on (a)*
Digitalis	Thiazide diuretics	Toxicity increased
	Steroids	Toxicity increased
	Quinidine	Toxicity increased
	Calcium	Toxicity increased
	Sympathomimetic amines	Arrhythmias increased
	Propranolol	Arrhythmias decreased
	Potassium	Toxicity decreased
	Antacids, oral	Digoxin absorption decreased

Table 4.3: *Preparations and dosage of cardiac glycosides*

Glycoside	Dose		Preparations available
	Digitalizing	Maintenance (oral)	
Oral preparations			
Digoxin	1-1.5 mg	0.25-0.75 mg	Tablets 0.25 and 0.5 mg
Digitoxin	1.2-1.5 mg	0.1-0.2 mg	Tablets 0.05, 0.1, 0.15 and 0.2 mg
Lanatoside C	6.0 mg	1.0 mg	Tablets 0.5 mg
Parenteral preparations			
Digoxin	0.5-1.0 mg IV	0.25-0.75 mg	Injection IV 0.5 mg/2 ml ampoule
Digitoxin	1.2 mg IV	0.1-0.2 mg	InjectionIV 0.2 mg/ml, 1 ml and 2 ml ampoules
Deslanoside	1.2-1.8 mg (6-8 ml) IV	–	Inection IV 0.2 mg/ml 2 ml and 4 ml ampoules
Ouabain	0.5 mg IV	–	Injection IV 0.5 mg in 2 ml ampoules

INTRACTABLE HEART FAILURE

The ideal drug for management of CHF should: (i) **increase ventricular performance;** (ii) **decrease filling pressure;** and (iii) **increase cardiac output by decreasing afterload.** Cardiac glycosides accomplish the first two objectives, but not the last one.

Vasodilators and **positive inotropic agents** are used as alternative or additional drugs in the treatment of CHF.

Vasodilators

A large number of patients of CHF fail to respond to conventional therapy (digitalis glycosides and diuretics), in such cases use of vasodilators significantly improves haemodynamic performance:

1. **Arteriodilators:** Hydralazine, minoxidil, phentolamine, nifedipine, diltiazem.
2. **Venodilators:** Isosorbide dinitrate, nitroglycerin.
3. **Combined arterio-venodilators:** Captopril, enalapril, nitroprusside, prazosin.

Positive Inotropic Agents

Amrinone and Milrinone

Amrinone (Inocor) is the first of a new class of **positive inotropic agents** that are unlike the cardiac glycosides. It is a potent inotropic vasodilator. **Amrinone** and **milrinone**, its close structural analogue are **phosophodiesterase inhibitors**, an action which results in increased intracellular concentration of cyclic adenosine monophosphate (c-AMP) which facilitates the contraction of the myocardial muscle. These agents have been classified as **non-glycoside, non-catecholamine positive inotropic drugs.**

Glucagon, a polypeptide hormone produced by the alpha-cells of islets of Langerhans has a ***potent positive inotropic activity*** in addition to its hyperglycaemic action.

Dopamine and **dobutamine**, both potent inotropic agents, have also been used for the short-term management of intractable CHF. Both these drugs ***stimulate*** $\boldsymbol{beta_1}$***-receptors in the heart*** and increase the cardiac output.

4.4 ANTIARRHYTHMIC DRUGS

Cardiac arrhythmias are defined as disorders of **rate, rhythm, origin** or **conduction** of impulse within the heart.

The Genesis of Arrhythmias

Cardiac rhythm disturbances are the result of altered impulse generation (**automaticity**), altered impulse propagation (**conductivity**), or both factors acting together.

Automaticity Defect (Ectopic Impulse Generation)

Normally the sinoatrial (SA) node, the pacemaker has the highest degree of automaticity, and is responsible for normal sinus rhythm. When the SA node is suppressed as in some bradyarrhythmias, other specialized conduction tissue with automatic properties takes up the role of the pacemaker. Such a site is known as an **ectopic focus**, and the cells exhibit an increased tendency to depolarize during diastole.

Conductivity Defect (Altered Impulse Propagation)

Some arrhythmias may be attributed to a defective transmission of the cardiac action potential. Simple slowing in the rate or ventricular contraction follows **AV blockade** or **bundle branch block.**

Effects of Potassium

The level of extracellular potassium is of critical importance and regulates both ***automaticity*** and ***conductivity***. Normal cardiac rhythm is the result of minimal automaticity, and optimal conductivity.

Classification of Antiarrhythmics

Five drugs have been commonly employed in the management of arrhythmias, namely, **quinidine**, **procainamide**, **propranolol**, **lidocaine** and to a lesser extent **phenytoin.**

Based on their **primary mode of action** these drugs fall into four classes (I-IV).

Class I: This class is subdivided into three subclasses:

IA : **Quinidine, procainamide, disopyramide.**

IB : **Lignocaine, Phenytoin, Tocainide, Mexiletine.**

IC : **Flecainide, Encainide, Propafenone.**

Class II: Antisympathetics: Propranolol, acebutolol, metoprolol, atenolol, sotalol.

Class III: Amiodarone, bretylium, sotalol.

Class IV: Calcium channel blockers: Verapamil, diltiazam.

The above drugs are used to treat *tachyarrhythmias.* Agents used to treat *bradyarrhythmias* are:

i. **Sympathetic agonist:** Isoprenaline.
ii. **Parasympathetic antagonist:** Atropine.

Individual Drugs

Class IA

Quinidine

Quinidine is the dextro-rotatory isomer of quinine, obtained from the bark of the cinchona tree.

Pharmacological actions: Quinidine has direct actions on the cardiac cell membrane which alter the **automaticity, excitability, conduction velocity** and **effective refractory period**. In addition, quinidine has indirect atropine like (anticholinergic) effects. *Quinidine lengthens the effective refractory period.*

Mode of action: It abolishes ectopic pacemaker activity. The **conduction velocity is decreased, and the refractory period is prolonged.** The reduction in potassium efflux may be responsible for the increase in the duration of the action potential observed with quinidine.

Pharmacokinetics: Orally administered quinidine is readily absorbed into the blood where about 80 percent is bound to plasma proteins. Peak plasma concentrations are reached in 2 to 4 hours. It is largely *hydroxylated* in the liver and excreted through the kidneys. The half-life of the parent compound is between 5 to 7 hours.

Toxicity: The common toxic manifestations are diarrhoea, nausea and vomiting. **Cinchonism** may occur in a dose-related manner and consists of tinnitus, headache and blurring of vision. **Hypersensitivity** to quinidine occurs rarely. *Haematologic abnormalities* like thrombocytopenic purpura may occur.

Therapeutic uses: The major clinical uses of Quinidine are in the treatment of **atrial fibrillation, atrial flutter,** and **paroxysmal supraventricular tachycardia.**

Dosage

1. *Quinidine sulphate*: 200 to 300 mg orally 3 to 4 times daily.
2. *Quinidine hydrochloride*: 200 mg IV or IM injected slowly. Parenteral use of Quinidine is dangerous.

Procainamide Hydrochloride

Procainamide differs from the local anaesthetic procaine simply in the replacement of the ester linkage in the molecule by an amide linkage. This feature has made procainamide more stable in the body.

Pharmacological actions: The electrophysiologic properties, and antiarrhythmic actions of procainamide are ***similar*** to those of quinidine, except that procainamide has a definite direct depressant effect on the SA node.

Pharmacokinetics: Procainamide is well absorbed from the gastrointestinal tract, peak concentrations are reached in 1 to 2 hours. Normally between 45 and 60 percent is excreted unchanged via the kidney. The half-life is usually between 2 and 4 hours.

Toxicity: The toxic effects on the heart are similar to those of quinidine.

Therapeutic uses: The usefulness of procainamide parallels that of quinidine. It is primarily used to **suppress ventricular ectopy in cases of ventricular arrhythmias.**

Dosage: *Procainamide hydrochloride*: Initially 1 to 1.25 g orally followed by 250 to 750 mg every 4 to 6 hourly depending upon the disorder. IM 0.5 to 1 g; IV 50-100 mg every 3 to 5 hours upto 1000 mg under ECG monitoring.

Disopyramide Phosphate

Disopyramide is a newer antiarrhythmic agent, with actions similar to those of quinidine and procainamide.

Class IB

Lidocaine Hydrochloride

Lidocaine (lignocaine) is a local anaesthetic, useful in the treatment of ***ventricular tachycardia and abnormalities of rhythm occurring after myocardial infarction.*** Lidocaine differs from quinidine and procainamide in its mode of action as it **decreases the duration of the action potential. It enhances conduction velocity, and increases membrane responsiveness**. Lidocaine is now the drug of choice in managing **acute ventricular arrhythmias** when a rapid onset of antiarrhythmic action is required.

Pharmacokinetics: Lidocaine is given intravenously. It is metabolized in the liver, with less than 10 percent of the dose excreted unchanged in the urine. The plasma half-life of a single injection is very short (15 minutes).

Toxicity: Lidocaine is a relatively safe drug, but *bradycardia* and *hypotension* can occur. Toxicity is usually expressed on the central nervous system, leading to drowsiness, paresthesias, disorientation, convulsions, behavioural disturbances, and increased irritability.

Therapeutic uses: Lidocaine is used in the emergency treatment of **ventricular tacharrhythmias following myocardial infarction**. It may also be used for treating **digitalis-induced arrhythmias.**

Dosage: Lidocaine hydrochloride 50-100 mg is administered intravenously as a loading dose, followed by an IV infusion of 1-4 mg/minute.

Phenytoin Sodium

Phenytoin (diphenylhydantoin) is an antiepileptic drug. The main use of phenytoin is confined to ***digitalis-induced arrhythmias.***

The major actions of phenytoin resemble those of lidocaine.

Therapeutic uses: Phenytoin is used in the treatment of paroxysmal tachycardia, and other **arrhythmias associated with digitalis intoxication.** For dosage schedule see **Table 4.5.**

Tocainide

Tocainide, a close structural analogue of lidocaine, is resistant to gastric acid and little affected by first-pass hepatic metabolism. Its mode of action is similar to that of lidocaine. It is used for the treatment of ventricular arrhythmias, like **premature ventricular contractions, ventricular tachycardia,** and **unifocal** or **multifocal couplets.**

Mexiletine

Mexiletine is an orally effective antiarrhythmic, and is similar to **lidocaine** and **tocainide** in its actions. Mexiletine is used for treating various ***ventricular arrhythmias***.

Class IC

Flecainide

Flecainide is an orally effective antiarrhythmic that possesses **membrane stabilizing activity,** and has local anaesthetic properties. **Ventricular refractory period is prolonged.** Flecainide is mainly used in the treatment of **life-threatening ventricular arrhythmias.**

Encainide

Encainide **increases the ratio of the effective refractory period to the action potential duration.** Encainide is used for life-threatening arrhythmias like **sustained ventricular tachycardia.**

Class II

Propranolol

Acebutolol

Almost all beta-blockers have significant antiarrhythmic activity. Amongst them, **propranolol** and **acebutolol** are the agents which have been

Table 4.5 : *Dosage, therapeutic uses, and toxicity of commonly used antiarrhythmic drugs*

Generic name	Dosage	Therapeutic uses	Toxicity
Quinidine sulphate	Orally 200-300 mg 3 or 4 times daily	Premature atrial and ventricular contraction (PACs, PVCs); paroxysmal atrial tachycardia (PAT); atrial fibrillation and flutter.	Hypotension, cinchonism vomiting, diarrhoea, drug rash, haemolytic anaemia, thrombocytopenia, asystole, heart block
Procainamide HCl	IV: 50-100 mg, every 3-5 hrs, upto 1 g. Oral: 3-6 g/day in 6 divided doses	Premature ventricular contractions and ventricular tachycardia; recurrent ventricular arrhythmias following myocardial infarction	Hypotension, respiratory arrest, heart block, AV or intraventricular block, ventricular fibrillation
Lidocaine HCl	IV: single IV bolus dose of 50-100 mg, followed by continous IV injection 1-4 mg per min	PVCs; ventricular tachycardia in patients following acute myocardial infarcation and in cases of digitalis intoxication	Hypotension, respiratory arrest, seizures, heart block
Phenytoin sodium	IV: 5-10 mg/kg by slow IV injection. Oral: 100-400 mg orally in divided doses	Atrial and ventricular tachycardia, specially in digitals intoxication	Gingival hyperplasia, drowsiness
Propranolol HCl	Oral: 10-30 mg 3 or 4 times daily. IV: 1-3 mg at a rate of not more than 1 mg/min with ECG monitoring	Supraventricular and ventricular arrhythmias specially those induced by catecholamines, or pheocromocytoma	Hypotension, heart block, cardiac failure, bronchospasm, altered carbohydrate metabolism

used to treat a variety of arrhythmias specially **exercise-induced arrhythmias,** or those associated with **excessive sympathetic** or **circulating catecholamine levels.**

The beta-blockers **competitively** antagonize the action of adrenergic agents, specifically on the heart (beta$_1$-receptors). The antiarrhythmic activity is attributed to *two* actions: (i) *blockade of cardiac beta-adrenoceptors*; and (ii) *membrane stabilizing activity*, also labeled as *quinidine-like activity*. The direct effects of propranolol resemble those of quinidine and procainamide.

Propranolol is used for the following arrhythmias: *exercise-induced ventricular tachycardia, supraventricular tachyarrhythmias* (atrial fibrillation, atrial flutter, paroxysmal atrial tachycardia); *tachyarrhythmias of digitalis intoxication; tachycardias due to thyrotoxicosis or excessive catecholamine activity during anaesthesia*, and persistent premature ventricular extrasystoles. The usual oral dose is 10-30 mg 3 or 4 times daily. IV propranolol is reserved for life-threatening arrhythmias in a dose of 1-3 mg at a rate of 1 mg/minute.

Class III

Amiodarone

Amiodarone is an orally effective agent reserved for ***life-threatening ventricular arrhythmias***, refractory to other agents. It possesses both

alpha- and **beta-blocking actions**. The peripheral vascular resistance is reduced. Automaticity is decreased causing marked bradycardia and sinus arrest.

Bretylium

Bretylium, an adrenergic neurone blocker was originally introduced as an antihypertensive, but later was found to have antiarrhythmic activity. Currently it is used exclusively as an alternative drug for the emergency control of serious ventricular arrhythmias. *The ventricular fibrillation threshold is increased.*

Class IV

Verapamil

Verapamil inhibits the influx of calcium through the cardiac cell membrane into the cardiac cell. It ***slows AV conduction,*** and ***increases the P-R interval***. It also produces peripheral vasodilatation. Verapamil has been used in **atrial flutter** and **fibrillation with rapid ventricular rate, and supraventricular tachyarrhythmias**. **Side effects** include hypotension and it ***should not*** be administered simultaneously with beta-blockers. Verapamil may be given orally in a dose of 80 mg three or four times daily. Verapamil 1 mg/min upto 10 mg intravenously is the drug of choice for an attack of atrial tachycardia.

Digitalis

The digitalis glycosides have complex **direct** and **indirect** effects on the heart. The factors responsible for the antiarrhythmic activity of digitalis are: (i) ***lengthening of AV nodal conduction time*** and ***refractory period*** due to its vagotonic and direct effects; (ii) ***shortening of the atrial refractory period*** due to vagal stimulation; (iii) ***shortening of the ventricular muscle refractory period*** by a direct action; and (iv) ***enhancement of myocardial contractility***.

In **atrial flutter** or **fibrillation**, digitalis is used to slow the ventricular rates. It may be used to terminate **supraventricular tachycardia** and **sinus tachycardia**.

Digitalis can induce almost any cardiac rhythm disorder leading to serious ventricular fibrillation. The drugs most commonly used to treat severe digitalis-induced arrhythmias are ***lidocaine***, ***phenytoin*** and ***propranolol***.

Drugs for Bradyarrhythimias

Isoprenaline Hydrochloride

Isoprenaline stimulates the beta-adrenoceptors in the heart, blood vessels and bronchioles. It has a ***non-selective action*** and acts as an agonist for both $beta_1$ (heart) and $beta_2$ (blood vessels, brochioles) adrenoceptors.

Isoprenaline is used in patients with **second- or third degree AV block** where it can effectively maintain the heart rate and cardiac output prior to insertion of a pacemaker. It is useful in emergency treatment of **Stokes-Adams seizures,** and for **severe propranolol-induced myocardial depression**.

Atropine Sulphate

Atropine is a cholinergic blocking agent, and it blocks the myocardial cholinergic (muscarinic type) receptors. It is used to treat certain **reversible bradyarrhythmias** which accompany acute myocardial infarction like sinus bradycardia. Atropine may be used in cases of **sinoatrial arrest, vasovagal syndrome**. For these conditions initially 0.4 to 1 mg of atropine is given intravensouly and repeated every 1 to 2 hours.

4.5 ANTIANGINAL DRUGS

Angina pectoris manifests itself in the form of a dramatic and terrorizing ***retrosternal pain*** often of a 'crushing' nature. This ischaemic pain may last for several seconds, and terminate on rest (angina of effort). At a cellular level it is the result of ***deficient myocardial perfusion***, inadequate to meet the oxygen need of the myocardium. This oxygen supply-demand imbalance is the basis for the pathophysiology of angina.

TYPES OF ANGINA PECTORIS

1. **Classic, stable angina:** It is termed as 'exertional angina' or 'angina of effort'.
2. **Classic, unstable angina:** Chest pain occurs even at rest, ischaemia is severe. The person is at high risk of myocardial infarction.
3. **Vasospastic (Prinzmetal's variant) angina:** Myocardial ischaemia is the result of **coronary vasospasm,** pain is prolonged, and may develop during activity or rest.

When a branch of the coronary artery is occluded, and the myocardium supplied by it dies, it is known as **myocardial infarction.**

CLASSIFICATION

I. Nitrates and nitrites

a. **Relief of anginal pain**
   Nitroglycerin (Glyceryl trinitrate).

b. **Prevention of anginal attacks**
   Pentaerythrityl tetranitrate
   Erythrityl tetranitrate
   Mannitol hexanitrate
   Isosorbide dinitrate
   Isosorbide mononitrate.

c. **Treatment of cyanide poisoning**
   Sodium nitrite.

II. Agents for prevention of anginal attacks

a. **Beta-blockers**
   Propranolol, Nadolol, Atenolol, Metoprolol

b. **Calcium channel blockers**
   Verapamil, Nifedipine, Diltiazem

c. **Antiplatelet agents**
   Dipyridamole, Aspirin.

III. Other measures

a. **Antianxiety drugs,** e.g., Diazepam.

b. **Induction of myxoedema** with radioiodine or antithyroid drugs.

Nitrates and Nitrites

Nitroglycerin and *amyl nitrite* were the first members of this group to be used as coronary vasodilators more than 100 years ago.

Pharmacology and Mode of Action

The basic action of the nitrites is a **direct relaxation of the smooth muscles.** All types of blood vessels are dilated, and the coronary arteries share this generalized vasodilatation. Though there is a moderate reflex tachycardia **the end result is reduced cardiac work**. There is evidence that nitroglycerin may cause a **beneficial redistribution of coronary blood flow.**

These agents also relax the musculature of the ***bronchi***, the ***gall bladder,*** and the ***biliary tract***, ***uterus***, the ***stomach*** and the ***intestines.***

Lately, the organic nitrates are thought to involve the **nitrate receptors** in the vascular smooth muscle.

Adverse Reactions

1. The usual side effect is sudden **hypotension**. Light headedness, dizziness, flushing of the face, throbbing headache and fainting, and a complete **nitrite syncope** might occur.
2. **Tolerance** is developed rapidly.
3. **Methaemoglobinaemia.**

Therapeutic Uses

1. In **angina pectoris** to relieve or prevent anginal pain.
2. In **refractory biliary colic** and **bronchial asthma** as antispasmodics.
3. In abdominal cramps of **lead colic.**
4. In **trigeminal neuralgia.**
5. In **Raynaud's disease** and **trophic ulcers** topical application of nitroglycerin may provide useful local vasodilation.
6. In **cyanide poisoning.**

Treatment of Cyanide Poisoning

The lethal action of cyanide is due to its **inactivating the enzyme cytochrome oxidase.** Thiosulphate reacts with cyanide to produce **stable thiocynate.** A suggested regimen is an under:

1. **Sodium nitrite** 0.3 to 0.5 g dissolved in 10 to 15 ml of water is injected intravenously over 3 to 4 minutes. *Amyl nitrite inhalations* may be given every 2 minutes for 30 seconds.
2. **Sodium thiosulphate** 12.5 g in 50 ml of water given intravenously over 10 minutes.
3. **Oxygen inhalation** or even a blood transfusion may have to be given.

Specific Agents

Glyceryl Trinitrate (Nitroglycerin)

It is administered in doses of 0.3 to 0.6 mg **sublingually**. The onset of action is within 2 to 5 minutes and the duration of action is about 30 minutes. *It is advisable to direct the patient to expel the undissolved tablet from the mouth as soon as relief is obtained.*

Currently nitroglycerin is available in many dosage forms:

(i) **Nitroglycerin sublingual tablets** (0.15, 0.3, 0.4, 0.6 mg)–dose 0.3-0.6 mg under the tongue; (ii) **Nitroglycerin translingual oral spray** (0.4 mg/metered dose)–one to two sprays onto oral mucosa; (iii) **Nitroglycerin transmucosal** (controlled release buccal tablets 1, 2, 3 mg)–dose 1 tablet placed in buccal pouch; (iv) **Nitroglycerin injection** (0.5, 0.8, 5.0, 10 mg/ml)–dose 5 mcg/min IV infusion, increase upto 20 mcg/min; (v) **Nitroglycerin topical ointment** (2%)–dose half-inch strip of ointment applied by spreading over 6×6 inch area of the skin, do not rub in, increase by half-inch increments; and (vi) **Nitroglycerin transdermal systems** (Transderm Nitro–2.5, 5, 10, 15 mg/24 hours) apply one patch to a non-hairy skin area once in 24 hours.

Amyl nitrite: It is a volatile liquid available in small breakable ampoules (pearls) containing 0.3 ml of the drug. The pearl is cracked between the folds of a handkerchief, and the vapours inhaled.

Long-Acting Nitrates

Pentaerythrityl tetranitrate in a dose of 20-60 mg tid has been claimed to reduce the severity and frequency of anginal attacks in about one-third of patients.

Isosorbide dinitrate is given as a 5 mg *sublingual* tablet, and is effective within 5 minutes. It is used for prophylaxis or treatment of anginal attacks.

Isosorbide–5–mononitrate is used for the prophylaxis of angina pectoris, and as an adjunct in congestive heart failure. *Dose* initially 20 mg bid, tid or 40 mg bid, upto 120 mg daily in divided doses, if required.

Beta-Adrenoceptor Blockers

The agents approved for treatment of angina pectoris include **propranolol, nadolol** and **atenolol**. These agents markedly **reduce myocardial oxygen demand.** The haemodynamic effects responsible for the beneficial effects of beta-blockers are a **decreased heart rate**, **blood pressure,** and **myocardial contractility**, all of which **reduce cardiac workload.** Propranolol blocks the oxygen wasting effects of catecholamines.

Propranolol: The initial dose is 10-20 mg tid or qid, dosage may be increased to optimal levels which may range from 80 to 160 mg/day.

Nadolol: Nadolol has a long half-life (18-24 hours), and may be used as a ***once a day dosing schedule***. Initial dosage is 40 mg, which may be increased by 40-80 mg increments every 3 to 7 days.

Atenolol: Atenolol is a long-acting ($t_{½}$ 6-9 hours) *cardioselective* beta-blocker with actions similar to those of propranolol. The usual dose is 50 mg once daily. *Metoprolol*, another *cardioselective* beta-blocker may also be used for prophylaxis of angina in a dose of 50-100 mg bid or tid orally.

Calcium Channel Blockers

Calcium channel blockers are a group of drugs that **reduce intracellular calcium transfer**, thereby reducing contractility of the muscle cell. The three clinically important agents are **verapamil, diltiazem** and **nifedipine.** They act specially on the **nodal tissue** in the heart, and the arterial smooth muscle. These sites of action account for most of the clinical applications of calcium channel blockers namely **angina pectoris** (classical and variant), **supraventricular arrhythmias, hypertension** and **peripheral vascular disease.** All three agents benefit angina of effort acting through a mixture of mechanisms: (i) all increase coronary blood flow; (ii) **Diltiazem** has negative chronotropic effect and reduces afterload; (iii) **verapamil** has a mild negative inotropic effect and decreases afterload; and (iv) the major effect of **nifedipine** is to reduce afterload.

Pharmacology and Mode of Action

Verapamil is a papaverine derivative; **nifedipine** is a dihydropyridine derivative; and **diltiazem** is a benzothiazepine derivative. Despite marked structural differences they all **block the slow Ca^{++}channel selectively** in the heart muscle and smooth muscle with varying potencies.

Electrophysiology

Verapamil slows AC conduction and prolongs the ERP within the AV node. Verapamil can **restore normal sinus rhythm in patients with paroxysmal supraventricular tachycardias (PSVT).**

Haemodynamics: Calcium antagonists dilate the coronary arteries and arterioles both in normal and ischaemic regions of the myocardium, and inhibit coronary artery spasm. This increases myocardial oxygen delivery in patients with **vasospastic (Prinzmetal's or variant) angina.** All three of the conventional calcium channel blockers decrease coronary vascular resistance, and increase coronary blood flow.

Calcium antagonists ***reduce arterial blood pressure*** at rest and at a given level of exercise by dilating peripheral arterioles, and thereby reducing total peripheral resistance (afterload) against which the heart works. Such an unloading of the heart accounts for their effectiveness in **chronic stable angina.**

Therapeutic Uses

The uses of calcium antagonists in cardiovascular diseases are summarized in **Table 4.6.**

Contraindications and Precautions

Verapamil and dilitazem are contraindicated in **sick sinus syndrome,** except in the presence of a functioning ventricular pacemaker. Other contraindications are **second or third degree AV blocks** and **hypotension** (systolic below 90 mmHg). *Hypersensitivity* to nifedipine has been reported.

Adverse Reactions

Verapamil is the best tolerated calcium antagonist. **Constipation** is the most common side effect. Headache, vertigo, weakness, nervousness, pruritus, flushing and gastric disturbances may occur.

Nifedipine may cause headache, tachycardia, dizziness, fatigue, nausea, oedema, flushing, orthostatic hypotension, and precipitates CHF.

Dilitazem may cause bradycardia, dizziness, headache, flushing, and dryness of mouth. Hypersensitivity reactions have been reported. CHF, AV conduction defects, and sinus arrest occur rarely.

Drug Interactions

Concomitant use of calcium antagonists and beta-blockers is risky, as the cardiac function can be adversely affected because of the combined depressant effects on the myocardial contractility and AV conduction.

Felodipine: Felodipine has a *more selective effect on smooth muscle cells* of resistance vessels than nifedipine and Verapamil. This drug also has a marked **diuretic effect** secondary to increased **natriuresis.** The potassium level remains unchanged. There is an increase in cardiac output upto about 50 percent.

Haemorheology, i.e., the study of the flow properties of blood and its interaction with the vascular system has received professional attention lately. **Felodipine** enhances red cell deformability or flexibility, i.e., the ability of the red blood cells to change their shape in response to mechanical force or stresses is increased.

Therapeutic uses: Felodipine lowers blood pressure without any change in renin levels. In **hypertensive emergencies** it is given in a dose of 0.01 to 0.04 mg/kg IV, over 20 to 120 minutes.

Short-term **side effects** include headache, diarrhoea and flushing in some patients. Long-

Table 4.6 : *Calcium antagonists and cardiovascular disorders*

Drug	Indications	Dosage
Verapamil	1. Supraventricular tachycardia (SVT)	1. IV bolus 5-10 mg, repeated after 10 minutes, then 0.005 mg/kg/min, if needed.
		2. IV infusion 1 mg/min to a total of 10 mg/min to a total of 10 mg.
	2. Atrial flutter/fibrillation	80-120 mg tid increasing 80-120 mg qid
	3. Prophylaxis of SVT, angina of effort, angina at rest, and hypertrophic cardiomyopathy	Orally 80-120 mg Orally 80-120 mg tid increasing to 80-120 mg qid.
Nifedipine	1. Angina of effort, angina at rest, Prinzmetal's angina	Orally 30-80 mg in 3 to 4 divided doses.
	2. Hypertension, acute left-ventricular failure	Orally, 10 mg 2 to 4 times daily; 10 mg sublingually 6 hourly.
Diltiazem	1. Supraventricular tachycardia (SVT)	IV 0.15-0.25 mg/kg given over 2 minutes.
	2. Atrial flutter/fibrillation	IV 0.15-0.25 mg/kg given over 2 minutes.
	3. Prophylaxis of SVT, angina of effort and at rest, Prinzmetal's angina	Oral 30-90 mg tid increasing to qid

term use may lead to ***ankle oedema***, but without weight gain as felodipine has a potent diuretic effect.

To *conclude*, the beta-blockers and calcium antagonists have a somewhat similar spectrum of therapeutic usefulness. In **supraventricular tachyarrhythmias**, the most used agent for both IV and oral routes is **Verapamil**, followed by **dilitazem.** In **ventricular arrhythmias** complicating coronary artery spasm, all calcium antagonists are effective.

ANTIPLATELET AGENTS

Dipyridamole

Dipyridamole is a potent non-nitrate coronary vasodilator used in the long-term prophylactic therapy of angina pectoris. Dipyridamole **inhibits adenosine deaminase**, thereby increasing the levels of adenosine and other vasodilatory nucleotides. It also **blocks the action of phosphodiesterase**, resulting in an increased level of cyclic-AMP, causing coronary vasodilation. Increased cyclic- AMP also **reduces platelet aggregation.** Dipyridamole promotes development of collateral circulation.

Therapeutic uses: Dipyridamole either alone or in combination with aspirin has been used to prevent **transient ischaemic attacks**, and protect against further **thromboembolic complications.** Other uses include prevention of thromboembolism associated with **ischaemic heart disease, and prevention of coronary bypass graft occlusion.**

Dipyridamole is administered orally as tablets (25, 50, 75 mg). The usual dosage is 25-50 mg bid or tid orally. It is a well tolerated drug.

DRUG MANAGEMENT OF ANGINA PECTORIS

1. Treat the cause, if possible, e.g., anaemia, syphilis.
2. Weight reduction and change in life style.
3. **Nitroglycerin** to be taken before exercise that is expected to induce angina.
4. **Beta-adrenoceptor blockade:** Propranolol is given continuously.
5. The **long-acting organic nitrates** may be used for prophylaxis.
6. **Sedation** may help if anxiety is a factor.
7. Smoking should be discouraged.
8. In severe cases a**nticoagulant therapy** should be considered.
9. **Control of plasma lipids.**
10. Severe angina, unresponsive to drug treatment is an indication for **surgical bypass grafting** of the affected coronary arteries.

DRUG TREATMENT OF ACUTE MYOCARDIAL INFARCTION

i. **Pain:** Morphine, pethidine.
ii. **Arrhythmias:** Lignocaine.
iii. **Pump failure:** Digitalis, glucagon.
iv. **Cardiogenic shock:** Mephentermine, dopamine.

The use of drugs for the prophylaxis of arrhythmias in the absence of any rhythm abnormality is controversial. **Lignocaine, quinidine**, and **procainamide** have been tried. Treated patients have fewer arrhythmias. The **anticoagulants** may be used for one month for the prevention of recurrence of myocardial infarction.

The most important factor to be managed is the extreme apprehension and pain in the patient. To allay anxiety **diazepam** produces adequate sedation. **Intravenous morphine** or **pethidine** are the drugs of choice for analgesia with 10 mg of morphine being equivalent for 75 mg of pethidine.

For the secondary prevention of reinfarction drugs like **aspirin, sulphinpyrazone** and **beta-adrenoceptor blockers** have been employed. **Low-dose heparin therapy** has recently been shown to reduce the incidence of deep vein thrombosis, and consequent pulmonary embolism. **Oxygen** is given to most patients with complicated MI.

To conclude, drugs employed in the treatment of angina pectoris exert one or more of the following effects: **increase in coronary blood flow; decrease in cardiac work; and improvement in myocardial efficiency.**

4.6 DRUG THERAPY OF SHOCK

Shock is a state of ***acute circulatory failure*** in which the cardiac output is inadequate to provide normal tissue perfusion. The symptoms are particularly related to the hypoperfusion of vital organs like the **brain, heart , kidneys, liver** and **lungs** manifested as a **clouded sensorium, oliguria** and **cardiac arrhythmias**.

THE PERIPHERAL CIRCULATION

The total blood volume is about 5 litres, and this amount is pumped by the heart once each minute. The stoke volume is about 70 ml per beat, ejected about 72 times each minute. Only about 15 percent of the blood volume lies in the arterial bed, and variations in arterial calibre have little effect on vascular capacity. The arterioles are called **resistance vessels.** Normally they are widely open to permit free perfusion of tissues.

Most of the circulating blood volume (over 70%) lies on the venous side, in the venules. Hence, the venous system is called the **capacitance system.** The veins are less muscular, with a large diameter and offer a low resistance. Failure of venous tone would lead to pooling of blood in the venules and capillaries, resulting in a fall in cardiac output. Such a condition is labeled as **peripheral circulatory failure.**

To *summarize*, whatever the cause of shock, the constant haemodynamic defect ***is a reduction in the perfusion of tissues, precipitated by a fall in cardiac output.*** Impaired tissue perfusion leads to *hypoxaemia*, *metabolic acidosis*, *lactic acidaemia* and *hyperkalaemia*. If this state of **reversible shock** continues, the patient passes into a state of **irreversible shock.**

HAEMODYNAMIC PATTERNS IN SHOCK

1. **Inadequate venous return:** The cardiac output is lowered. For the management, first **proper replacement of fluids** is necessary.
2. **Low systemic vascular resistance:** Patients of **septic shock, shock following myocardial infarction**, shock of **head injury**, and **chemical toxicity** exhibit this pattern.
3. **High systemic vascular resistance:** The systemic vascular resistance is high, and the cardiac output is low, causing tissue hypoperfusion. Patients in **shock following myocardial infarction, septic shock**, and shock following **cardiac surgery** fall in this category.

DRUG THERAPY OF SHOCK

The treatment of shock may be divided into **primary therapy** for the presumed cause, and **secondary therapy** for the correction of the haemodynamic disturbance. The following drugs are employed:

1. Sympathomimetic amines.
2. Alpha-Adrenoceptor blocking agents.
3. Corticosteroids.
4. Oxygen.
5. Cardiac glycosides.
6. Glucagon.
7. Dextrans.

Sympathomimetic Amines

They exert their cardiovascular effects by acting on the ***beta$_1$-adrenoceptors*** in the heart, ***alpha-*** and ***beta$_2$-adrenoceptors*** in the blood vessels, and ***dopamine receptors*** in the renal, mesenteric, coronary, and cerebral vascular beds. When shock is due to inadequate circulating blood volume, ***blood*** or ***plasma volume expanders*** should be administered first and later the sympathomimetics may be used to improve tissue perfusion.

The sympathomimetic amines used in the treatment of shock are ***noradrenaline, adrenaline, dopamine,*** and the synthetic compounds ***isoprenaline, metaraminol,*** and ***dobutamine.***

Noradrenaline: In the shock syndrome with high peripheral resistance, noradrenaline induces further vasoconstriction, and is rarely helpful or rather it is harmful.

Adrenaline: The use of adrenaline is restricted to anaphylactic shock.

Dopamine increases renal and mesenteric blood flow possibly by acting on the dopamine receptors. It is most useful in treating oliguric patients with low or normal peripheral vascular resistance. Dopamine is employed in the management of **cardiogenic, septic,** and **traumatic shock.**

Isoprenaline has a beta-adrenergic action both on the heart and periphery. It is helpful in patients of shock with high peripheral vascular resistance.

Dobutamine is a synthetic catecholamine and acts primarily on the beta$_1$-receptor, with less pronounced actions on beta$_2$- and alpha-receptors. Dobutamine has been used in patients with **severe congestive heart failure,** and in **patients following cardiac surgery.**

Adverse Reactions

Therapeutic doses of sympathomimetic amines may cause restlessness, headache, pallor, dizziness, precordial pain, and palpitation. Overdosage can induce convulsions, cerebral haemorrhage and tachyarrhythmias leading to fatal ventricular arrhythmias.

Alpha-Adrenoceptor Blocking Agents

Alpha-blocker therapy must follow adequate replacement of fluid volume. Phenoxybenzamine is the agent usually employed in cases of **traumatic** or **surgical shock.** Phenoxybenzamine has to be administered cautiously in a dose of 1 mg/kg body weight IV slowly well diluted in a volume of 50 ml 5 percent glucose.

Corticosteroids

Some authorities consider that massive doses of corticosteroids are useful in shock as they cause **vasodilatation**, and a **positive inotropic effect**, thereby improving tissue perfusion. In cases of *septic shock* they may decrease the sensitivity to endotoxins.

Oxygen

Oxygen *increases the cardiac output,* and tissue oxygenation can be significantly improved. Oxygen is necessary in patients who have arterial hypoxaemia, which usually occurs in **cardiogenic shock. Positive pressure ventilation** may be required to maintain adequate oxygen exchange.

Cardiac Glycosides

Cardiac glycosides improve myocardial contractility, raise the cardiac output, and improve tissue perfusion, specially in cases of *congestive heart failure.*

Dextrans

Low molecular weight dextran (Mol Wt. 40,000), also known as Dextran 40, is available as a 10 percent solution in either isotonic saline or 5 percent dextrose in water for intravenous use. Thereby it **improves the microcirculation.** Thus dextran 40 may be employed in cases of shock to improve tissue perfusion.

CLINICAL APPLICATIONS

Shock is generally classified according to its aetiology, and there are **four** main types: (i) Hypovolaemic; (ii) Cardiogenic; (iii) Septic; and (iv) Anaphylactic shock.

Hypovolaemic Shock

Hypovolaemic shock results from external or internal loss of blood, plasma or water *following haemorrhage, trauma, burns, protracted vomiting or diarrhoea.* Therapy consists of **appropriate fluid replacement using saline, plasma or blood, and correction of acidosis.**

Cardiogenic Shock

The most common cause of cardiogenic shock is **acute myocardial infarction (AMI)**, although myocardial depression also occurs in other forms of shock. There is a failure of the heart as a pump, i.e., 'pump failure'.

Therapy consist of relief of pain and anxiety. **Oxygen** administration antagonizes tissue hypoxia, and acidosis. The use of **cardiac glycosides** (digoxin) with caution is rational. **Phenoxybenzamine** may be employed in selected cases. **Vasodilator drugs** (sodium nitroprusside) may be useful in patients with severe pump failure.

Septic Shock

Bacterial shock requires **immediate intensive antibiotic therapy,** and adequate circulating volume should be maintained. **Sympathomimetic amines** should be used with **fluid replacement,** and controlled by monitoring the central venous pressure. **Dopamine** is preferred. **Corticosteroids** have been advocated to suppress the systemic reactions to endotoxins.

Anaphylactic Shock

In anaphylactic reactions there is extrema vasodilatation and increased capillary permeability. *Treatment consists of:* (i) prompt administration of **adrenaline** to act as a vasoconstrictor, and for relaxing the smooth muscle. A dose of 0.5 ml of a 1:1000 solution is given intramuscularly or 0.1 ml of 1:1000 solution diluted in 10 ml of saline is injected intravenously; (ii) **Antihistamines** like diphenhydramine are administered; (iii) **Corticosteroids** are administered for their anti-inflammatory and antiallergic actions; and (iv) treat hypoxia by **oxygen** inhalations and **positive pressure respiration**, if required. Simultaneously the fluid and electrolyte balance should be taken care of.

To **summarize,** the two basic aims in the therapy of shock are: (i) to *eliminate the initiating cause* (primary therapy); and (ii) *to correct the haemodynamic derangements (secondary therapy)* allowing time for specific therapy to be effective or physiologic improvement to take place.

Drugs Acting on the Haemopoietic System

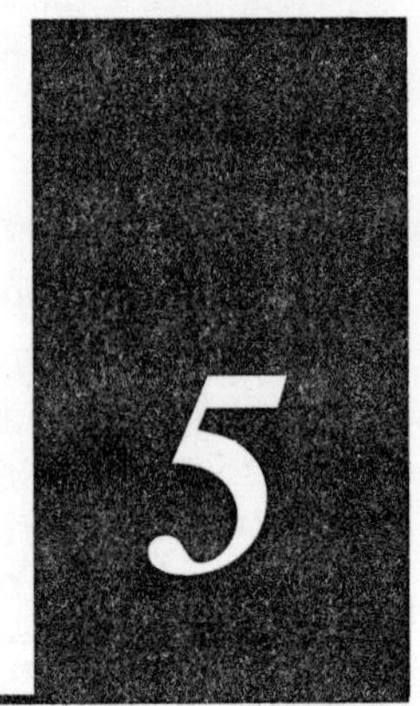

5.1 HAEMATINICS

Haematinics are agents used for the prevention and treatment anaemias. In anaemia there is some deficiency in the **quality,** or in the **quantity** of blood, the common factor being a diminished oxygen-carrying capacity of the blood, leading to diminished tissue oxygenation. Anaemias can be divided into: (a) ***microcytic hypochromic*** (iron-deficiency anaemia); (b) ***megaloblastic or macrocytic hyperchromic*** (megaloblastic anaemia); (c) ***aplastic;*** and (d) ***haemolytic*** anaemias.

SYNTHESIS OF HAEMOGLOBIN

Haemoglobin is formed in the red bone marrow. The total available tissue in the body for haemopoiesis is 1400 g. The life span of erythrocytes is about 120 days. Interestingly about 10^{12} erythrocytes are produced daily, and during a human life span about 1 ton of erythocytes are released into the blood stream.

Haemoglobin is a ***metalloporphyrin,*** and the metallic atom is iron in the ferrous state (Fe^{++}). This porphyrin is designated as **haem**. Folic acid and vitamin B_{12} are capable of increasing the rate of haem synthesis in the red cells.

The essential raw material for haemoglobin synthesis is: (i) ***iron;*** (ii) ***pyrrole groups*** for porphyrin synthesis; and (iii) ***amino acids*** for globin synthesis. In addition an adequate diet, providing traces of ***copper***, ***manganese***, ***cobalt salts***, ***pyridoxine***, ***riboflavin*** and ***protein*** is essential.

Most anemias are due to the deficiency of one or more of the following:

Iron

Folic acid (Pteroylglutamic acid)

Vitamin B_{12} (Cyanocobalamin).

IRON

The human body contains about 3.5 g of iron of which about 2/3 is contained in the blood, and the reminder is stored (as ferritin and haemosiderin) in the bone marrow, spleen and muscles. The iron requirement ranges between 0.5-1.0 mg daily for adult males and postmenopausal women. During pregnancy and lactation there is an increase in the iron requirement to 2.5-3.0 mg daily.

Iron Absorption, Distribution and Excretion (Ferrokinetics)

Iron is widely distributed in foodstuffs, including ***meat, leafy vegetables, pulses, wheat, oat meal, eggs*** and ***chocolate.***

Iron in foodstuffs is mostly in the **ferric** form, but gastric acid reduces it to the **ferrous** state which is more readily absorbed. The ferrous iron passes through the mucosal cell directly into the blood stream, where it is bound to **transferrin** and carried to the storage sites.

In the mucosal cell the excess of ferrous iron is re-oxidized to the ferric state, which is insoluble and combines with the protein **apoferritin** to form a complex called **ferritin.** Ferritin is a storage form of iron.

Ferritin releases iron (Fe^{+++}) into the circulating blood which is bound to a globulin known as **transferrin.** In this form it is carried to the storage depots from where it is utilized for erythropoiesis.

Therapeutic Uses

The chief indication of iron therapy is **iron-deficiency anaemia**, which is the result of severe or chronic haemorrhage, malignancy, infection, nutritional deficiency, pregnancy, lactation or parasitic infestations (specially ankylostomiasis).

IRON THERAPY

Oral iron preparations: The old preparation ferrous sulphate is as effective as any of the later and more expensive preparations:

Ferrous sulphate hydrated	0.3 g tid
Ferrous sulphate exsiccated	0.2 g tid
Ferrous gluconate	0.6 g tid
Ferrous fumarate	0.2 g tid

The ***slow release*** and ***chelated forms of iron*** are also available, and they cause less of gastrointestinal upsets and are better tolerated.

Parenteral iron preparations: Usually oral iron therapy is adequate to treat the anaemia. Parenteral therapy is only required when there is: (i) intolerance to oral therapy; (ii) improper iron absorption from the intestines; (iii) malabsorption syndromes; (iv) inadequate response; or (v) severe iron-deficiency anaemia.

Intramuscular Preparations

Iron dextran injection (Imferon)–Contains elemental iron 50 mg/ml. The dose is 1-4 ml daily by deep intramuscular injection

Intravenous Preparation

Iron dextran injection–It is the same as the intramuscular preparation except that it is without preservatives. The initial dose should be limited to 25 mg, and daily increments upto 100 mg per day may be given slowly intravenously.

Toxicity of Iron

Therapeutic doses may cause nausea, abdominal discomfort, and either constipation or diarrhea. High oral doses can cause serious gastrointestinal irritation, and necrosis of the mucous membrane and shock leading to **acute iron poisoning.** The symptoms include pallor, lassitude, haematemesis, and cardiovascular collapse.

Treatment of acute iron poisoning is:(i) administration of raw eggs and milk to help in binding iron in the gut; (ii) **Desferrioxamine** (Desferal) 1-2 g IM every 12-hourly. It is an iron chelating agent and forms a non-toxic complex which is excreted in the urine; and (iii) **Calcium disodium edathamil** may be used, if desferrioxamine is not available.

On prolonged parenteral iron overdosage, the body is unable to excrete the excess of iron, and it is accumulated in the body, leading to **haemochromatosis,** i.e., deposition of haemosiderin in the liver and other organs.

FOLIC ACID

Folic acid (pteroylglutamic acid) is a member of the B complex group of vitamins. It is present in ***yeast, green vegetables,*** and ***liver,*** and is capable of curing megaloblastic anaemias. The daily requirement is 50-100 mcg, and rises to about 200 mcg in pregnancy. Folic acid deficiency leads to **macrocytic hyperchromic anaemias.**

Mode of action: Folic acid itself is inactive. In the body it is converted to *folinic acid*, which is its active form. Folinic acid further participates in the production of purines and pyrimidines leading to the ***synthesis of deoxyribonucleic acid*** (DNA), and thus regulates cells division.

Therapeutic Uses

Folic acid is used in the prevention and cure of *megaloblastic anaemias* due to folate deficiency:

1. Nutritional megaloblastic anaemia.
2. Megaloblastic anaemia of pregnancy.
3. Megaloblastic anaemia in infancy and childhood.
4. Megaloblastic anaemia associated with alcoholism and liver disease.
5. **Malabsorption syndromes:** In sprue, coeliac disease and steatorrhoea.

6. Chronic haemolytic states.
7. **Drug-induced megaloblastic anaemias.**
8. Megaloblastic anaemia of malignant disease.
9. Aplastic or hypoplastic anaemias.
10. Some cases of agranulocytosis.

Iron and folic acid combinations are used to treat ***dimorphic anaemias*** which are common in India.

Dose: Synthetic folic acid 10-30 mg orally daily is usually given. The dose for prophylaxis is 50-100 mcg/daily.

Toxicity: Folic aid is non-toxic in man. It should never be used as sole drug in the treatment of pernicious (Addisonian) anaemia.

VITAMIN B_{12} (CYANOCOBALAMIN)

Vitamin B_{12} is mainly employed in the treatment of *pernicious anaemia* (Addisonian anaemia).

Sources: Vitamin B_{12} is the most potent of the known vitamins. Rich sources of cyanocobalamin are ***organ meats, lamb and beef liver, kidney and heart.*** Egg yolk, fish and some cheeses also have a moderate amount. The daily dietary requirement ranges from 0.6 to 1.2 mcg. The total vitamin B_{12} store in the human adults is about 5 mg, mostly in the liver.

Pernicious anaemia: This is a vitamin B_{12} deficiency disease, due to the lack of a specific substance secreted by the normal gastric mucosa. This substance is a glycoprotein called the **'intrinsic factor'** of Castle. This intrinsic factor is essential for the intestinal absorption of the dietary **'extrinsic factor'**, which is vitamin B_{12} itself.

Mode of action: Vitamin B_{12} and folic acid play an important role in the biochemical processes of **methylation** and **transmethylation,** leading to synthesis of nucleic acids. A deficiency of vitamin B_{12} interferes with normal folate metabolism and induces a ***functional folate deficiency***. Clinically folic acid or vitamin B_{12} alone can cure **sprue** and allied disorders, but both are required together to relieve **pernicious anaemia. Vitamin B_{12} relieves both neurological and haematological disturbances in pernicious anaemia.**

Pharmacokinetics: The absorption of vitamin B_{12} from the gut is unreliable as there is a deficiency of the stomach intrinsic factor.

Therapeutic Uses

1. **Pernicious (Addisonian) anaemia.**
2. **Malabsorption syndromes:** In coeliac disease, sprue and idiopathic steatorrhoea.
3. **Neurological conditions:** Vitamin B_{12} has been employed in high doses of 1mg or more daily in cases of **trigeminal neuralgia, toxic/diabetic/alcoholic neuritis**, and other **nutritional neuropathies.**
4. **Psychiatric disorders:** Disorders during old age may favourably respond to vitamin B_{12} therapy.

Preparations and Dosage

Hydroxycobalamin: It is given in a dose of 100 mcg IM every 3 days for 7 to 10 doses. The maintenance dose is 1000 mcg every 2 to 4 months, given lifelong.

Toxicity

The cobalamins are usually well tolerated. Rarely allergic reactions may occur. Their use as 'tonics' must be avoided.

Erythropoietin

Erythropoietin is a glycoprotein produced by the peritubular cells in the proximal tubule of the kidney. In the bone marrow erythropoietin is produced by the macrophages, and functions as a ***growth factor inducing the differentiation of stem cells into erythrocytes.*** It stimulates proliferation, maturation and haemoglobin formation in the erythrocytes.

Therapeutic uses: Erythropoietin is very effective in the treatment of **anemia of chronic renal failure**. It is also effective in the treatment of anaemia associated with **acquired immunodeficiency syndrome (AIDS),** specially in the patients on zidovudine (AZT) therapy, and anaemia associated with **cancer chemotherapy**.

Dosage: Recombinant human erythropoietin

is available as epoetin alfa (Epogen, Eprex) in buffered saline containing human albumin in single dose vials of 2000,4000, or 10,000 units for IV or SC injection. The recommended initial dose is 50-100 units/kg three times a week in patient with chronic renal failure. The dosage can be increased by increment of 25 units/kg at monthly intervals. No significant allergic reactions have been observed with erythropoietin use.

To conclude, **iron** therapy is employed for iron deficiency anaemias. **Folic acid** and/or **cobalamins** are employed for treating megaloblastic anaemias. Shotgun therapy with antianaemic preparations must be avoided. The place of ***anabolic steroids*** (nandrolone, oxymetholone) in the therapy of **aplastic anaemia** remains controversial.

5.2 ANTICOAGULANTS AND HAEMOSTATIC AGENTS

In man coagulation and fibrinolysis are in state of ***dynamic equilibrium.*** In both systems an inactive precursor is converted into the active substance, inhibitors being present to prevent excessive activity (**Fig. 5.1**).

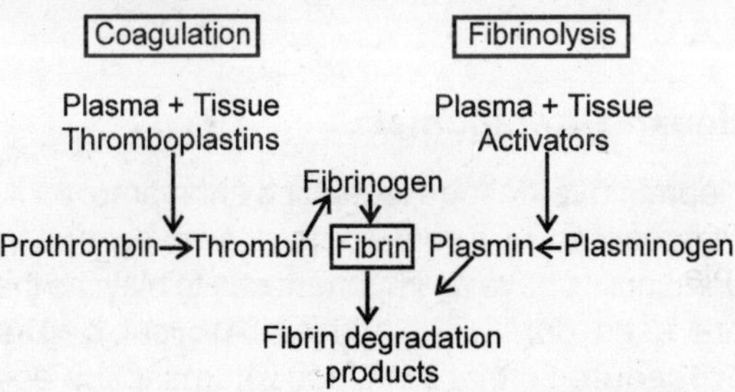

Fig. 5.1: *The dynamic equilibrium of coagulation and fibrinolysis.*

The end result of this dual process is that **thrombin** and **plasmin** are simultaneously active at the site of fibrin formation. The fibrin degradation products themselves have important actions in haemostasis with platelet function, and also have direct anticoagulant effect.

Anticoagulants are employed in the prevention and treatment of ***deep venous thrombosis, myocardial infarction, pulmonary embolism, and other thromboembolic disorders***.

MECHANISM OF HAEMOSTASIS

Whenever there is an injury to the blood vessel wall, **a primary mechanism** operates to form a **platelet plug**, followed by the **secondary mechanism** of haemostasis or **blood coagulation,** which operates to form the **fibrin clot**.

The primary mechanism of haemostasis resulting in the formation of the *platelet plug* is shown in **Fig. 5.2**.

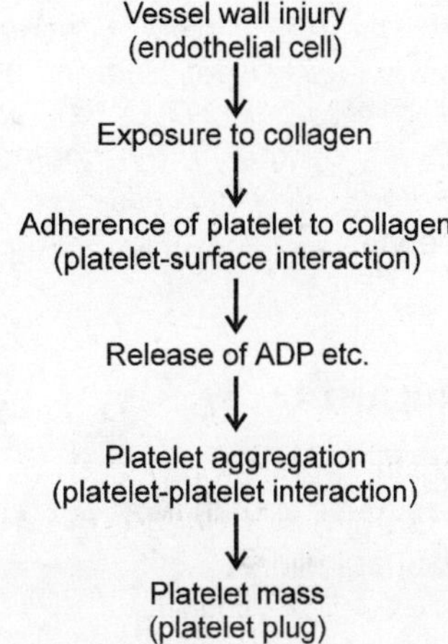

FIG. 5.2: *The primary mechanism of haemostasis*

MECHANISM OF BLOOD COAGULATION

Blood coagulation is the secondary mechanism of haemostasis. Currently this is based on the *Macfarlane's Cascade theory.*

The cascade theory consists of: (i) the '**intrinsic system**', and (ii) the '**extrinsic system**'. The final steps of the two systems are the same (**Fig. 5.3**).

To simplify, the **intrinsic system** requires all factors in blood and damaged platelets to form **thromboplastin,** and simultaneously the **extrinsic system** utilizes tissue factor, factor V, and factor VII to generate **thromboplastin**. Further, thromboplastin and calcium **convert prothrombin to thrombin**, and **thrombin converts fibrinogen to fibrin**. Finally fibrin mesh

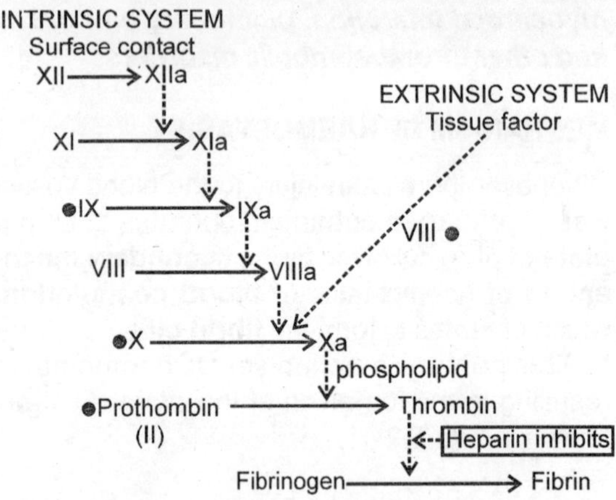

Fig. 5.3 : *Mechanism of blood coagulation. The 'cascade' system (simplified), showing the sites of action of major anticoagulant drugs. a = activated; ● = reduction of synthesis by coumarins and indanediones (oral anticoagulants).*

entraps the erythrocytes and leucocytes to form the **clot.**

ANTICOAGULANTS

The anticoagulants commonly used are: (i) **Direct acting**, like heparin; and (ii) **Indirect acting**, like warfarin and phenindione.

CLASSIFICATION OF ANTICOAGULANTS

1. **Intravenous anticoagulant (directly acting)**
   Heparin.
2. **Oral anticoagulants (Indirectly acting)**
   - *Coumarin derivatives*
     Warfarin (Coumadin)
     Acenocoumarin (Sintrom).
   - *Indanedione derivative*
     Phenindione (Dindevan).

INTRAVENOUS ANTICOAGULANT

Heparin

Heparin largely occurs in the mast cells around the blood vessels. Commercially heparin is prepared from ox lung, and standardized on animal blood.

Mode of action: Heparin inhibits clotting both *in vivo* and *in vitro*. In solution it carries a strong **electronegative charge** which is responsible for its interaction with basic proteins needed for clotting. Heparin with an alpha-globulin forms a complex, which has a powerful **antithrombin activity.** This chiefly accounts for its anticoagulant activity, **prolonging the clotting time of blood.** In addition, heparin has an **antithromboplastin effect.**

Heparin *reduces lipaemia* following a fatty meal by causing a redistribution of plasma lipoprotein fractions.

Dose: Heparin is ineffective orally. It has to be injected intravenously or subcutaneously. It is usually given in a dose of 10,000 to 12,500 I.U. (100 mg = 10,000 I.U). The plasma $t_{½}$ is 50 minutes (low dose) and 120 minutes (high dose). The injections should be repeated every 4 to 6 hours.

Control of therapy: The **clotting time** should be maintained above 15 minutes (normal 5 to 7 minutes), i.e., about twice the normal. It should be measured before start of heparin therapy, and later once daily before an injection is due.

Adverse effects: Haemorrhagic tendency may develop due to prolonged clotting time of blood.

Long-term heparin treatment may cause **osteoporosis.** Hypersensitivity reactions may occur.

Heparin Antagonists

Heparin overdosage lasts for a short time, as it is metabolized in a few hours. However, heparin antagonists have an important role to play, as they are used during the **extracorporeal bypass procedure** so that the blood returns to the body with normal coagulability.

Protamine sulphate, a protein obtained from *fish sperm* is strongly basic, and nullifies the anticoagulant action of heparin which is acidic. It is given intravenously and neutralizes an equal weight of heparin.

ORAL ANTICOAGULANTS

The **coumarins** and **indanediones** are derivatives of 4-hydroxycoumarin, and indane-1, 3-dione respectively. They are active orally and only *in vivo*.

Mode of action: The coumarins and indanediones act by r*educing the synthesis of prothrombin (Factor II) factors VII, IX and X* (**Fig. 5.3**). The normal synthesis of these four factors requires vitamin K. *The anticoagulant effect on an average takes 36-48 hours to build up.*

Pharmacokinetics: These agents are well absorbed on oral administration, and peak levels occur in 2-3 hours (**Table 5.1**). In the blood they are largely bound to plasma protein. The coumarins and indanediones cross the placenta and predispose to foetal and neonatal bleeding.

Control of therapy: Quick's one stage '*prothrombin time*' or Quick time is determined to regulate the dose. A satisfactory control is obtained with the *patient's prothormbin time maintained 2 to 3 times normal* (normal about 12 seconds). Initially the prothormbin time should be measured daily till it is stabilized, and later may be checked once monthly.

Adverse effects: Bleeding may occur due to an overdose, specially in the renal and alimentary tracts. **Subdural** and **intracerebral haematomas** may occur. Patients with liver disease or vitamin K deficiency are specially prone to these complications. Other adverse reactions include **skin rashes, blood dyscrasias, jaundice** and **vomiting.**

Vitamin K as Antidote

Vitamin K_1 (water soluble) may be administered in a dose of 100-200 mg IV. On IV administration the prothrombin time return to normal in 3 to 5 hours, and on oral administration within 12 hours. *Vitamin K preparations do not antagonize heparin effect.* In a serious emergency fresh **whole blood transfusion** may be given.

Therapeutic Uses of Anticoagulants

1. **Venous thromboembolism.**
2. **Arterial thrombosis.**
3. **Deep venous thrombosis and pulmonary embolism.**
4. **Acute myocardial infarction:** Anticoagulant therapy may be of benefit if started within 3 days of the episode. The duration of therapy is usually 2-4 weeks.
5. **Atrial fibrillation.**
6. **Acute coronary insufficiency and angina pectoris:** These patients may benefit, but routine use is not advocated.
7. **Cerebrovascular disease:** There is inconvulsive evidence whether the anticoagulants are useful in transient ischaemic attacks (TIA).
8. **Retinal vein or artery thrombosis.**

Table 5.1 : *Oral anticoagulants, their dosage and therapeutic profile*

	Dose*		Anticoagulant effect			Therapeutic Profile
Drug	Initial (mg/day)	Maintenance (mg/day)	Onset (hrs)	Peak (hrs)	Duration (days)	
Coumarins						
Warfarin sodium**	30-50	2.5-25	2-12	36-48	4-5	Intermediate
Acenocoumarin	16-28	2-12	12-24	36-48	1-2	Short
Indanediones						
Phenindione	200-300	25-200	8-12	24-28	1-4	Short

* Because of long $t_{1/2}$ and indirect mode of action, if dosage is to be changed, it should be every 5-7 days, when a steady-state is attained.

** Warfarin sodium can be used in a dose of 50 mg IV or IM.

9. **Vascular surgery:** Anticoagulants may be useful both during and after surgery.

Contraindications

In disorders with a bleeding tendency, like **haemorrhoids, ulcerative colitis, hepatic diseases,** and **blood diseases** the anticoagulants are contraindicated. **Hypertension** increases the risk of cerebral haemorrhage. *Severe haematuria* may occur if the kidneys are previously damaged.

Drug Interactions

As the oral anticoagulants are bound to plasma proteins, any other drug with a higher affinity for proteins would displace them, leading to an increased sensitivity and toxicity, even when the dose of the anticoagulant given is well within the therapeutic limits.

Drugs enhancing anticoagulation: Sulphonamides, clofibrate, ethacrynic acid, methylphenidate, anabolic steroids and quinidine.

Drugs diminishing anticoagulations: Barbiturates, phenytoin, griseofulvin, vitamin K.

HAEMOSTATIC AGENTS

Haemostatics are agents used to arrest bleeding, or to control oozing from minute blood vessels by the formation of an **artificial clot**, or by providing a matrix which facilitates clotting. They are ineffective in combating bleeding from large arteries and veins. Since they are ultimately absorbed from the site of application, they are known as **absorbable haemostatics.**

Absorbable Haemostatics

1. **Gelatin sponge:** It is used to control capillary bleeding. It is a surgical sponge which is left in place after the closure of the operative wound.
2. **Oxidized cellulose:** It is surgical gauze or cotton, specially treated to promote clotting by a reaction between haemoglobin and cellulosic acid.
3. **Human fibrinogen:** Fibrinogen with thrombin solution can be used locally to induce clotting.
4. **Fibrin foam:** It is used as a mechanical agent to promote blood clotting. It is applied directly to the bleeding area.
5. **Russel's viper venom:** It has a strong thromboplastin activity, and may be used in cases of haemophilia. It is applied locally and should never be injected.
6. **Thrombin:** It is obtained from bovine plasma, and should be only used topically. It can be used in the form of a solution or powder with *gelatin sponge*, or *fibrin foam*.
7. **Adrenaline:** It is useful in **epistaxis.** It stops bleeding by causing local vasoconstriction when the bleeding nostril is packed with gauze soaked in adrenaline solution.

Systemic Haemostatics

Systemic agents for checking bleeding are less well established. The antifibrinolysins (**aminocaproic** and **tranexamic acid**, **ethamsylate** and **naftazone**) have been claimed to reduce capillary bleeding when given systemically.

5.3 FIBRINOLYTIC AND ANTIPLATELET DRUGS

The blood has an inborn capacity of dissolving intravascular clots by means of its **fibrinolytic system**. Agents which promote fibrinolysis are designated as **fibrinolytics** or **thrombolytics**.

FIBRINOLYTIC DRUGS

The fibrinolytic system works through fibrinolysin (also called plasmin) which is a proteolytic enzyme with a marked affinity for fibrinogen or fibrin. The working sequence of this system is detailed in **Fig. 5.4**.

The drugs acting on the fibrinolytic system can be divided into: **plasminogen activators**, and **plasminogen inhibitors.**

PLASMINOGEN ACTIVATORS

Streptokinase

Streptokinase is derived from β-haemolytic strepto

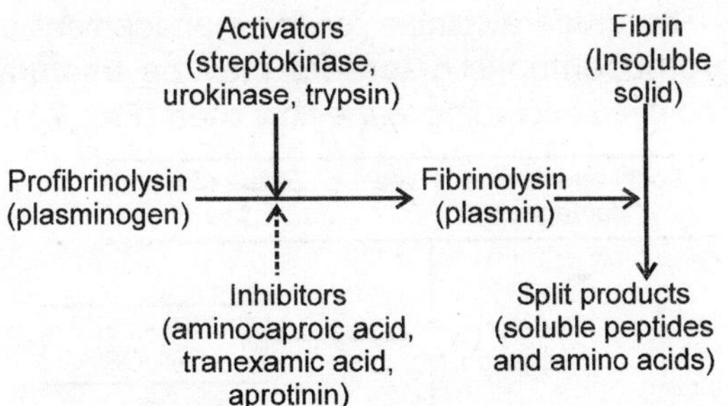

Fig. 5.4: *Fibrinolytic system, its activators and inhibitors.*

cocci, and it acts as a plasminogen activator leading to fibrinolysis. It can be used in **deep vein thrombosis, pulmonary embolism,** or **central retinal vein thrombosis**. It has been used in **myocardial infarction** with success.

It is given by intravenous infusion upto a loading dose of 500,000 units by an infusion pump over 30 minutes. This is followed by an infusion of 100,000 unit hourly. To control therapy the *thrombin time* is maintained 2 to 4 times normal.

Urokinase

Urokinase is a plasminogen activator, related to streptokinase, physiologically occurring in *human urine*. It is extremely expensive. Urokinase can be used in patients allergic to streptokinase.

PLASMINOGEN INHIBITORS (ANTIFIBRINOLYTIC DRUGS)

Aminocaproic Acid

Aminocaproic acid inhibits competitively the activation of plasminogen to plasmin. It is a specific **antidote** for an overdose of a fibrinolytic agent. It is used sometimes to control **haemophilia.** It has also been used in the treatment of haemorrhage due to **severe trauma, major surgery,** in **obstetric complications, leukaemias** and **hepatic cirrhosis.**

The usual dose is 5 g initially (orally or IV), followed by 1.25 g per hour till bleeding stops. Aminocaproic acid may promote *disseminated intravascular clotting.*

Tranexamic Acid

Like aminocaproic acid tranexamic acid may also *enhance the tendency towards intravascular coagulation.* It is administered IV (divided daily doses of 1.5-3.0 g) or orally (divided daily doses of 1.0 or 1.5 g), and is available as 500 mg tablets or injection (100, 250 mg).

ANTIPLATELET DRUGS

The **antiplatelet drugs** also known as **platelet aggregation inhibitors,** possess diverse structures and actions. They are used for the treatment of thrombosis occurring in disorders like **myocardial infarction,** and **cerebrovascular stroke,** and **transient cerebral ischaemic attacks.**

BASIS OF ANTIPLATELET DRUG THERAPY

Out of the many approaches to thrombosis prevention, **two** are most noteworthy:

i. **Inhibition of cyclo-oxygenase in platelets:** Aspirin, sulphinpyrazone, and indomethacin.
ii. **Elevation of cyclic adenosine 3'5'-monophosphate levels in platelets:** Dipyridamole.

INDIVIDUAL DRUGS

Out of the many drugs which affect platelet function only **aspirin, dipyridamole** and **sulphinyrazone** would be dealt in further detail.

Aspirin

Aspirin ***irreversibly inactivates the enzyme cyclo-oxygenase,*** and thus interferes with the production of cyclic endoperoxides, thereby inhibiting platelet aggregation.

Clinically aspirin has proved effective in doses of 300 mg daily. Higher doses should not be given as they nullify the beneficial effect.

Dipyridamole

Dipyridamole ***elevates endogenous c-AMP*** levels by inhibiting phosphodiesterase and ***inhibits platelet aggregation.*** **Thus it has a synergistic**

action when used in combination with aspirin. The suggested dosage schedule for combination therapy is **dipyridamole** 100 mg daily, plus **aspirin** 500 mg daily. *The precaution is that very high doses of aspirin antagonize dipyridamole effect.*

Sulphinpyrazone

Sulphinpyrazone essentially is a *uricosuric agent.* It inhibits platelet aggregation by ***reversibly inactivating cyclo-oxygenase,*** and thereby leading to the inhibition of prostaglandin and thromboxane A_2 synthesis in the platelets. This drug has been tried in cases of myocardial infarction. The usual dose employed is 600-800 mg daily.

Therapeutic Uses

The antiplatelet drugs have been variously employed, singly or in combination for:

i. ***Prevention of myocardial infarction*** and **reinfarction.**
ii. Myocardial ischaemia and angina pectoris.
iii. Transient cerebral ischaemia and stroke.
iv. Postoperative venous thrombosis.
v. Haemodialysis, arteriovenous shunts, prosthetic heart valves and arterial surgery.
vi. Microvascular disorders.
vii. Organ transplant rejection reactions.

Adverse effects: ***Bleeding complications*** might develop, but are mild and manageable.

Ticlopidine

Ticlopidine reduces platelet aggregation by inhibiting the ADP pathway of platelets. It inhibits binding of fibrinogen to platelets. Ticlopidine also reduces the viscosity of whole blood. The use of ticlopidine is restricted to ***patients intolerant to aspirin for prevention of strokes, transient ischaemic attacks, unstable angina, CABG, secondary prophylaxis of myocardial infarction, and percutaneous transluminal coronary angiography (PTCA).*** The **dose** is 250 mg bid with or after meals.

The drugs available for the management of thromboembolic disorders may be usefully employed according to the flow chart (**Fig. 5.5**).

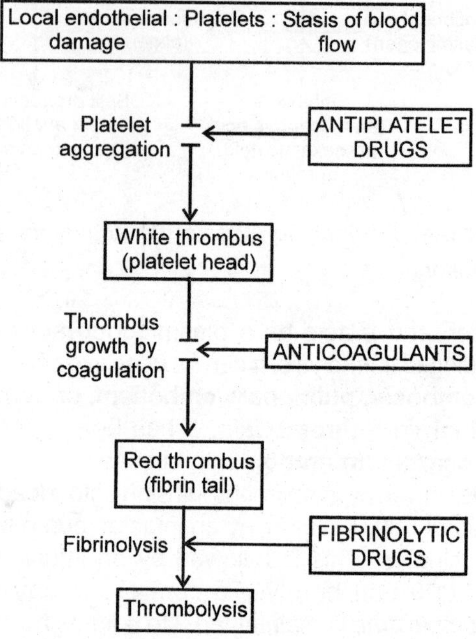

Fig. 5.5: *Points of therapeutic application of antiplatelet, anticoagulant, and fibrinolytic drugs in various phases of thrombus formation.*

Antiplatelet drugs should be employed mainly before the formation of the **white thrombus** to inhibit platelet aggregation. The **anticoagulants** prevent the deposition of fibrin in the thrombus, and retard thrombus growth. The **fibrinolytic drugs** attempt to remove deposited fibrin from the **red thrombus** leading to thrombolysis.

5.4 HYPOLIPIDAEMIC AGENTS

Cholesterol is a lipid. It is synthesized from acetate in many tissues of the body. The basic scheme for its synthesis is **Acetate→Mevalonate→ Squalene→Lanosterol→Cholesterol.** It is highly fat soluble with a limited water solubility, and it localizes itself in the lipid regions of cell membranes.

Lipids exist in the blood mainly as **cholesterol** and **triglycerides.** In addition there are smaller amounts of phospholipids, fatty acids and fatty acid esters. Free fatty acids (FFA) are bound to plasma albumin, while other lipids form complexes with proteins (albumin, globulins). These lipoproteins differ in **density, composition** and **size**, and are separable by **electrophoresis.** Based on their electrophoretic density patterns they mainly are: (i) **chylomicrons;** (ii) very low density lipoproteins (**VLDL**); (iii) low density lipoproteins (**LDL**); and (iv) high density lipoproteins α – lipoproteins (**HDL**). The WHO has classified hyperlipidaemias into Types I, IIa, IIb, III, IV, and V, depending on their lipoprotein and lipid profile.

ATHEROSCLEROSIS

Atherosclerosis is a metabolic disorder characterized by faulty transport, distribution and deposition of lipids. It is influenced by multiple factors. The concept that atherosclerosis is necessarily associated with hypercholesterolaemia, and subsequent formation of **atheromatous plaques** in the intimal walls of the arteries is accepted. This disorder mainly affects the large and medium sized arteries, namely, the **cerebral, coronary, vertebral** and **renal** arteries. The important clinical complications are **coronary heart disease, cerebrovascular disease,** and **peripheral vascular disease.**

Many authorities agree that any person whose plasma cholesterol level is higher than 200 mg/dl, and whose plasma triglyceride level exceeds 150 mg/dl has sufficient hyperlipaemia to require attention. Adults have elevated levels due to *improper diet, excessive alcohol intake, hypothyroidism, diabetes mellitus, or an inherited trait.*

HYPOLIPIDAEMIC DRUGS

The available drugs are:

i. Predominantly effective in *hypertriglyceridaemias*:
   Fibric acid derivatives: Clofibrate, Gemflbrozll, Fenofibrate, Bezafibrate.
ii. Predominantly effective in *hypercholesterolaemia*:
   Bile acid-binding resins: Cholestyramine, Colestipol.
   HMG-CoA reductase inhibitors: Lovastatin, Atorvastatin, Fluvastatin, Pravastatin, Simvastatin, Rosuvastatin.
iii. **Miscellaneous drugs:** Nicotinic acid, Dextrothyroxine, Safflower oil, Gugulipid.

Fibric Acid Derivatives

Their main action is to ***decrease serum triglycerides***, but they also ***reduce LDL-cholesterol,*** and ***raise HDL-cholesterol***.

Fibric Acid Derivatives

Clofibrate

Clofibrate is used in patients with *hypertriglyceridaemia* or *hypercholesterolaemia* to reduce the respective blood levels. Clofibrate can cause serious toxicity.

Mode of action: Clofibrate probably ***inhibits hepatic cholesterol synthesis***, and decreases, the rate of lipoprotein release from the liver.

Side effects: Nausea, gastrointestinal upset, drowsiness, headache and dizziness may occur. Weight gain, pruritus, skin rashes, alopecia, leucopenia, and agranulocytosis have been reported. A rise in transaminases may occur. Hypoglycaemia can occur in some patients.

Therapeutic uses: Clofibrate is useful in hyperlipidaemia types III, IV and V, but is less effective in type II.

Dose: Upto 2 g daily in 4 divided doses depending on the patient's response.

Gemfibrozil

Gemfibrozil is a *structural analogue of clofibrate,* and shares many of its pharmacologic and toxicologic properties. It has a variable effect on cholesterol. It may also increase the HDL fraction, and the ratio of HDL cholesterol to total cholesterol.

Gemfibrozil is used in the treatment of *types IV and V hyperlipoproteinaemia* in patients with high serum triglyceride, and a definite risk of pancreatitis. The **adverse effects** include GI distress, skin rash, musculoskeletal pain, blurred vision, anaemia and leucopenia. It may enhance the effect of oral anticoagulants. The **recommended dosage** is 1200 mg a day in 2 divided doses, 30 minutes before meals.

Fenofibrate

Fenofibrate is a relatively newer agent. It has the same indications as gemfibrozil. The **usual dosage** is 100 mg orally after each meal.

Bezafibrate

Bezafibrate induces appreciable reduction in plasma triglycerides, VLDL, and LDL cholesterol. HDL levels are raised.

Mode of action: It increases the activity of *lipoprotein lipase*, and several other enzymes. It promotes the effect of anticoagulants in patients of hyperlipoproteinaemia.

Indications: All forms of hyperlipidaemias resistant to diet control; and secondary hyperlipidaemias associated with diabetes mellitus, gout, and chronic renal failure.

Dose: 200 mg tid reduced to bid as maintenance.

Adverse reactions include GI upset, myalgia, muscle cramps, headache, nausea, anorexia, alopecia, leucopenia, and decreased libido.

BILE ACID BINDING RESINS

Cholestyramine

Colestipol

Cholestyramine is the chloride salt of a quaternary ammonium anion-exchange resin, which in the intestinal lumen binds bile acids, exchanged for chloride. This insoluble ***resin complex is not absorbed***, and thus it promotes the fecal excretion of bile acids which would have been otherwise largely reabsorbed from the intestines.

Cholestyramine may be used in doses of 4g thrice daily in hyperlipidaemia type II. However, it is mainly used for the r***elief of pruritus due to biliary tract obstruction.*** **Side effects** include constipation, diarrhoea, heart burn or nausea.

Lately the anion-exchange resin **colestipol** has been introduced which is similar in action to cholestyramine. It is given orally in a dose of 12-25 g/day in 3 or 4 divided doses.

HMG CoA Reductase Inhibitors

Lovastatin

Lovastatin is isolated from a strain of *Aspergillus terreus.* Compared to many other hypolipidaemic drugs it is well tolerated in majority of patients.

Lovastatin is an inactive lactone. In the body it is hydrolyzed to a beta-hydroxy acid form which is a ***potent inhibitor of HMG CoA reductase,*** an enzyme that catalyzes the conversion of HMG CoA to mevalonate, a **rate-limiting step** in the biosynthesis of cholesterol. It does not adversely affect steroidogenesis. It is mainly used in the treatment of *familial hypercholesterolaemia (types IIA and IIb).* The recommended starting dose is 20 mg (20 mg tablets) once a day with the evening meal. **Side effects** include headache, GI distress, myalgia, increased serum transaminases, blurred vision, and peripheral neuropathy.

Simvastatin

Simvastatin, a HMG CoA reductase inhibitor is a ***prodrug*** which is bioactivated in the liver to form the active *beta hydroxyacid derivative.* This inhibits the conversion of HMG-CoA to mavalonic acid by inhibiting the enzyme HMG-CoA reductase, the ***rate limiting step*** in the synthesis of cholesterol. Simvastatin reduces total cholesterol, LDL cholesterol, and triglycerides. It increases HDL cholesterol. *Indications*: It is used in cases of primary hypercholesterolaemia with elevated LDL and increased risk of coronary artery disease not responding to dietary measures. *Adverse reactions* include myopathy, myalgia, rhabdomyolysis (idiopathic myoglobulinuria) with acute renal failure. In addition headache, nausea, abdominal pain, hypersensitivity, lens opacities, blurred vision, sexual dysfunction, and depression may occur.

Other reductase inhibitors, namely **atorvastatin, fluvastatin** and **pravastatin** have actions and uses similar to lovastatin and simavastatin.

Nicotinic Acid

Nicotinic acid when administered in large doses of 1.5 to 8 g daily, lowers plasma triglyceride and cholesterol levels. Probably *it acts by inhibiting the release of free fatty acids from adipose tissue, and inhibits cholesterol synthesis in the liver.* It has been found effective in hyperlipidaemia types II, III, IV and V . The **side effects** include flushing of the face, dizziness, pruritus, gastrointestinal upset, and liver dysfunction which occur at a fairly high frequency. Thus the usefulness of nicotinic acid as a hypolipidaemic agent is limited.

Dextrothyroxine

The dextro-isomer of thyroxine *increases the rate of oxidation or hydroxylation of cholesterol to bile acids in the liver, and promotes the biliary excretion of cholesterol.* This lowers the blood cholesterol level. Dextrothyroxine may be effective in hyperlipidaemia types II and III, but the **side effects** due to general metabolic stimulation including angina pectoris and arrhythmias, seriously limits its use.

Safflower Oil

This fixed oil is extracted from the seeds of safflower, *Carthamus tinctotius.* It contains linoleic acid (unsaturated fatty acid), and mixed saturated fatty acids. *Safflower oil reduces serum cholesterol when used instead of saturated fats (animal fats).* Safflower oil is available as a 65 percent emulsion of the oil, and may be used as a cooking medium.

Gugulipid

Gugulipid is an Indian indigenous medicine. It is a mixture of sterones obtained from *gum guggul* (used in the Ayurvedic system of medicine). It is moderately effective in cases of *hypercholesterolaemia* and *hypertriglyceridaemia. Dose:* One tablet (25 mg) thrice daily.

Other agents like b-sitosterol, oestrogens, neomycin, and aminosalicylic acid also possess hypolipidaemic action, but are not used therapeutically.

Fish Oils

Cold water fish oils rich in *omega-3 marine triglycerides,* namely *eicosapentaenoic acid* and *docosahexaenoic acid* when ingested are useful in cases of severe *hypertriglyceridaemia.* Such preparations may also be used for their *antiplatelet* action.

5.5 BLOOD AND PLASMA VOLUME EXPANDERS

Anaemias caused by **hypoplasia** or **aplasia** of the bone marrow can only be managed by blood transfusions. Similarly, in the management of **haemorrhagic shock** whole blood transfusion has no better substitute.

A search for suitable plasma substitutes has been rewarding. The plasma substitute *must have the qualities of plasma itself,* i.e., (i) its osmotic pressure should match with that of blood; (ii) it should be metabolized and excreted without toxic effects; (iii) it should be non-antigenic; and (iv) it should be compatible with the elements of blood.

Plasma volume expanders are agents which may overcome the imbalance in conditions of shock, and tide over the critical period until the ideal material is available, or the patient recuperates. The agents available are: (i) Blood and its elements; and (ii) Macromolecular colloidal solutions.

BLOOD AND ITS ELEMENTS

Citrated Whole Human Blood

Human blood is collected from healthy donors under aseptic conditions. It is **mandatory** to ensure that the donors are free from AIDS (Acquired immunodeficiency syndrome), or viral hepatitis B infection, as blood transfusion is a mode of transmission of these diseases. Due care is taken to reduce haemolysis during storage. The usual anticoagulant used for preservation is ***acid citrate dextrose*** (ACD) solution. Whole human blood is stored soon after collection and mixing with anticoagulant, in sterile containers at a temperature of 4° to 6°C. Material with signs of haemolysis should not be used.

Whole human blood is used to replace blood volume and elevate oxygen carrying capacity following blood loss due to surgery or severe haemorrhage. The haemoglobin concentration of blood is raised by about 1 g/100 ml by transfusion of 540 ml of whole blood. Due precautions should be taken to properly match the blood to avoid dangerous blood transfusion reactions.

Packed Red Cells

Packed red cells are used in severe forms of anaemia which do not usually require a simultaneous restoration of blood volume. It also reduces the danger of circulatory overload, and pulmonary oedema. Packed red cells are separated from citrated whole blood and cannot be safely stored for longer than 24 hours at a temperature of 10°C.

Dried Human Plasma

This is prepared by drying a sterile pool of supernatant fluid from quantities of whole blood. It is stored below 25°C in an atmosphere of nitrogen in sterile containers, protected from light. **Dried human plasma** is completely soluble in water for injection, and should be used immediately after reconstitution. There is a danger of transmitting ***viral hepatitis type B*** which must be kept in mind.

Human Serum Albumin

Human serum albumin is a sterile solution of the serum albumin fraction of blood from healthy donors. It is used in the management of **shock, hypoproteinaemia,** and **oedema of nephrosis.** Human albumin (5 and 20%) is available as a sterile, pyrogen-free solution for IV use, dried human albumin fraction is also available.

MACROMOLECULAR COLLOIDAL SOLUTIONS

Polygeline

Polygeline is a polymer from degraded gelatin, and is available as a sterile pyrogen-free solution for IV use. It can replace upto 70-80 percent of circulating plasma. It can be used in all forms of **oligaemic shock, burns,** and **endotoxic shock.** It has also been employed for **preoperative haemodilution,** and **perfusion of isolated organs.** Hypersensitivity reactions can occur.

Dextran 70 and Dextran 75

The dextran used clinically is a complex polysaccaride obtained by the action of *Leuconostoc mesentroides* on sucrose. *The average molecular weights are 70,000 for dextran 70, and 75,000 for dextran 75.* The usual dose is about 50 ml of a 6 percent solution infused intravenously at a rate of 20-40 ml /minute. Dextran solutions may cause allergic reactions. Dextrans 70 and 75 are ***mainly used to restore and maintain the blood volume.*** Their advantages over whole blood are their wide availability, lack of incompatibility problems, and their use has no danger of transmitting viral hepatitis or AIDS.

Dextran 40

This preparation is popularly designated as *low molecular weight dextran* (Mol. Wt. 40,000). It is available as a 10 percent solution in dextrose, or sodium chloride injection. It is known that dextrans disrupt aggregation of red cells and have a **"desludging action"** in the blood vessels. Dextran 40 is primarily used for the **prevention** and **therapy of venous thrombosis.** There are claims that dextran 40 also improves capillary microcirculation by its **desludging** action.

Hetastarch

Hetastarch is a synthetic polymer prepared from **amylopectin.** Its actions are similar to dextran and can be used for blood volume expansion.

Hetastarch is available as 6 percent solution in sodium chloride 0.9 percent injection. The usual dose is 500-1000 ml, upto a maximum of 1500 ml daily.

To conclude, agents are available to make up for the lost blood volume, and for maintaining optimal fluidity, and osmotic pressure of blood.

Drugs Acting on the Genitourinary System

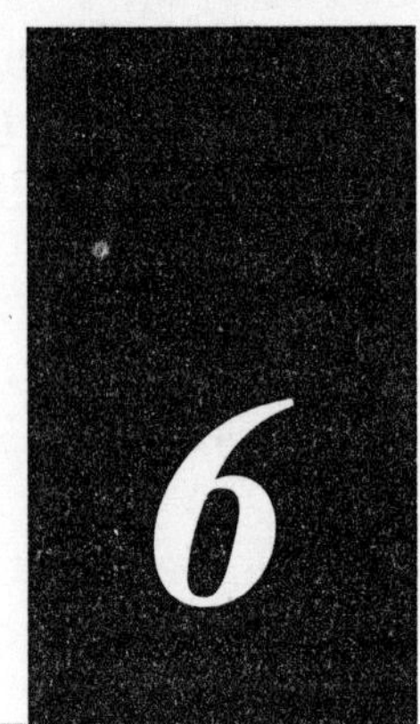

6.1 FLUID AND ELECTROLYTE BALANCE

Next to oxygen, water is most important to life. The volume and composition of the body fluids varies within a narrow range from day to day, there being a state of balance between the intake and elimination from the body. A balance between *water, electrolytes* and *acid-base content* of the body is extremely important for **homeostasis** (**Fig. 6.1**).

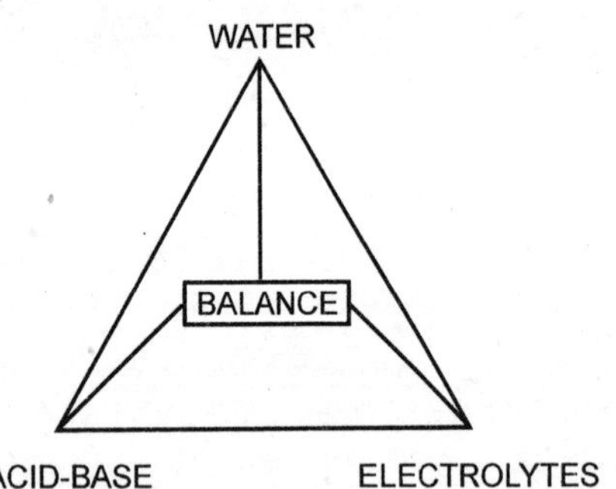

Fig. 6.1: *The triangle of homeostasis*

Disturbances in fluid and electrolyte metabolism involve four major properties, namely, *volume, osmolality, hydrogen ion concentration* (pH), and *specific ion concentrations.*

WATER BALANCE

The prime importance of water is evident by the fact that 45-65 percent of body weight in man is water, i.e., about 42 litres is the total body water (TBW). The total volume of water is divided into **two** major compartments: **the extracellular fluid** (ECF) compartment, and the **intracellular fluid** (ICF) compartment. Almost all cell membranes are freely permeable to water.

ELECTROLYTE BALANCE

Electrolytes are inorganic salts present in solution as charged ions (cation$^+$, positive; anion$^-$, negative). They maintain the osmotic pressure, which maintains the volume of the solvent water. An **isotonic solution** is one which exerts a physiological osmotic pressure, and causes no passage of water across the cell membrane.

A **molar solution** (M) contains a mole/litre. For a monovalent substance (Na^+, K^+, Cl^-) **normality**, i.e., the concentration in mEq/l equals the molarity, whereas for divalent substances (Ca^{++}, SO_4^{--}) normality will be half molarity. **Molarity** is applicable to any soluble substance the molecular weight of which is known.

The **sodium pump** which is an active chemical pump in the cell membrane, continuously extrudes Na^+ from the cell, and K^+ is transported inwards.

The 0.9 percent saline solution is isotonic to body fluid, and is usually termed 'normal saline'.

COMPOSITION OF BODY FLUIDS

There are marked differences in the composition of the **extracellular** and **intracellular fluid.**

Table 6.1: *Average daily water intake and output in a healthy adult*

Intake	ml	Output	ml
Water drunk	1500	Urine output	1600
Water in food	750	Faecal water	50
Water from metabolism of food	250	Water lost in expired air : Insensible and sensible persipiration	850
Total	2500		2500

Sodium is the major cation in the *extracellular fluid,* with **chloride** and **bicarbonate** as the major anions in ECF. In contrast, the major cations in the *intracellular fluid* are **potassium** and **magnesium,** with very little sodium, and the main anions are **phosphate** and **protein** with **very little bicarbonate**.

Physiological or normal hydration of the body is maintained by a balance between the water **intake** and the **output** in a healthy individual (**Table 6.1**).

ACID-BASE BALANCE

In the ECF the pH is normally maintained with remarkable constancy, at about 7.4 in arterial blood, and about 7.35 in venous blood and interstitial fluid. pH values of arterial blood below 7.4 are classified as **acidosis**, and a pH value above 7.4 is classified as **alkalosis**.

An excess of CO_2 produces ***acidosis*** which stimulates the respiratory centre to eliminate the CO_2 in the expired air, correcting the acidosis. Whereas, in ***alkalosis*** the CO_2 level of ECF is reduced, the respiratory centre is depressed causing temporary apnoea which restores the body fluid pH to normal.

ACID-BASE DISTURBANCES

Alkalosis and acidosis are disturbances of the acid-base balance. The induced disturbance may be compensated or uncompensated (**Table 6.2**).

In simple terms, **acidosis** denotes a decrease in pH (rise in H^+), and ***alkalosis*** denotes an increase in pH (fall in H^+) of the extracellular fluid. These changes are the result of **respiratory** or **metabolic** abnormalities.

Table 6.2 : *The acid-base disturbances*

Acid-base disturbance	*Bicarbonate content (plasma)*	*pH*
Compensated alkalosis	Increased	Unchanged
Uncompensated alkalosis	Increased	Rises
Compensated Acidosis	Decreased	Unchanged
Uncompensated acidosis	Depleted	Falls

Potassium

Potassium is the major intracellular cation. It is also found in low but critical concentration in the extracellular fluid. Its concentration varies from 3.4 to 5.6 mEq/litre in health. Potassium plays an important role in *muscle contraction, enzyme action, nerve conduction,* and *cell membrane function.* The myocardial excitability, conduction and rhythm are markedly affected by the concentration of K^+ in ECF.

Hypokalaemia

Diuretic therapy is the most common cause of hypokalaemia. Hypokalaemia manifests as a depression of the ST segment, and a lowering of the T-wave in the electrocardiogram (ECG), and a prominent U wave which may be biphasic (**Fig. 6.2**).

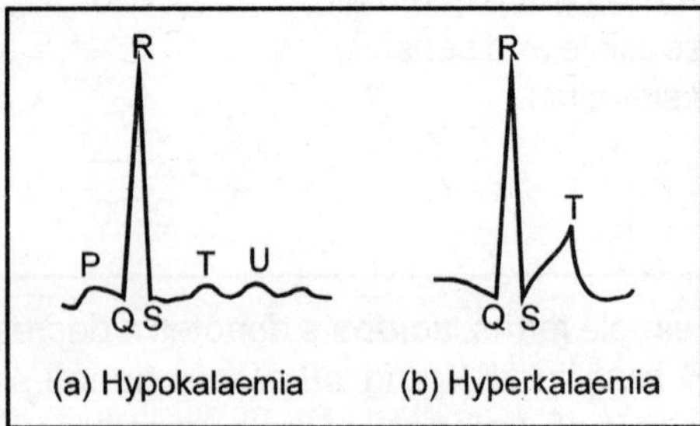

Fig. 6.2: *The electrocardiogram in potassium*

Hyperkalaemia

Hyperkalaemia is usually the result of *inefficient potassium excretion by the kidneys* due to impaired renal function, or due to large amounts of K^+ ingested in diet. The extracellular concentration of K^+ increases, and the ECG manifests an absence of P-wave, and tall T-waves, ventricular fibirillation and cardiac arrest (**Fig. 6.2**).

Calcium

Calcium levels in the blood range between 10 to 10.5 mg/dl. In the blood it exists in two forms, half of it bound to protein as **non-diffusible** calcium, and the other half as **diffusible** calcium in chemically complexed and ionized form. The serum calcium level is controlled by opposing effects of two hormones—**parathormone** and **calcitonin,** both exerting their major effect on bone which is the calcium depot.

Magnesium

Magnesium is an important activator ion participating in many enzyme actions, including those requiring ATP or other nucleotides as co-enzymes. The normal plasma level is 1.5-2.5 mEq/litre.

Hypomagnesaemia

Magnesium deficiency is encountered in chronic alcoholism with delirium tremens, starvation, diarrhoea, malabsorption, vigorous diuresis, hypoparathyroidism, and renal tubular damage. It is manifested as CNS hyperirritability.

Hypermagnesaemia

Magnesium excess results from renal insufficiency, and the inability of the kidney to excrete magnesium. Occasionally magnesium sulphate when used as a cathartic may produce toxicity in the presence of impaired renal function.

Ammonia Imbalance

In cases of advanced and complicated cirrhosis the blood ammonia level is elevated leading to a ***portal systemic encephalopathy***, which is a metabolic disorder of the central nervous system.

Peritoneal Dialysis Solutions

These special solutions are used to remove urea, creatinine, uric acid, serum electrolytes, and excess of body fluids and toxins from the body. They are indicated in **acute** and **chronic renal failure, intractable oedema, hyperkalaemia, hypercalaemia,** and **poisoning with dialysable agents**. Peritoneal dialysis is a specialized technique, and both overhydration and hypovolaemia should be avoided.

6.2 DIURETICS

Diuretics are commonly defined as drugs that increase the amount of urine produced by the kidneys. A ***precise definition*** is that diuretics are agents which augment the renal excretion of **sodium,** and either **chloride** or **bicarbonate** primarily, and water excretion secondarily. The term '**saluretic**' is used to describe a drug that increases the renal excretion of sodium and chloride ions.

Physiologically fluid exchange is controlled by the balance between the ***blood colloid osmotic (oncotic) pressure, and the hydrostatic pressure along the capillary system*** (**Fig. 6.3**). But due to an abnormal pressure relationship **more** of fluid leaves the capillary system at the arterial end, and **less** of it returns at the venous end resulting in **oedema.**

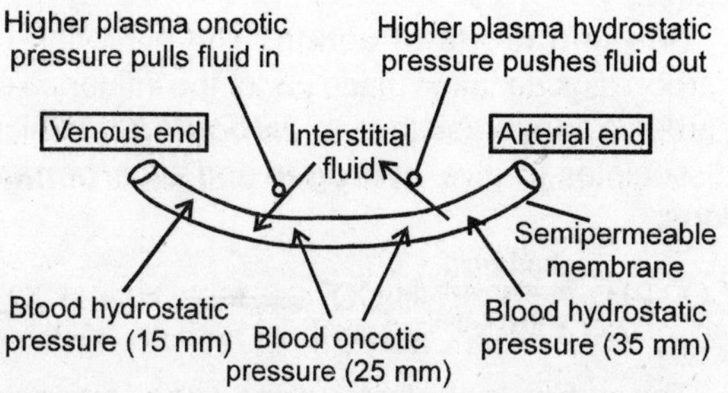

Fig. 6.3: *The normal capillary system of fluid exchange.*

RENAL REGULATION OF WATER AND ELECTROLYTE BALANCE

The kidney is primarily a regulatory organ. It adjusts the amount of fluid and essential chemicals in the ***intracellular*** and ***extracellular*** fluid compartments. The major functions of the kidney are:

1. Excretion of the *nitrogenous waste products of protein metabolism.*
2. Maintenance of *acid-base equilibrium,* and
3. Maintenance of *sodium, potassium, chloride* and *bicarbonate ions* in a proper balance.

The functional unit of the kidney is the **nephron,** and the above three functions are carried out by the complex process of urine formation, which consists of the production of an **ultrafiltrate of plasma** in the glomeruli, *reabsorption* and *secretion of electrolytes,* and *other solutes* in the tubules, and a *passive diffusion of water* and *solutes* according to the concentration gradients caused by the active transfer of sodium and chloride ions across the tubules.

CLASSIFICATION OF DIURETICS

Although these drugs vary in their chemical structure and mechanisms of action, almost all of them **interfere with the tubular reabsorption of sodium**. A classification of diuretics is presented in **Table 6.3**.

Table 6.3: *The diuretic agents*

Class	*Total daily dose (mg)*
I. Benzothiadiazides and relate compounds	
The thiazides	
Hydrochlorothiazide	25-100*
Related compounds	
Chlorthalidone	50-100
Indapamide	2.5-5.0
II. High-ceiling or loop diuretics	
Furosemide (Lasix)	20-80 20-40 mg IV 0.5-2.0
Torsemide	5-20
Ethacrynic acid	25-50 50-100 mg IV
III. Carbonic anhydrase inhibitor	
Acetazolamide	250-500
IV. Potassium-sparing diuretics	
Spironolactone	25-100
Triamterene	100-200
Amiloride	50-100
V. Osmotic diuretics	
Mannitol	50-100 g IV in 15-20% solution 40-120 g IV in 4% solution
Glycerin (Glycerol)	1-1.5 g/kg
VI. Methylxanthines	
Aminophylline	250-500 mg IV slowly

* Daily dosage in mg orally, unless otherwise mentioned

INDIVIDUAL AGENTS

Benzothiadiazides (Thiazides)

The prototype agent, **chlorothiazide** was introduced in 1958, and became widely used as an orally effective agent. The thiazides are related chemically to the *sulphonamides,* but have no antibacterial activity.

Site and mode of action: Their main action is ***to block the active reabsorption of sodium (Na^+) and chloride (Cl^-)*** with water in the distal tubule by inhibition of Na^+/K^+-adenosine triphosphatase (ATPase). This limits the energy supply for active transport in the tubule. They have a **saluretic action.**

Toxicity: The thiazides may cause dizziness, weakness, fatigue, and leg cramps. But the major side effects of thiazides are **hypopotassaemia, hyperuricaemia,** and **aggravation of diabetes mellitus. Hyperuricaemia** may precipitate gout in susceptible patients. **Caution** is specially required in patients with severe hepatic or renal damage, as the thiazides may induce *hepatic coma or renal failure.* Rarely thiazides may cause skin rashes, leucopenia, thrombocytopenic purpura, and agranulocytosis.

High-Ceiling or Loop Diuretics

Furosemide, torsemide and **ethacrynic acid** have been labelled as "high-ceiling" or "loop-diuretics" because they inhibit the *sodium* and *chloride* reabsorption in the thick segment of the ascending limb of the loop of Henle, as well as in the proximal convoluted tubule, and the distal diluting site. Thus they are **potent** diuretics.

Site and mode of action: There is an increased urine volume with loss of Na^+, K^+ and Cl^-. The Cl^- loss induces **hypochloraemic alkalosis,** and K^+ loss may provoke digoxin intoxication. **Unlike most other diuretics, the loop diuretics continue to be effective even in the presence of electrolyte and acid-base imbalance, and nitrogen retention.**

Toxicity: A rapid reduction in extracellular fluid volume can result in a cardiovascular collapse, with associated hypokalaemia and **hypochloraemic alkalosis**. A **potassium-sparing diuretic** or **potassium supplements** are indicated in digitalized or cirrhotic patients. Furosemide and ethacrynic acid may cause **azotaemia, hyperuricaemia, hypomagnesaemia,** and **hyperglycaemia.** Acute pancreatitis, **agranulocytosis,** and **thrombocytopenia** have been reported. Dose-related **reversible ototoxic effects** like tinnitus, hearing impairment, and rarely deafness can occur.

Carbonic Anhydrase Inhibitor

Acetazolamide is a sulphonamide and is the prototype carbonic anhydrase inhibitor. Carbonic anhydrase inhibitors have a limited use as diuretics.

Site and mode of action: The hydration of carbon dioxide takes place under the influence of carbonic anhydrase to form ***carbonic acid*** which dissociates to give ***hydrogen*** and ***bicarbonate ions***:

$$CO_2 + H_2 \underset{\text{anhydrase}}{\overset{\text{carbonic}}{\rightleftharpoons}} H_2CO_3 \rightleftharpoons H^+ + HCO_3^-$$

The sodium is eliminated along with bicarbonate ions and the water in which they are dissolved. **The urine become alkaline.** Ultimately these agents lead to a build up of acidity in the interstitial fluid, and **metabolic acidosis** results which initiates *compensatory mechanisms* and diuresis ends. Thus, the diuretic effect of acetazolamide is ***self-limiting.***

Therapeutic uses: The carbonic anhydrase inhibitors are ***rarely used as primary diuretics,*** because their action is weak and self-limiting. Their combination with thiazides has a **synergistic** effect. Acetazolamide has been used with benefit in cases of **premenstrual tension, migraine** and **acne vulgaris.**

Toxicity: Paresthesias and drowsiness are common with large doses. **Hepatic coma** or **pre-coma** may be precipitated in cases of hepatic cirrhosis. **Renal calculus formation** may occur due to the alkaline urine leading to precipitation of calcium phosphate crystals. Acetazolamide may have a goitrogenic effect. Hypersensitivity reactions, arganulocytosis, and other blood dyscrasias may occur.

Potassium-Sparing Diuretics

The potassium-sparing diuretics, **spironolactone, triamterene** and **amiloride** interfere with sodium reabsorption at the distal exchange sites and promote sodium excretion while **potassium is conserved.** Their major use is in conjunction with the *thiazides* or *loop diuretics*.

Spironolactone

Spironolactone is an **aldosterone antagonist**. Aldosterone is an adrenal mineralocorticoid responsible for the maintenance of electrolyte balance in the body. It stimulates the sodium pump inducing sodium reabsorption and potassium loss. Spironolactone antagonizes this tubular effect of aldosterone, leading to **sodium and water loss in the urine, and potassium is conserved.**

Therapeutic uses: Spironolactone is generally used in combination with other diuretics, and has been specially useful in cases of **congestive heart failure, hepatic cirrhosis, and nephrotic syndrome.**

Toxicity: Spironolactone may induce **hyperkalaemia,** specially if diuretic therapy is accompanied by high potassium intake. Minor side effects like drowsiness and rashes may occur. It may cause **gynaecomastia, androgen-like side effects** and **gastrointestinal upset. Menstrual disturbances** may occur in women.

Traimterene

Triamterene is a **nonsteroidal** compound which produces a spironolactone-like effect by acting on the distal tubule to increase Na^+, Cl^- and HCO_3^- loss, and conserve K^+. But it is not an aldosterone antagonist. Triamterene is employed in combination with a thiazide or loop diuretic in the management of oedema associated with **congestive heart failure, cirrhosis** or **nephrotic syndrome.**

Amiloride

Amiloride is an organic base and has renal actions like triamterene. Its mode of action is incompletely understood. It has no *aldosterone antagonistic activity*.

Osmotic Diuretics

Osmotic diuretics are *non-electrolytes.* **Mannitol, urea, glycerol** and **isosorbide** are four osmotic diuretics which are freely filtered through the glomerulus, and are insignificantly reabsorbed from the tubules.

Site and mode of action: Under normal condition Na^+ and Cl^- are reabsorbed in the proximal tubule, and since the tubule is permeable to water, there is a ***passive back diffusion*** of water. Such a process keeps the tubular fluid isosmotic. This continues till the major fraction of the glomerular filtrate is reabsorbed. In the presence of a *non-reabsorbable solute* like *mannitol* and *urea* the overall osmotic relationship within the proximal tubule remains almost unaltered. Thus **back diffusion of water does not take place, and less of sodium is reabsorbed**.

Mannitol

This osmotic diuretic is administered intravenously and is useful for the **prophylaxis of acute renal failure**. It is also used to **reduce intraocular pressure and vitreous volume prior to ocular surgery**; to **reduce intracranial pressure in patients of cerebral oedema;** and to promote **excretion of toxic substances.** Headache, nausea, chills, lethargy and confusion may occur. There may be a feeling of constriction or pain in the chest. **Congestive heart failure** and **pulmonary oedema may occur.**

Glycerol

Glycerol is of particular use prior to ophthalmological procedures to **reduce intraocular pressure**. It is given orally in a dose of 1 to 1.5 g/kg usually as a 50 percent solution. The intraocular pressure falls within an hour and the effect continues till 5 hours.

Methylxanthines

The xanthines have a weak diuretic activity. **Aminophylline** (theophylline ethylenediamine) is the most used member. The diuresis is partly a result of cardiac stimulation, better renal haemodynamics, and an increased glomerular filtration rate (GFR). In addition there is a direct action on the tubule, and **sodium reabsorption is inhibited together with an increased Cl^- and water loss.** Aminophylline is used in the management of **acute pulmonary oedema.**

THERAPEUTIC USES OF DIURETICS

For the management of oedematous states three approaches are available: (i) **treat the primary cause**; (ii) **suppress renal tubular reabsorption of salt and water** by diuretics; and (iii) **reduce the intake of sodium salts** which is achieved by a low-salt diet.

1. **Congestive heart failure (CHF):** In an emergency like acute pulmonary oedema, intravenous **furosemide** may be given. In less severe cases, **hydrochlorothiazide** may be used.
2. **Essential hypertension:** The thiazides usually serve as primary antihypertensive agents.
3. **Hepatic cirrhosis with ascites:** Potassium-sparing diuretics like **spironolactone** may be employed.
4. **Nephrotic syndrome:** Dietary sodium restriction may be combined with **thiazides,** adding **spironolactone** to control secondary hyperaldosteronism.
5. **Chronic renal failure:** A loop diuretic like **furosemide** may be useful.
6. **Acute oliguric renal failure:** Mannitol may be employed.
7. **Acute glomerular nephritis:** The hypervolaemia and oedema associated with acute glomerular nephritis is sometimes treated successfully with **furosemide.**
8. **Cerebral oedema:** Oral **glycerol** may be given a trial. Intravenous **mannitol** is usually preferred as a short-term therapy.
9. **Glaucoma:** The carbonic anhydrase inhibitors (acetazolamide) may be used.
10. **Intraocular surgery:** The osmotic diuretics (glycerol, mannitol) are used to reduce intraocular pressure, prior to ocular surgical procedures.
11. **Diabetes insipidus:** The thiazides exhibit **paradoxical antidiuretic action** in patients with *diabetes insipidus*.

COMPLICATIONS OF DIURETIC THERAPY

1. **Metabolic acidosis:** Acetazolamide, may lead to a metabolic acidosis.
2. **Alkalosis:** The thiazides and loop diuretics cause excessive Cl^- ion loss with retention of bicarbonate.
3. **Hypokalaemia:** Loop diuretics, thiazides or carbonic anhydrase inhibitors cause an excessive loss of K^+ via the urine.
4. **Hyperkalaemia:** High levels of plasma K^+ can be the result of hypovolaemia or administration of K^+ sparing diuretics.
5. **Dilutional hyponatraemia:** The loop diuretics or thiazides may cause such a situation.
6. **True hyponatraemia:** The **loop diuretics** or **thiazides** may cause an excessive salt loss (low salt syndrome).

REFRACTORY OEDEMA

Diuretics are likely to lose their efficacy due to factors like: **hyponatraemia, reduction in glomerular filtration rate, hypocholraemic alkalosis,** and **other electrolyte and acid-base imbalances**. Extracellular fluid composition should be readjusted. **Corticosteroids** are sometimes helpful in refractory oedema of cirrhosis liver with ascites.

6.3 DRUGS ACTING ON THE UTERUS

The uterine smooth muscle (myometrium) has its own **inherent rhythm** of contraction and relaxation independent of its nerve supply. In the non-gravid uterus, during the menstrual cycle, the rhythm is influenced by two hormones: (i) **oestrogens**, in the first half of the cycle induce contractions of low amplitude and high frequency; and (ii) **progesterone**, in the second half of the cycle induces contractions of greater amplitude and lower frequency. At the onset of menstruation the contractions become stronger, and sometimes cause pain and discomfort (dysmenorrhoea).

The progesterone production increases through the course of a pregnancy, and is responsible for maintaining the uterus in a non-excitable state. As pregnancy advances these contractions become stronger and more regular till **during labour they are painful, rhythmic, and regular with periods of relaxation in between**. The intensity, duration, and frequency reaches its maximum during the **second** and **third stages** of labour. After a short interval of rest the contractions return, and lead to the **separation** and **expulsion of the placenta,** and then the **involution of uterus** takes place, and the uterus returns to almost its non-gravid shape and size within a period of six weeks.

The drugs acting on the uterus can be classed into two groups:

1. Uterine stimulants (Oxytocics or Ecbolics).
2. Uterine relaxants (Tocolytics).

UTERINE STIMULANTS

Oxytocics or **ecbolics** are drugs which stimulate uterine contractions indirectly or directly, and help in the expulsion of its contents.

i. **Indirect Oxytocics:** These drugs induce pelvic congestion, and stimulate uterine activity, e.g., purgatives.
ii. **Direct Oxytocics:** Oxytocin, ergometrine, and prostaglandins.

Oxytocin

Oxytocin is a **polypeptide hormone** obtained from the posterior pituitary gland. **The sensitivity of the uterus to oxytocin increases with advancing pregnancy**.

Oxytocin concentration is highest in the second stage of labour. It causes **fundal contraction**, and **dilatation of the cervix**. Oxytocin is also released in response to **sucking** by the baby, and helps in **expression of milk,** and also in the **involution of the uterus** during the postnatal period.

Oxytocin causes a **direct** stimulation of the uterine muscle, favouring formation of contractile **actomyosin**. Oxytocin is destroyed when ingested orally, hence it has to be given parenterally.

Therapeutic Uses

1. **Induction of labour:** For induction 2 to 5 units of oxytocin in 1000 ml of 5 percent dextrose injection may be given by slow IV drip.
2. **Hypotonic uterine inertia.**
3. **Retained placenta and postpartum haemorrhage:** Oxytocin 2 to 5 units may be given subcutaneously, IM, or in the form of a drip.
4. **Oxytocin challenge test :** This is one of the tests to determine foetal well being in high risk obstetrical patients.
5. **Engorged breasts:** For let down of milk from engorged breasts 5 units oxytocin may be given IM before expression of breast milk manually or by a breast pump.
6. **Incomplete abortion**.

Oxytocin is not administered to women with a previous history of uterine surgery, or cesarean section, or when the uterus is overdistended as rupture of the uterus can occur. Oxytocin should only be administered by a well trained staff.

Ergometrine

Ergot is the product of a fungus ***Claviceps purpurea*** which grows on rye and other grains. **Ergometrine is the only alkaloid used as an oxytocic**. Ergometrine and its semisynthetic derivative **methylergometrine** are extensively used as oxytocics.

Ergometrine acts directly on the uterine smooth muscle, and increases the frequency and duration of uterine contractions. **These contractions are superimposed on a tonic contraction with no relaxation in between**.

Therapeutic Uses

1. **To prevent and control postpartum haemorrhage**.

2. **Involution of the uterus.**
3. **Incomplete abortion.**

Contraindications: The use of ergot alkaloids in pre-eclampsia, hypertension, coronary artery disease, and thrombophlebitis is contraindicated.

Toxicity: Side effects are uncommon with ergometrine and methylergometrine. Cramp-like pains may occur. Overdoses are likely to cause **peripheral gangrene**.

Preparations and Dosage

1. **Ergometrine maleate:** Injection 0.25 mg/ml IM or IV. Maximum dose 1 mg. Orally 0.5 mg tablets three times a day.
2. **Methylergometrine maleate:** Injection 0.2 mg/ml IM or IV. Orally 0.25 to 0.5 mg two or three times daily.
3. **Oxytocin and ergometrine injection:** Available as synthetic oxytocin 5 units and ergometrine 0.5 mg in 1 ml. Usually given IM in the third stage of labour.

Prostaglandins

The prostaglandins are **long-chain fatty acids,** and derive their name from their high concentration in seminal fluid. They are found almost in all tissues.

Two prostaglandins **dinoprost tromethamine** (PGF_2 alpha) and **dinoprostone** (PGE_2) possess oxytocic activity.

Mode of action: There is evidence that PGF_2 alpha causes an increase in the free calcium (Ca^{++}) level in the myofibril. As a consequence there is an **increase in the free Ca^{++} levels intracellularly, triggering contraction of the myofibril.**

Therapeutic uses: Both, **dinoprost tromethamine** (PGF_2 alpha) and **dinoprostone** (PGE_2) can be employed for **induction of therapeutic or elective abortion, and induction of labour.**

Toxicity: The side effects are mainly gastrointestinal, like nausea, vomiting and diarrhoea. They may cause a *tetanic contraction of the uterus.*

UTERINE RELAXANTS (TOCOLYTIC AGENTS)

The term 'tocolysis' was first used in 1966, derived from the Greek, *tocos* = birth, and *lysis* = dissolution. Thus **tocolytic** agents include all drugs inhibiting labour.

Ethyl Alcohol

Ethyl alcohol is sometimes administered intravenously for its sedative and analgesic effect, and has been found to **reduce uterine contractions during premature labour.** For this 50 ml of 95 percent ethyl alcohol is mixed with 450 ml of 5 percent dextrose in distilled water to give a 9.5 percent alcohol solution.

Beta-Adrenoceptor Stimulants (Beta-Agonists)

Isoxsuprine Hydrochloride

Isoxsuprine is a smooth muscle relaxant. It acts by stimulating the beta-adrenoceptors. It relaxes the uterine muscle and also improves cerebral and peripheral blood circulation.

Isoxsuprine is used to inhibit **premature labour** and to manage **tetanic uterine contractions**, and **toxaemia** of pregnancy. It can be administered orally, intramuscularly, or as an IV drip. Initial dose is 80 mg in 250 ml of 5 percent dextrose IV followed by 0.1 to 0.2 mg/min until uterine relaxation is obtained.

Ritodrine Hydrochloride

Ritodrine is a **more specific $beta_2$-adrenoceptor stimulant** (causing uterine and bronchial relaxation), and produces fewer cardiovascular reactions. It *relaxes the uterus* and delays the onset of labour. It is administered as an IV drip at a rate of 50 mcg/minute, gradually increased by 50 mcg/minute every 10 minutes (not to exceed 400 mcg /min), until adequate relaxation is obtained, Ritodrine can also be administered intramuscularly or orally. *Side effects* include tachycardia and hypotension.

Other beta-agonists like *fenoterol*, *terbutaline* and *salbutamol* have also been tried for inhibiting uterine activity.

Magnesium Sulphate

High concentrations of magnesium depress uterine activity. Magnesium sulphate is used as an **intravenous infusion** in the management of pre-eclampsia to prevent convulsions, and to inhibit uterine contractions.

Various other drugs like **progesterone**, *pethidine* and *promethazine* have been used to inhibit uterine motility with limited success. As a last resort, **inhalation anaesthetics like ether,** and **halothane** can be used to suppress uterine contractions.

DYSMENORRHOEA

In dysmenorrhoea there are *cramp-like painful contractions of the uterus*, more so at the onset of menstruation. Currently it is thought that the **prostaglandins** are involved in this disorder, and substances which inhibit the synthesis of PGs like **aspirin** and **indomethacin** may be of some use.

Belladonna alkaloids (atropine and other cholinergic blocking agents) in ***combination with aspirin and codeine*** have been tried to treat severe dysmenorrhoea. Lately, the calcium antagonist, **nifedipine** has been tried for *dysmenorrhoea* and management of *preterm labour.*

Drugs Acting on the Endocrine System

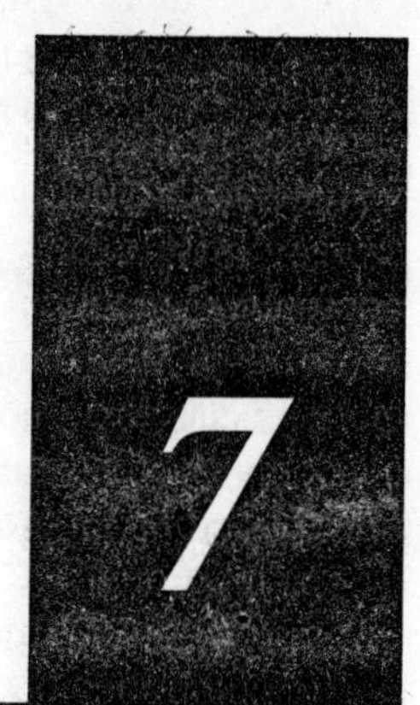

7.1 HYPOTHALAMIC AND PITUITARY HORMONES

Messages are carried by two well defined systems: (i) the **hormonal system** in which the chemical messengers (hormones) are produced by special glands, released into the blood stream, and **slowly** act upon the target cells in the body, and (ii) **the nervous system** in which messages travel across the body in milliseconds.

Hormones are chemical substances produced endogenously by endocrine glands, and certain nerve cells. They are carried by the blood throughout the body, and influence the activity of specific **target** tissues and organs.

The **pituitary gland** is placed at the base of the brain, and is connected to the hypothalamus by the pituitary stalk. It consists of an **anterior lobe** (adenohypophysis), and a **posterior lobe** (neurohypophysis).

The **anterior lobe** comprises of six or seven different types of cells which synthesize, store, and secrete **trophic hormones** regulating other endocrine glands. The hormones of the anterior pituitary are: the **thyroid stimulating hormone** (thyrotrophin, TSH), **adrenocorticotrophic hormone** (corticotrophin, ACTH), **follicle stimulating hormone** (FSH), **luteinizing hormone** (LH), **prolactin** (PL), **growth hormone** (somatotrophin, STH, GH), and **melanocyte stimulating hormone** (MSH).

REGULATION OF ANTERIOR PITUITARY SECRETION

The anterior pituitary gland has been traditionally termed as the *master of the endocrine system*. However, more recently this regulatory role has been attributed to the hypothalamus. Thus, the secretion of the trophic hormones from the anterior pituitary gland is controlled in two ways: (i) by the **hypothalamus;** and (ii) by **feedback** of hormones from the endocrine target glands.

Hypothalamic Control

The secretion of hormones from the anterior pituitary is controlled by the *hypothalamo-pituitary neurohormones*. They are also called **hypothalamic releasing** or **release inhibiting hormones.**

Feedback Control

The trophic hormone producing and secreting activity of the anterior pituitary is also influenced by the hormones of the respective target glands, i.e., by a **feedback** from the glands which it influences (**Fig. 7.1**).

HYPOTHALAMIC HORMONES

TRH promotes the secretion of TSH from the anterior pituitary. The neurohormone CRF controls ACTH secretion.

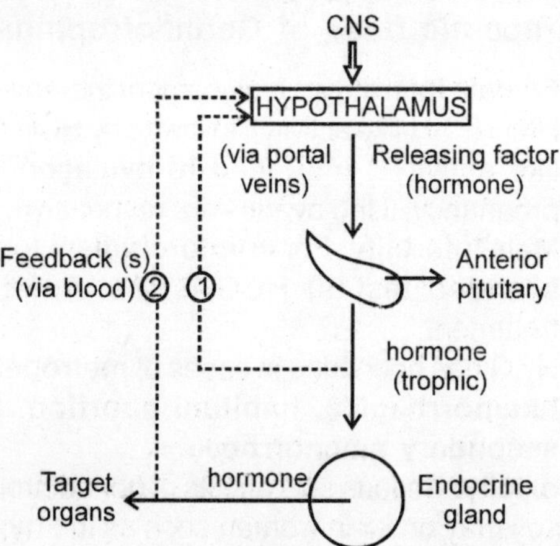

Fig. 7.1: *The negative feedback control of the anterior pituitary secretion. Environmental or endogenous stimuli act upon the hypothalamus, which secretes specific releasing factors conveyed to the anterior pituitary. As a result specific trophic hormones are released-higher the blood level of the trophic hormone, less of it is released (feedback 1). The trophic hormone induces its target endocrine gland to secrete specific hormone(s). The raised blood level of this specific hormone also suppresses the trophic hormone release through the hypothalamus (feedback 2).*

The mechanism of the differential release of FSH and LH is poorly understood. **Dopamine** is a stimulatory, and **serotonin** is an inhibitory neurotransmitter in the release of the gonadotrophin releasing hormone.

ANTERIOR PITUITARY HORMONES

Thyroid Stimulating Hormone (TSH, Thyrotropic Hormone, Thyrotrophin)

The TSH controls the activity of the thyroid gland by regulating the uptake of iodide by the gland. The hormones of the thyroid gland (thyroxine, triiodothyronine) exert a **negative feedback** effect which controls the secretion of TRH by the hypothalamus, and TSH by the anterior pituitary.

The main use of TSH (Thytropar) is as a **diagnostic agent** to differentiate between ***primary*** and ***secondary*** hypothyroidism due to pituitary failure.

Adrenocorticotrophic Hormone (ACTH)

The ACTH is released into the systemic circulation in response to the neurohormone, **corticotrophin releasing hormone** (CRH). The ACTH stimulates the adrenal cortex to increase the production of glucocorticoids mainly, and sex hormones to some extent. These adrenocortical steroids released into the blood control the secretion of CRH from the hypothalamus, and ACTH from the anterior pituitary by a **negative feedback** mechanism.

Actions: The site of action of ACTH is the **zona fasciculata** and **zona reticularis** of the adrenal cortex, of which it causes a hyperaemia and hypertrophy. ACTH stimulates the synthesis and secretion of the glucocorticoids cortisol, and corticosterone mainly, and to some extent the secretion of androgens.

Mode of action: ACTH first binds to specific **receptors** on the membrane of the adrenocortical target cells. This hormone receptor complex activates the membrane enzyme, adenylate cyclase. This, in turn, *promotes the formation of the intracellular cyclic nucleotide, cyclic adenosine 3'-5'-monophosphate (c-AMP)*. This second messenger then stimulates the enzymatic reactions that catalyse the steps in the biosynthesis of both adrenocortical protein, and adrenocortical steroid hormones.

Therapeutic Uses

1. Used **diagnostically** to determine whether adrenal insufficiency is due to pituitary or adrenal failure.
2. Used **therapeutically** to treat non-endocrine disorders like status asthmaticus, anaphylactic shock, rheumatic, and collagen disease.
3. ACTH is claimed to have special advantages over adrenocorticoids in the therapy of *multiple sclerosis, ulcerative colitis, infantile convulsions, and severe myasthenia gravis.*

Contraindications: Tuberculosis, azotemic nephritis, acute psychosis, active peptic ulcer, congestive heart failure, and diabetes mellitus.

Toxicity: Long-term administration of ACTH

induces suppression of ACTH production; exacerbation of diabetes mellitus; hypertrophy of the adrenal medulla; oedema; hypertension; and difficulty in withdrawing the drug. In addition there may be rounding of facial contour, mild hirsutism, acne, menstrual irregularities, and hypopotassaemic alkalosis. Hypersensitivity reactions may occur.

Preparation: ACTH may be given by injection or infusion.

Short-acting Preparation

Corticotrophin injection Usual dose is 25-40 units IM, or SC 6 hourly, or 10-25 units diluted in 500 ml of 5 percent glucose given by slow IV infusion over 8 to 24 hours.

Long-acting Preparation

Corticotrophin gelatin injection: Usual dose 25-40 units IM or SC every 24-72 hours.

Corticotrophin zinc injection: Dose 20-60 units IM or SC every 24-72 hours.

Synthetic corticotrophin preparation.

Tetracosactrin: Dose 0.25-0.75 mg IM or IV.

Gonadotrophins

The anterior pituitary stimulates the ovary by means of two gonadotrophins: **follicle stimulating hormone** (FSH) is responsible for the development of the ovarian follicle; and **luteinizing hormone** (LH) is the stimulus to ovulation, and later it maintains the corpus luteum. Their cyclic activity regulates the menstrual cycle.

Human menopausal gonadotrophin (HMG) is prepared from the urine of postmenopausal women. It is used to **induce ovulation** in infertile women having anovular ovaries.

In **males**, the FSH stimulates **spermatogenesis,** and the LH is identical with the interstitial cell stimulating hormone (ICSH) which stimulates the testicular Leydig cells to produce **testosterone.**

A third pituitary hormone **prolactin** (PL) acts in humans on the female breast only and not on the gonads.

Therapeutic Uses of Gonadotrophins

1. **Female infertility:** Replacement therapy with HMG (FSH-like activity), followed by HCG (LH-like activity) may lead to ovulation and pregnancy, if the ovaries are responsive.
2. **Male infertility:** For **cryptorchidism** (undescended testes) HCG is the preferred treatment.
3. HCG has been tried in cases of **metropathia haemorrhagica, habitual abortion,** and **secondary amenorrhoea.**

Toxicity: Serious side effects of gonadotrophin therapy may occur in women such as the **hyperstimulation syndrome.** This occurs due to an exaggerated oestrogen response, characterized by abdominal pain, nausea, distention and ovarian enlargement. Additional complications can be multiple pregnancy, ovarian rupture with haemoperitoneum.

Preparations and Dosage

1. **Human menopausal gonadotrophin injection (HMG):** A sterile solution is prepared immediately before use containing 75 IU FSH, and 75 IU LH in 1 ml of normal saline. One injection of HMG is given IM daily for 9 to 12 days, and is followed one day after the last injection by an injection of HCG.
2. **Human chorionic gonadotrophin injection (HCG):** The solution is prepared freshly and injected in a dose of 500 to 5000 IU IM according to the indication and regimen chosen.
3. **Serum gonadotrophin injection (PMSG):** PMSG is extracted from the serum of pregnant mares, and used for its FSH activity. The powder contains not less than 100 IU per mg. It has the same use as HMG.

Prolactin

Prolactin acts upon the oestrogen and progesterone primed mammary gland and initiates milk production (lactogenic action).

The infant's suckling of the mother's breast stimulates further secretion of ***prolactin*** and

oxytocin from the posterior pituitary, and the latter is responsible for the 'let down' of milk.

Bromocriptine

The semisynthetic ergot alkaloid **bromocriptine** has a specific dopamine receptor agonist action. It lowers prolactin release by activating dopamine receptors on the pituitary cells. Bromocriptine is used for **galactorrhoea, suppression of puerperal lactation, hyperprolactinaemia, hypogonadism,** and **restoring fertility in women.** It is also being tried in cases of **acromegaly** and **parkinsonism.**

Human Growth Hormone (Somatotrophin, STH, GH, HGH)

The *growth hormone* from the anterior pituitary promotes the growth of body tissues.

The deficiency of HGH leads to **hypopituitary dwarfism.** On the other hand hyperfunction leads to **acromegaly, gigantism,** and other forms of **hyperpituitarism.** Recently ***bromocriptine*** has been employed in the treatment of acromegaly.

The HGH stimulates cartilage growth (chrondrogenesis), and therefore promotes the growth of the skeletal system. It has a **protein anabolic action**. It has a **diabetogenic action.**

The growth hormone is species specific, and only that of human origin is active in man.

Therapeutic uses: Human growth hormone (HGH) is used in the management of growth disorders, particularly dwarfism. HGH therapy may be useful in certain phases of **renal failure, bone marrow hypoplasia, juvenile spontaneous hypoglycaemia, and to antagonize catabolism in response to burns or severe trauma.**

Toxicity: HGH can precipitate diabetes and severe ketoacidosis develops in diabetic patients even after a single dose. Antibodies to HGH may develop in some patients.

POSTERIOR PITUITARY HORMONES

The posterior pituitary stores: The **antidiuretic hormone** (ADH or vasopressin), and **oxytocin.** These hormones are carried to the posterior pituitary via the **neurohypophyseal tract**, and stored in the nerve terminals.

Antidiuretic Hormone (ADH, Vasopressin)

ADH modulates the tubular reabsorption of water. It is secreted from the nerve terminals in response to a decrease in plasma volume, increased osmolarity of blood, stress, coitus, and drugs like nicotine, barbiturates and morphine. When osmolarity is increased, (dehydration), ADH secretion is increased, and conversely reduction in osmolarity (overhydration) inhibits the release of ADH. **Alcohol inhibits the release of ADH.**

The deficiency of ADH is the cause of **diabetes insipidus** also designated as ***central diabetes insipidus*** (ADH responsive). In contrast **nephrogenic diabetes insipidus** (ADH resistant) is a rare hereditary disorder. Diabetes insipidus is characterized by the *excretion of large volumes of sugar free dilute urine,* and an increased osmolarity of blood.

Mode of action: The ADH via the blood reaches the kidney, and ***activates the adenylcyclase system*** and thus involves c-AMP which is known to enhance the permeability of the collecting tubule, leading to an ***increased water permeability***. The urine volume decreases.

The oral hypoglycaemic sulfonylurea, *chlorpropamide* has an antidiuretic action in patients with central diabetes insipidus.

The **thiazide diuretics** are effective in **nephrogenic diabetes insipidus.** The thiazides may also be used in central form of the disease.

Therapeutic Uses

1. **Diabetes insipidus**.
2. Vasopressin has a **spasmogenic** action and may be used in the management of **postoperative abdominal distension** and **paralytic ileus**. Vasopressin infusion may be employed to control bleeding from **oesophageal varices**, **bleeding peptic ulcers,** and **cirrhotic patients.**

Toxicity: The antidiuretic effect of vasopressin may lead to **water retention** and **hyponatraemia** (water intoxication). Vasopressin causes coronary constriction, may precipitate **angina pectoris, cardiac arrhythmias,** and **myocardial infarction.**

Preparations

1. **Posterior pituitary powder:** The dose is 5 to 40 mg administered topically (intranasal) as a snuff.
2. **Vasopressin injection** (Pitressin): Dose 5 to 10 units SC or IM three or four times daily.
3. **Vasopressin tannate injection** (Pitressin tannate in oil): It is a long-acting preparation. Dose 2.5 to 5 units every 1 to 3 days.
4. **Lysine vasopressin:** Administered intranasally as a spray, and each spray contains 2 units of activity.
5. **Desamino arginine vasopressin** (Desmopressin, DDAVP): The usual dose is 2.5 to 15 mcg intranasally twice daily.

Oxytocin

Oxytocin contracts the smooth muscle of the nipple and causes a flow of milk (let down). Suckling by the infant releases oxytocin which is responsible for **milk ejection**, and in addition **facilitates the contraction of the uterus, prevents postpartum haemorrhage,** and **hastens restoration of the uterus to its pregravid state (Chapter 6.3).**

Clinically **oxytocin** is the drug of choice for the **induction of labour at term**, and **vasopressin** is the drug of choice for the management of **central diabetes insipidus.**

7.2 THYROID HORMONES AND ANTITHYROID DRUGS

The main function of the thyroid gland is to synthesize, store, and secrete **thyroxine** (T_4) and **triiodothyronine** (T_3), under the control of **thyrotrophic hormone** (TSH) from the anterior pituitary. These hormones are essential for normal energy metabolism, body growth, and mental development. It also secretes the hypocalcaemic hormone **calcitonin.**

THYROID HORMONES

Biosynthesis, Release and Transport

The following steps are involved:

1. *Uptake of iodide* (iodide trapping).
2. *Oxidation of iodide* to free iodine and *iodination of tyrosine.*
3. Formation of thyroxine, and triiodothyronine by *coupling of iodotyrosines.*
4. *Proteolysis of thyroglobulin* and release of thyroxine and triiodothyronine into the blood.

Thyroglobulin stores T_3 and T_4 in the gland. These two hormones are released into the blood by diffusion. In the body cells thyroxine is converted (deiodinated) to *triiodothyronine* which is the *active form* of the hormone. Only the free forms of the hormones are active.

Control of Release

The plasma levels of thyrotrophin (TSH) control the rates of synthesis and release of T_4 and T_3. A **negative feedback mechanism** ensures physiological hormone levels within a narrow limit (**Fig. 7.2**).

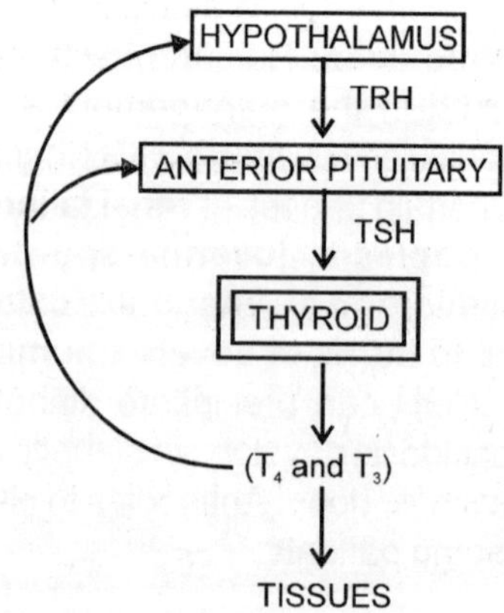

Fig. 7.2: *Control of the thyroid hormone production. TRH =thyrotrophin-releasing hormone; TSH = thyroid stimulating hormone; T_4 = thyroxine; T_3 = triiodothyronine).*

Actions

The actions of thyroid hormones may be summarized as under:

i. Increased calorigenesis and raised BMR.
ii. Increased carbohydrate and protein metabolism.
iii. Increased cholesterol turnover (hypolipidaemic effect).
iv. Increased heart rate, contractility and cardiac output.
v. Increased calcium mobilization from bone.
vi. Synergism with the action of catecholamines on the cardiovascular system, and carbohydrate metabolism.
vii. Regulation of water and electrolyte balance.
viii. Normal development of the nervous system.
ix. Essential for normal body growth, development and reproduction.

Mode of Action

High affinity binding sites (receptors) for T_3 and T_4 in the nucleus, mitochondria and plasma membrane of cells, suggest multiple sites of action. Thyroid hormones bind to *receptors* on cell surfaces increasing the uptake of glucose and amino acids. They also enter the cells to interact with material resulting in **increased synthesis of RNA**, leading to accelerated protein synthesis.

Therapeutic Uses

1. **Thyroid deficiency states:** Used in the treatment of **myxoedema** in adults, and **cretinism** in children.
2. **Hypothyroidism secondary to anterior pituitary destruction (Simmonds' disease).**
3. **Chronic thyroiditis (Hashimoto's disease), nontoxic and nodular goitre.**
4. **Hyperlipidaemia.**

Toxicity

The toxicity of thyroid preparations resembles the manifestations of hyperthyroidism like **hyperirritability, insomnia, nervousness, tachycardia, palpitation, arrhythmias, angina pectoris, polyphagia,** and **emaciation.** They may also lead to hypertension.

Preparations

The following preparations are available:

i. **Thyroid USP:** Various tablet strengths from 15 to 30 mg are available. Dose 30 to 250 mg daily orally.
ii. **Thyroglobulin (Proloid):** Tablets ranging from 15 to 300 mg are available. Average dose is 150 mg.
iii. **Levothyroxine sodium:** Average dose is 150 mcg daily. Range 50 to 300 mcg daily.
iv. **Liothyronine sodium:** It is the sodium salt of synthetic triiodothyronine (T_3). It has a rapid onset of action, and a short duration of action. It is the drug of choice in an emergency situation like *myxoedema coma.* Dose 5 to 100 mcg daily orally. Injectable preparation for intravenous use is also available (20 mcg ampoules).
v. **Liotrix (Thyrolar):** It is a 4:1 mixture of the synthetic sodium salt of T_4 and T_3 (levothyroxine sodium and liothyronine sodium). It is orally effective.

THYROTROPHIN (TSH) AND THYROTROPHIN–RELEASING HORMONE (TRH)

Thyrotrophin or TSH is an anterior pituitary hormone that stimulates production of thyroid hormones. It is used in tests of thyroid function. **Thyrotrophin releasing hormone** or TRH is a hypothalamic hormone. TRH may be useful as a diagnostic agent to assess the pituitary reserve.

IODINE AND THYROID FUNCTIONS

A minute amount of iodine intake (100 mcg daily) is necessary for the normal synthesis of the thyroid hormones. Except in 'goitre belts' (geographical regions in which iodine deficiency goitre is prevalent due to the washing out of iodides from the soil) man receives a sufficient supply of iodine from **vegetables** and **animal muscle meat.** Specially **sea fish** is a rich source of iodine. Lack of ingested iodine leads to ***thyroid follicular proliferation and thyroid hypertrophy.*** This cycle of events was based on extensive work done by Marine. A prolonged repetition of this **Marine cycle** would lead to large goitres in the people living along the goitre belts.

Prophylaxis of Iodine-Deficiency Goitre

Iodine intake may be increased by the administration of:

i. **Lugol's iodine:** It contain 5 percent iodine, and 10 percent potassium iodide in water. Lugol's iodine (0.2 to 0.5 ml orally daily) is administered.
ii. **Iodized table salt** may be used.

Toxicity of Iodine

Severe **hypersensitivity reactions** like angioedema, swelling of the larynx, and multiple cutaneous haemorrhages may occur. On continued administration chronic iodine poisoning or 'iodism' may set in. It is marked by coryza, conjunctivitis, laryngitis, bronchitis, urticaria and vesication.

ANTITHYROID DRUGS

In **hyperthyroidism** there is an excessive secretion and hyperactivity of the thyroid hormones. The management of thyrotoxicosis depends on the use of **antithyroid drugs, radioactive iodine** and/or **surgical removal of part of the thyroid gland.**

CLASSIFICATION

The following classification is based on their *mode of action*:

1. **Inhibitors of thyroxine synthesis**
   Propylthiouracil
   Carbimazole
2. **Drugs that destroy thyroid tissue**
   Radioactive iodine
3. **Antiadrenergic drugs**
   Propranolol
   Guanethidine
4. **Drugs with uncertain mode of action**
   Potassium iodide
   Sodium iodide
   Lugol's iodine.

Inhibitors of Thyroxine Synthesis

Thioamides

Propylthiouracil, a thioamide, is the prototype in the group, and has replaced the parent compound thiouracil. It **inhibits the synthesis of the thyroid hormones,** but does not inactivate or interfere with the action of the already formed and stored thyroxine in the gland. **Carbimazole** is as effective as propylthiouracil.

Mode of Action

These antithyroid drugs inhibit the formation of thyroxine mainly by interfering with: (i) the **iodination** of tyrosine; and (ii) the **coupling** and **condensation** of the iodotyrosines.

Therapeutic Uses

1. **Hyperthyroidism** (Graves disease).
2. Preparation of the thyrotoxic patient for surgical treatment.

Contraindications

As the thioamides cross the placenta, they can cause **foetal goitre.** Their use should be minimized in pregnancy. They should not be used in lactating mothers as they are concentrated in milk.

Toxicity

They have a **goitrogenic action.** Allergic reactions may occur. A **hypothyroid state** may be induced. Severe **leucopenia** and **agranulocytosis** have been reported. *Carbimazole* is claimed to produce fewer adverse effects.

Dosage and Preparations

Propylthiouracil 50-100 mg every 8 hourly.
Carbimazole 5-10 mg every 8 hourly.

Drugs that Destroy Thyroid Tissue

Radioactive Iodine (I^{131})

Several radioactive isotopes of iodine are available, but radioiodine I^{131} is most used. It has a half-life of 8.04 days, and emits **beta** and **gamma** radiations. I^{131} accumulates in the thyroid gland. The destructive action of I^{131} on the thyroid gland is induced by beta radiations.

Mode of Action

The biological activity of I^{131} is attributed to **ionizing beta radiations** which destroy the functional and regenerative capacity of the thyroid cells within few weeks of administration. **The follicular cells are necrosed, followed by fibrosis.**

Therapeutic Uses

1. Selected cases of **hyperthyroidism**.
2. **Thyroid carcinomas with multiple metastases.**
3. **Diagnostic uses:** Radioiodine uptake studies are useful for **localization of metastatic deposits** in lungs and bones.

The **advantages** of I^{131} are that mortality is low, control is complete, recurrence uncommon, and it has a convenient (oral) mode of administration. The **disadvantages** are that radioiodine has a slow onset of action, and during this time the patient may need propranolol or propylthiouracil therapy. Hypothyroidism may occur.

Contraindications

I^{131} is contraindicated during **pregnancy** and **lactation,** in **large toxic nodular goitres,** and in **severe thryrotoxic cardiovascular disease.**

Toxicity

I^{131} may produce **mild pain and tenderness in the thyroid area, acute swelling of the thyroid gland, radiation thyroiditis,** and **bone marrow depression**. Overdosing may lead to **hypothyroidism.** Late adverse reaction occurring after years of treatment is thyroid **carcinoma**.

Preparations and Dosage

Sodium Iodide I^{131} is available as a solution or in capsules containing I^{131} suitable for oral or intravenous administration.

The usual total dose works out to 4,000 to 10,000 microcuries, or 4 to 10 millicuries (1000 microcuries = 1 millicurie).

Antiadrenergic Drugs

Propranolol, the beta-blocker may be used as adjunct to antithyroid therapy to control the adrenergic mediated symptoms like **tachycardia, palpitation** and **hypertension.** Propranolol in addition relieves anxiety and tension. Propranolol has found a special use in thyroid crisis. Propranolol reduces the peripheral conversion of T_4 to T_3.

Drugs with Uncertain Mode of Action

Iodide

Iodide is used in the treatment of **iodine-deficiency goitre and this prevents endemic goitre and cretinism.** Paradoxically if iodide is administered to hyperthyroid patients, there is a reduction in the vascularity and swelling of the gland. The gland shrinks and the symptoms improve.

Mode of Action

High iodide content in blood inhibits thyroid hormone release. Ultimately the thyroid escapes this action, and a thyroid crisis may occur. This is designated as the **'escape phenomenon'.**

Therapeutic Uses

To prepare hyperthyroid patients for surgery potassium iodide 60 mg thrice daily is given for 14 days before operation.

DRUG THERAPY OF THYROTOXIC CRISIS

This crisis has become uncommon with the growing use of beta-adrenoceptor blockers in the preoperative treatment of thyrotoxic patients.

Plasmapheresis is an adjunct of therapy of thyroid crisis. The guidelines for drug therapy are:

1. **Correction of sympathetic over-activity:** Propranolol 40 mg 6-hourly or 2 mg IV 6 hourly.
2. **Correction of relative adrenal insufficiency** by administering hydrocortisone 200 mg IV.
3. **Blockade of further thyroid hormone synthesis and release:**
   i. *Sodium iodide* 1-2 g by slow IV infusion.
   ii. *Oral antithyroid drugs*: Neomercazole 100 mg stat, and maintenance dose of 15 mg tid for 72 hours.
4. Heart failure may require **digitalization** and **diuretics.**
5. **General measures:** Tepid sponging of the patient for hyperpyrexia, oxygen inhalations, and IV glucose infusion for severe dehydration.

To conclude, the mainstay for the management of hyperthyroidism is on the ***inhibitors of thyroxine synthesis*** (propylthiouracil, carbimazole), and *radioactive iodine*. Propranolol is used to allay the sympathetic mediated symptoms. ***Potassium iodide*** only controls thyrotoxic symptoms temporarily.

7.3 PARATHYROID HORMONE, CALCITONIN, VITAMIN D AND CALCIUM METABOLISM

The total calcium in the body is between 1000 and 1200 g, and 99 percent of it is in the bony skeleton. The normal calcium level in blood 10 to 10.5 mg/dl. In the blood it exits in two forms: (i) **non-diffusible** calcium (50%) which is protein bound; and (ii) **diffusible** calcium (50%), a part of which is complexed with phosphate and carbonate, and another part is ionized Ca^{++}.

Calcium metabolism in the body is mainly governed by two hormones, **parathormone** from the parathyroids, and **calcitonin** from the thyroid gland. In addition **vitamin D** and its metabolites regulate plasma calcium levels.

PARATHORMONE

The parathyroid hormone, parathormone (PTH) is a large polypeptide. It is obtained from bovine parathyroid extract. The chief physiologic role of PTH is the maintenance of **calcium homeostasis.**

Control of Release

Parathormone release is regulated by the Ca^{++} ion concentration in the blood. Release of PTH is stimulated by a fall, and inhibited by a rise in the ionized Ca^{++} levels of plasma. No effective control by the anterior pituitary has been demonstrated.

Actions

The major effects are exerted on the Ca^{++} transport in the (i) bone, (ii) kidneys, and (iii) intestines.

i. **Bone:** PTH leads to **resorption** of the bone, releasing calcium into the blood. PTH promotes osteoclastic activity, and depresses osteoblastic activity. The plasma calcium ion concentration is raised.
ii. **Kidneys:** PTH inhibits the renal tubular reabsorption of phosphate. This results in an increased phosphate clearance, and a **phosphaturia.** In addition PTH decreases calcium clearance.
iii. **Intestine:** In the presence of vitamin D it promotes the absorption of calcium from the intestines.

Mode of Action

Parathormone stimulates adenyl cyclase activity in the bone and kidney cells, leading to ***an increase in cyclic-AMP formation***, which regulates the intracellular calcium ion concentration.

Therapeutic Uses

Parathyroid injection is only used for the early control of tetany due to **hypoparathyroidism.** Once the tetany has been controlled the treatment is mainly dietetic and administration of vitamin D.

Dose

Parathyroid injection: 20 to 40 USP units twice daily subcutaneously or intramuscularly, but in emergencies it may be given intravenously. Dose range 40 to 300 units daily.

Toxicity

Overdosage with PTH causes **hypercalcaemia. Hypersensitivity reactions** may occur. Prolonged use of PTH can lead to **demineralization of bone,** and **metastatic calcifications** in the kidneys (nephrocalcinosis, urolithasis), and in other organs.

CALCITONIN (THYROCALCITONIN)

Calcitonin is secreted by the parafollicular cells (C cells) of the *thyroid gland.* The main action of calcitonin is to produce **hypocalcaemia** by inhibiting bone resorption, and by promoting the urinary excretion of calcium and phosphate. Calcitonin release is regulated by the ionized calcium concentration of blood perfusing the thyroid gland. The calcitonin products available for use are synthetic compounds that resemble the polypeptide hormones of **salmon calcitonin** and **human calcitonin.**

Mode of Action

Calcitonin produces hypocalcaemia possibly by ***decreasing osteoclastic activity***, and **increasing osetoblastic activity** in the bone. Thus it inhibits bone resorption and antagonizes the action of PTH.

Therapeutic Uses

The use of calcitonin in **hypercalcaemic states** is limited, due to its short duration of action, and rapid development of resistance. **Salmon calcitonin** has been used with some success in **Paget's disease** and in **osteoporosis.**

Dose: Salmon calcitonin 40 to 160 units daily by subcutaneous, intramuscular, or intravenous injection. **Human calcitonin** is initially given in a dose of 0.5 mg/day.

Toxicity

Inflammatory reactions may be caused at the site of injection. It may produce mild hypocalcaemia, but does not produce tetany. Circulating antibodies form to salmon calcitonin, and its efficacy declines.

Vitamin D

Vitamin D designates a group of related sterols active against **rickets.** The effects of vitamin D (cholecalciferol) are mainly due to its more potent metabolites formed in the liver and kidneys. **Dihydrotachysterol** (AT_{10}) is a synthetic compound chemically related to calciferol. **It is used to correct hypocalcaemia of hypoparathyroidism, and to treat acute, chronic and latent forms of parathyroid tetany.** It has also been employed in cases of **vitamin D-resistant rickets** and **osteomalasia.**

Mode of Action

In the **bone** vitamin D maintains the stores of calcium in the mitochondria. In the **kidneys** the vitamin D metabolites increase calcium reabsorption from the proximal tubules. In the **intestines** the vitamin D metabolites promote the absorption of calcium.

Toxicity

Hypervitaminosis D is characterized by generalized decalcification of bones, hypercalcaemia, hyperphosphataemia, hypercalciuria and metastatic calcification.

Etidronate

Etidronate is a nonhormonal substance (bisphosphonate) that reduced the rate of bone turnover. It adsorbs onto the surface of **hydroxyapatite crystals,** disrupting the formation, growth, and dissolution of these crystals. The accelerated bone turnover in *Paget's disease* is slowed down, and bone pain and incidence of fractures is reduced.

Etidronate is used in the treatment of moderate to severe **Paget's disease and hypercalcaemia of malignancy.** The dose is 5 to 10 mg/kg/day for upto 6 months. Retreatment is needed on reactivation of the disease.

Hypoparathyroidism

Hypofunction of the parathyroid gland may be due to an accidental removal of the gland during thyroid surgery, or due to idiopathic hypoparathyroidism. The syndrome is known clinically as **tetany.**

Treatment

i. **Calcium gluconate:** In acute hypocalcaemia 10 to 30 ml of 10 percent calcium gluconate in 500 to 1000 ml of isotonic saline is administered intravenously.
ii. **Parathyroid injection:** In acute phases 100-200 units IV slowly, followed by 25 to 50 units IM 6 to 12 hourly is administered till the crisis is over.
iii. **Vitamin D**
   a. *Vitamin D_2* (calciferol or ergocalciferol) oily injection. Initially 400,000 IU IM daily, and a maintenance dose of 100,000 IU IM daily is given.
   b. *Dihydrotachysterol (AT_{10})* Initially 0.8 to 2.4 mg once daily orally, and for maintenance 200 mcg weekly to 1 mg daily orally is administered.
iv. *A calcium rich* and *phosphate poor* diet.

Hyperparathyroidism

Hyperfunction of the parathyroid gland may be due to diffuse hyperplasia of the glands, adenomas, carcinoma, and aberrant production of PTH.

Treatment

i. **Surgical removal** of the gland.
ii. **Intravenous saline infusion** to correct dehydration.
iii. Intravenous infusion of **0.1 M solution of dibasic sodium phosphate** to promote calcium excretion.
iv. **Disodium edetate (EDTA):** It chelates calcium. In an emergency 50 mg/kg in 500 ml saline may be given intravenously.
v. **Calcitonin** 5 to 25 mcg/kg may be of therapeutic value.
vi. **Glucocorticosteroids** may be tried.
vii. **Haemodialysis** may be of value when all other measures have failed.

Thus, effective pharmacotherapy for hyperparathyroidism is not available. Mainly the treatment is operative.

7.4 INSULIN AND ORAL HYPOGLYCAEMIC AGENTS

The external secretion of the pancreas is digestive in function, and the endocrine functions are performed by the **islets of Langerhans.** They are small highly vascularized masses of cells scattered throughout the pancreas.

The islets of Langerhans contain **four** types of secretory cells:

i. Alpha (A) cells, secrete **glucagon;**
ii. Beta (B) cells, secrete **insulin;**
iii. Delta (D) cells, secrete **somatostatin;** and
iv. PP (F) cells, secrete **pancreatic polypeptide**.

The insulin secreting beta-cells are the most numerous. The physiologic role of **glucagon** and **insulin** in the regulation of intermediary metabolism is well established.

Diabetes mellitus (DM) is a chronic metabolic disorder, resulting from insulin deficiency characterized by **hyperglycaemia, altered metabolism of carbohydrates, protein** and **lipids,** and **an increased risk of vascular complications.**

Predisposition to DM is **inherited**, although the genetic factors are complex. There are two recognized types of DM:

(i) **Insulin dependent** (Type I or juvenile onset; IDDM), and (ii) **Noninsulin dependent** (Type II or maturity onset; NIDDM), **Type I** usually occurs in nonobese persons before the age of 30 years. Circulating insulin is virtually absent. The **Type II** usually occurs after the age of 40 years, and obesity is a major risk factor. **Gestational diabetes** refers to the onset of glucose intolerance in women during pregnancy.

INSULIN

Insulin was first isolated in 1921 by Banting and Best, and used in the treatment of diabetes mellitus in 1922. It was completely synthesized in 1966.

The **pig** (porcine) insulin closely resembles human insulin, which may account for its low antigenicity. Recently **human insulin** has been successfully produced through *E.coli* by *recombinant DNA technique*, or by chemical modification of pork insulin.

Biosynthesis, Storage and Release

The **beta-cells** synthesize, store and release insulin. The normal pancreas contains about 200 units of insulin, and man secretes about 50 units daily.

Proinsulin is a transient intermediary in the synthesis of insulin. **Proinsulin** is derived from a larger precursor, **pre-proinsulin.** Conversion of proinsulin to insulin takes place in the beta-cells by proteolysis.

The most important factor controlling insulin secretion is glucose. An increase in blood glucose level promotes both synthesis, and release of insulin.

Transport, Metabolism and Excretion

Orally, administered insulin is rapidly proteolysed in the gut, hence oral administration is ineffective. It has to be given parenterally usually by *subcutaneous injection.* Insulin is taken up by the liver and kidney, where it is mainly degraded.

The plasma half-life of crystalline insulin injected subcutaneously is 40 minutes.

Actions

In DM there are disturbances in the metabolism of *carbohydrate, fat, protein, electrolytes* and *water.*

a. ***Carbohydrate metabolism***: Insulin deficiency produces two fundamental defects : (i) reduced entry of glucose into cells; and (ii) *increased release of glucose from the liver into circulation.* Both of these raise the blood glucose level (**hyperglycaemia**), and lead to the excretion of glucose in urine (**glycosuria**). In addition, in insulin deficiency there is an abnormally high rate of conversion of protein to glucose (**gluconeogenesis**). Insulin replacement facilitates entry of glucose into the cell. Further *insulin inhibits glycogenolysis, and gluconeogenesis.* This leads to a ***fall in the glucose content of the blood and tissues.***

b. ***Fat metabolism***: Insulin deficiency leads to a mobilization of fat from adipose tissue into the blood stream (lipaemia). The blood concentrations of triglyceride and FFA rise. The greater availability of FFA to the liver leads to an increased production of **acetoacetic** and **β-hydroxybutyric acid** (ketone bodies). These ketone bodies enter the blood, and produce a **metabolic ketoacidosis.** In diabetes the blood cholesterol level also rises.

c. ***Protein metabolism***: Insulin deficiency impairs protein synthesis, and promotes protein breakdown specially in the muscle. Increased protein catabolism leads to wasting. Insulin replacement has an **anabolic** effect.

d. ***Electrolytes***: Due to an increased protein breakdown, glycogenolysis, and tissue hypoxia, intracellular potassium (K^+) escapes into the extracellular fluid, and is lost in the urine. ***Insulin facilitates entry of potassium into the cells.***

e. ***Water***: As an osmotic consequence of glycosuria there is an extra loss of water from the body (polyuria). This leads to *dehydration* and *polydypsia.*

Mode of Action

The major effects of insulin are initiated by the attachment of the insulin molecule to a **specific insulin receptor** on the cell surface. This hormone receptor interaction is **reversible.**

Insulin lowers the c-AMP content in some tissues, perhaps by inhibiting the adenyl cyclase system. Insulin and glucagon are mutually **antagonistic.**

Preparations

Commercial insulin is extracted from the pancreas of **cattle** (bovine), and **pigs** (porcine). Preparations are adjusted to contain 40,80,100 or 500 units/ ml. Regular insulin (Crystalline insulin) is modified to form suspensions having varying particle sizes. The available preparations of insulin are detailed in **Table 7.1.**

All insulin preparations are usually given **subcutaneously.** Only insulin injection or regular insulin can be given **intravenously.** The insulins are marketed in 10 ml vials.

Newer Insulins

1. **Actrapid (Nusol):** It is a clear neutral solution of recrystallized porcine insulin. It acts faster than regular insulin.
2. **Rapitard (Biphasic insulin):** It is a cloudy mixture of actrapid (1 part), and insoluble crystals of bovine insulin (3 parts) buffered to pH 7. Its action is simiiar to **Lente insulin**, except that the onset of action is quicker, and the blood sugar control is smoother.
3. **Monotard:** It is **monocomponent insulin zinc suspension** containing highly purified insulin, and is claimed to be devoid of antigenic property.
4. **Human insulins:** Human insulins are highly purified insulins prepared by *recombinant DNA technique, or semisynthetically* using porcine insulin as starting material. Human insulins *are much less immunogenic than beef or pork insulins.*

Adverse Reactions and Precautions

1. **Hypoglylcaemia.**

Table 7.1 : *The characteristics of insulin preparations*

Type	Preparation	pH and appearance	Hours after subcutaneous inj. Onset of action	Maximal action	Duration of action	Can be safely mixed with	Time of injection	Time of hypoglycaemic risk
Fast-acting	Insulin injection (regular, crystalline insulin)	3.2 clear	1	2-3	5-7	All preparations	Before breakfast	Late morning
	Prompt Insulin Zinc suspension (SEMILENTE)	7.2 cloudy	1	4-6	12-16	LENTE	Before breakfast	Late morning to mid - afternoon
Intermediate-acting	Isophane insulin Suspension cloudy (NPH insulin)	7.2	2	8-12	18-24	Insulin injection	Before breakfast	Late morning to bedtime
	Insulin Zinc Suspension (LENTE)	7.2 cloudy	2-4	8-12	18-24	Insulin injection SEMILENTE	Before breakfast	Late afternoon to bedtime
	Globin Zinc insulin injection (Globin insulin)	3.4 clear	1-2	6-10	12-18	–	Before bedtime	Early morning
Long-acting	Protamine zinc insulin suspension (PZI)	7.2 cloudy	4-6	16-18	24-36	Insulin injection	At breakfast	During the night until breakfast time
	Extended zinc insulin suspension (ULTRALENTE)	7.2 cloudy	4-6	16-18	24-36	Insulin injection SEMILENTE	At breakfast	During the night until breakfast time

2. **Insulin allergy.**
3. **Insulin lipoatrophy.**
4. **Insulin presbiopia.**
5. **Insulin neuropathy.**
6. **Insulin resistance:** On prolonged insulin administration the daily requirement gradually rises due to the formation of **insulin antibodies.**
7. **Obesity.**

Every diabetic should carry an **identification card** containing related information which may be useful in managing an emergency.

Therapeutic Uses

1. **Diabetes mellitus.**
2. **Schizophrenia.**
3. **Anorexia nervosa:** Insulin improves the appetite, and there is a simultaneous gain in body weight.

PHARMACOTHERAPY OF DIABETES MELLITUS

All diabetics do not require insulin. Some patients of the maturity-onset type of the disease can be controlled on *diet* and *exercise* alone. However the following categories require insulin administration:

i. Juvenile diabetics, specially of more than 2 years duration.
ii. Older diabetics with maturity-onset diabetes.
iii. All diabetics with complications.
iv. Diabetic coma and precoma.
v. Primary or secondary failure of sulphonylurea therapy.
vi. During pregnancy to avoid the possible embryopathic activity of oral hypoglycaemic agents.
vii. Diabetics undergoing surgery.

DIABETIC COMA

Due to the lack of insulin there is a mobilization of fatty acids leading to formation of ***ketone bodies,*** and ***acidosis*** (**ketoacidosis**). There is a **hyperglycaemia** and **glycosuria** resulting in **dehydration** and **hypovolaemia.** The urine is loaded with ketone bodies and glucose. The blood glucose is raised to 600-800 mg%. During diabetic ketoacidosis an acute but temporary state of insulin resistance develops. **Therefore, high doses of Regular Insulin are needed.**

HYPOGLYCAEMIC COMA

In diabetics dangerous hypoglycaemia may occur due to missed meals, violent exercise, or due to an overdose of insulin. Symptoms are of two types: (a) **Cerebral** due to low blood glucose level there is confusion, depression, convulsions and visual disturbance; and (b) **sympathetic activation** due to adrenaline liberation there may be vasoconstriction, tachycardia, palpitation, tremors, pallor, sweating and piloerection. **Glucose** given orally can relieve symptoms, if given early.

GLUCAGON

Glucagon is a single chain polypeptide. It is synthesized, stored and secreted by the alpha-cells of the islets of Largerhans. **Glucose** is the major regulator of glucagon secretion. Hyperglycaemia inhibits, while hypoglycaemia stimulates the release of glucagon.

Mode of Action

Glucagon promotes glucose production (glycogenolysis) from liver glycogen via the stimulation the adenyl cyclase cell wall system, formation of c-AMP, and activation of hepatic phosphorylase. Activated phosphorylase breaks down glycogen to glucose which is released into the blood leading to a prompt hyperglycaemia.

Therapeutic Uses

1. Insulin hypoglycaemia.
2. Used with dextrose to cut short insulin induced hypoglycaemic coma.
3. It has been tried in **cardiogenic shock.**
4. Used in the **diagnosis** of insulinomas and pheochromocytomas.
5. May be used in the treatment of beta-blocker poisoning.

Adverse reactions: There may be slight nausea after large doses, and hypersensitivity reactions may occur.

Dose: Glucagon hydrochloride 1 mg IM, IV or SC.

ORAL HYPOGLYCAEMIC AGENTS

Oral hypoglycaemic agents are divided into two classes: (i) **Sulphonylueras;** and (ii) **Biguanides** (**Table 7.2**).

Sulphonylureas

The sulphonylureas are chemically related to the sulphonamides, but they have no antibacterial activity.

Pharmacological Actions

The sulphonylureas are readily absorbed from the gastrointestinal tract, appear in the blood within 1-2 hours, and peak levels are attained within 4-6 hours. They are partially protein bound and metabolized in the liver.

Sulphonylureas **lower blood glucose level** in non-diabetic and Type II diabetics. Almost simultaneously they **lower the plasma free fatty acid levels.** They are effective only in the presence of a functioning pancreas.

Mode of Action

The Sulphonylureas stimulate the beta-cell islet tissue to secrete insulin, i.e., they have an islet **beta-cytotropic** activity. They cause **degranulation** of the beta-cells. They also probably directly **inhibit hepatic glycogenolysis.** The sulphonylureas are ineffective in patients of Type I diabetes.

Toxicity

i. **Hypoglycaemia.**
ii. Allergic skin reactions.
iii. **Bone marrow depression.**
iv. Chlorpropamide is reported to induce cholestatic jaundice.
v. There is a likelihood of their inducing **embryopathy.**
vi. They are **goitrogenic.**
vii. Chlorpropamide may induce severe **intolerance** to alcohol similar to that caused by disulfiram.

Therapeutic Uses

i. **Maturity-onset diabetes mellitus.**
ii. **Insulin-resistant diabetes mellitus.**
iii. Chlorpropamide has been used in some cases of **diabetes insipidus.**

Biguanides

Metformin is the only biguanide available . It acts mainly by *decreasing gluconeogenesis,* and by *increasing peripheral utilization of glucose.*

Table 7.2 : *Prescribing details of oral hypoglycaemic agents*

Drug and class	Half-life (hours)	Duration of action (hours)	Tablet strength (mg)	Daily dose range	Dosage frequency
Sulphonylureas					
Chlorpropamide	30-36	60	100, 250, 500	0.1-0.5 g	Single
Glibenclamide	5	10-15	5	2.5-15 mg	Single/Divided
Glipizide*	2-4	24	5,10	5-40 mg	Single/Divided
Glimepiride*	18	24	1,2	1-6 mg	Single
Biguanides					
Metformin	3	5-6	500	1-1.5 g	Divided

* Second generation compounds

Metformin is used in *obese Type II diabetics* in whom exercise and diet have failed to control the disease. It may be effectively combined with sulphonylureas, insulin, acarbose or poiglitazone.

Side effects include anorexia, nausea, vomiting, diarrhoea, metallic taste, and rarely lactic acidosis.

NEWER ORAL HYPOGLYCAEMIC AGENTS

Thiazolidinedione Derivatives

Troglitazone

A new class of oral antidiabetics is emerging. It includes **troglitazone, ciglitazone, englitazone,** and **poiglitazone.** Their **mode of action** appears to be by enhancing the target tissue sensitivity to insulin.

Troglitazone lowers insulin resistance, and improves fasting and postprandial hyperglycaemia in patients with NIDDM. It provides an alternative for NIDDM therapy. ***Troglitazone*** has been approved by the FDA, USA for use in insulin-resistant patients who are receiving insulin. Troglitazone is available as 200 and 400 mg tablets.

Alpha-Glucosidase Inhibitor

Acarbose

Postprandial hyperglycaemia, and hyperinsulinaemia produce long-term complications of DM, namely *nephropathy, retinopathy,* and *neuropathy.* *Acarbose* is the first alpha-glucosidase inhibitor available in India. It has a direct effect on postprandial hyperglycaemic peak without producing hyperinsulinaemia, in contrast to other conventional oral hypoglycaemics.

In NIDDM insufficiently controlled with diet and exercise, acarbose is used as an *adjunct to conventional oral hypoglycaemics in patients with secondary sulphonylurea/biguanide failures, and certain types of lipoproteinaemias.* **Dose:** Initially 50 mg OD during the first week, 50 mg bid second week, and 50 mg third week. The dose is taken with the first mouthful of each meal. **Adverse reactions** include abdominal pain, nausea, flatulence, vomiting, diarrhoea, gastritis, stool discolouration, and rarely hepatitis with jaundice.

Guar Gum

Guar gum is a soluble dietary fibre obtained from Indian cluster beans (Guar). It is available in granular form. On oral administration it forms a viscous gel in the intestines, and decreases carbohydrate absorption, thereby reducing blood glucose levels.

Guar gum is used in *diabetes mellitus* as an adjunct to insulin or oral hypoglycaemic therapy. It reduces both fasting and postprandial blood glucose levels. It is given with or immediately before meals initially in a low dose (2.5 g/day), and gradually increased to 5 g stirred well in 150 ml of water 3 times daily. It is also used to slow gastric emptying in patients with *dumping syndrome.*

In patients of *hypercholestrolaemia* guar gum produces a modest reduction in plasma cholesterol and LDL-cholesterol. Products containing guar gum have been promoted as *slimming aids.* ***Adverse reactions*** include flatulence, diarrhoea and nausea. There is a risk of obstruction or rupture. *Caution:* Guar gum should not be ingested as dry granules.

Glucomannan

Glucomannan, a powdered extract from the tubers of *Amorphophallus konjac* is used to reduce food intake by inducing early satiety. It reduces the absorption of lipids and sugars. Clinically there is a reduction in blood glucose, and cholesterol levels. It is mainly used as an adjunct in obese patients with NIDDM, in a dose of 1 g stirred well in a glass of water for 10 minutes till it is fully dissolved, and taken ½ hour before meals upto 3 times daily. It has also been promoted as a *slimming aid.*

Adverse reactions include distension, nausea, vomiting and diarrhoea. Chronic use can cause vitamin deficiencies. **Caution:** Glucomannan should never be ingested in dry form, as it can cause an *oesophagal obstruction.*

With proper management of DM with **insulin, oral hypoglycaemics,** and **antibiotics** in addition to **exercise** and **diet regulation,** a diabetic can enjoy almost a normal life. Lately, the USFDA has approved

Exubera, a fast-acting powdered form of human insulin. It is administered by inhalation through the mouth to reach the lungs and the blood stream. It is an option for both Type I and Type II diabetes.

Exanatide is another new drug which facilitates the use of insulin by the body cells, protects pancreatic beta-cells, and induces satiety. It has actions similar to **GLP-1, a natural incretin hormone.** In addition, exanatide also reduces the production of glucagon. It is given in a dose of 5 or 10 mcg subcutaneously bid, an hour before breakfast and dinner to type II diabetics who have failed to respond to oral hypoglycaemics. It is not a substitute for insulin. *Side effects* include nausea, vomiting, and sometimes a rapid hypoglycaemia. Further clinical studies are in progress.

7.5 ADRENAL CORTICOSTEROIDS

The adrenal corticosteroids are amongst the most widely employed therapeutic agents. They are used either: (i) in **physiologic doses** as a replacement therapy to correct chronic adrenocortical insufficiency, or (ii) in **pharmacologic doses** to treat inflammatory conditions, allergic states, collagen disorders, and several other diseases.

PHYSIOLOGIC CONSIDERATION

The cells of the adrenal cortex are arranged in three zones: (i) the outer **zona glomerulosa** which secretes *aldosterone;* (ii) the middle **zona fasciculata;** and (iii) the inner **zona reticularis.** In man the cells of the zona fasciculata and zona reticularis function as a single unit and secrete **cortisol, corticosterone,** and small quantities of **male** and **female sex hormones.** The adrenal medulla is composed of chromaffin cells which secrete catecholamines (adrenaline and noradrenaline).

The natural steroid hormones produced and secreted by the adrenal cortex are divided into *three* main groups.

1. **Glucocorticoids:** These are **cortisol** (hydrocortisone) and **corticosterone.**
2. **Mineralocorticoids:** These are **aldosterone** and **deoxycorticosterone.**
3. **Sex hormones:** The **androgen** (dehydroepiandrosterone) secreted has weak masculinizing activity. **Progesterone** is formed as an intermediary in the synthesis of gluco- and mineralocorticoids, and only a **trace of oestrogen** is secreted.

BIOSYNTHESIS OF ADRENOCORTICOSTEROIDS

All steroid are derived from **cholesterol**. Cholestrol is converted into **pregnenolone**, the precursor of all steroid hormones. Four major classes of steroids are derived from pregnenolone– **oestrogens, progestogens, androgens and corticosteroids.**

The synthesis of cortisol is controlled by ACTH. Aldosterone is modulated by ***sodium potassium balance,*** and the **osmolarity of the extracellular fluid.**

REGULATION OF SECRETION

The biosynthesis and secretion of glucocorticoids is regulated by the **hypothalamo-pituitary axis**. ACTH is released from the anterior pituitary into the circulation in response to the **corticotrophin releasing hormone** (CRH), a neurohormone from the hypothalamus. Released ACTH stimulates the adrenal cortex to increase the production of mainly glucocorticoids. The released glucocorticoids (cortisol) exert a **negative feedback** effect on the hypothalamus, thereby regulating the further release of CRH, which regulates the synthesis and release of ACTH from the anterior pituitary.

CIRCADIAN RHYTHM OF PLASMA CORTISOL

The secretion of adrenal gland (cortisol), and anterior pituitary (ACTH) hormone does not occur at a steady rate, but varies at different times of the day. It follows a **circadian** rhythm , which is a 24-hour cycle. The human anterior pituitary in the usual sleep/wakefulness cycle starts producing larger amounts of ACTH after midnight. The plasma ACTH reaches its peak at about 6:00 AM. This induces the adrenal cortex to secrete large amount of glucocorticoids between 6.00 and 9.00 AM. During the day, the glucocorticoids secreted are used up and metabolized, and the **blood steroid level is the lowest in the late evenings.**

STRESS AND ADRENAL STEROIDOGENESIS

A **stressor** is an agent which attempts to alter the internal environment, e.g., physical injury, infection, high or low temperature, radiation injury, neuromuscular fatigue, emotions, noise, environmental pollutants, and so on. Stressors generally induce two type of syndromes: (i) the **local adaptation syndrome** (LAS) which is a local response; and (ii) the **general adaptation syndrome** (GAS) which could be a response to stressors when their action is prolonged, and irrespective of the agency the response would be the same. The GAS consist of three phases: (a) the **alarm** reaction; (b) the stage of **resistance;** and (c) the stage of **exhaustion.**

Usually the organism adapts itself to maintain **homeostasis.** But if the stress is excessive and prolonged, there may be **failure of adaptation**. At this stage the **diseases of adaptation** or **stress-induced diseases** set in. They include a large number of psychosomatic diseases, allergies, immunological disorders (autoimmune disease), and inflammatory disorders.

GLUCOCORTICOIDS

Physiological Actions

Cortisol and synthetic glucocorticoids affect the **carbohydrate, protein** and **lipid metabolism.**

Carbohydrate metabolism: The glucocorticoids increase the production of glycogen, mainly from non-carbohydrate sources, i.e., they promote **gluconeogenesis.** Cortisol inhibits glucose uptake by tissue leading to **hyperglycaemia** and **glycosuria,** i.e., **it has an anti-insulin action.** Excess of cortisol may lead to **'steroid diabetes'.**

Protein metabolism: The glucocorticoids affect protein metabolism in two ways: (i) by **catabolic** action they increase the rate of protein breakdown to amino acids; and (ii) by an **anti-anabolic** effect they decrease the rate of dietary amino acid incorporation into new protein molecules. There is muscle wasting, weakness, osteoporosis, thinning of skin, and retardation of growth. The lymphoid tissue is reduced.

Lipid metabolism: Cortisol excess causes a **redistribution of fat** in the body—the fat is withdrawn from the extremities and increased deposits occur on the trunk (**buffalo hump**).

Electrolyte and water metabolism: The endogenous glucocorticoids also possess some mineralocorticoid activity, similar to that of aldosterone. Cortisol promotes **sodium retention** and **potassium excretion** by the kidneys.

Pharmacological Actions

Anti-inflammatory activity: The corticosteroids (natural and synthetic) inhibit the inflammatory responses of body tissues to all kinds of noxious stimuli regardless of the cause, i.e., they exert a **non-specific anti-inflammatory action.**

Antiallergic activity: They **suppress immediate hypersensitivity reactions** by interfering with the steps in the process of release of histamine and kinins. **The delayed hypersensitivity reactions may be suppressed by corticosteroids through their ability to inhibit the immune response.**

Immunosuppressant activity: The corticosteroids **inhibit antibody formation,** and **antibody reactions**. The glucocorticoids are also used to prevent cell mediated immune reactions like the **graft rejection reaction.** There is a dramatic destruction of lymphocytes.

Effect on Organ Systems

Cardiovascular system: The corticosteroids exerts a **positive inotropic effect.** The **blood volume is increased** secondary to electrolyte and water retention. Prolonged corticosteroid administration is likely to cause **steroid induced hypertension.**

Central nervous system: They exert **indirect** effects through maintenance of plasma glucose, and electrolyte balance essential for CNS activity. The **direct** effects are poorly defined. With excessive amounts of glucocorticoids behavioural changes ranging from **euphoria** to **psychosis** can occur.

Gastrointestinal system: Glucocorticoids increase the secretion of gastric hydrochloric acid, pepsinogen, and pancreatic trypsinogen. They are **ulcerogenic.**

Urinary system: Cortisol increases plasma volume and filtration pressure, increasing the glomerular filtration rate. This leads to **water diuresis.**

Blood and haemopoietic tissue: Haematologic effects of glucocorticoids include decrease in lymphatic tissue, and in circulating lymphocytes, eosinophils and basophils, but there is an increase in neutrophils, platelets and erythrocytes. The reduction in lymphatic tissue, and lymphopenia is due to decreased lympathic activity (**lymphoregression**), and destruction of lymphocytes (**lympholysis**). The **clotting time is shortened** presumably due to the increased platelets.

Skeletal muscle: Excess of corticoids leads to **muscle wasting** due to catabolism.

Body growth: Large doses of glucocorticoids **retard or interrupt the growth of children**. Glucocorticoids inhibit cell division and **delay healing**.

METABOLISM AND EXCRETION

In the plasma cortisol is reversibly bound (95%) to an alpha globulin. Only free or unbound cortisol (5%) is active. Cortisol is taken up by the liver where it forms water soluble compounds which are excreted in the urine. A part of cortisol is metabolized and excreted in the urine as **17-ketosteroids**.

SYNTHETIC ADRENOCORTICOSTEROIDS

Molecular manipulation has met with appreciable success and synthetic compounds are available in which the **anti-inflammatory activity has been intensified, and the sodium retaining activity has been minimized.**

The first synthetic glucocorticoids were **prednisone** and **prednisolone.** They are 4 or 5 times more potent anti-inflammatory agents compared to cortisone and hydrocortisone, and the sodium retaining activity is much less. In compounds like **dexamethasone** and **betamethasone** the anti-inflammatory activity was increased and the salt-retaining effect was almost entirely eliminated.

Topically applied corticosteroids: When a local effect is desired, corticosteroids may be applied topically in various dosage forms (e.g. ointment, cream, lotion, aerosol, nasal spray, ophthalmic drops) or by intra-articular injection. *Fluorinated derivatives* (betamethasone, fluocinonide, halcinonide) are more potent than *non-fluorinated agents* (hydrocortisone, desonide), and are also less likely to cause sodium retention.

To **summarize**, modification of the structure of natural corticosteroids has produced compounds with the following properties:

1. Mainly glucocorticoid activity with significant mineralocorticoid actions–**Prednisone, prednisolone, cortisone**.
2. Glucocorticoid activity with high anti-inflammatory potency and insignificant mineralocorticoid action–**Dexamethasone, Betamethasone**.
3. Mineralocorticoid activity with insignificant glucocorticoid actions–**fludrocortisone**.

Mode of Action

The natural and synthetic glucocorticoids like other steroid hormones bind to **specific intracellular receptors** located in the cytoplasm of the target cells. Specific receptors have been clearly demonstrated for **cortisol, aldosterone, testosterone** and **oestradiol.** The **steroid-receptor *complex*** is transferred to the nucleus where it is bound to the chromatin. In the nucleus the steroid-receptor complex interacts with DNA, and stimulates the transcription of **new messenger RNA (m-RNA)**. These new proteins (enzymes) are responsible for the **glucocorticoid response** in the cells.

The corticosteroids exert a **non-specific anti-inflammatory action.** The corticosteroids also **stabilize the lysosomal membranes** in the cells preventing the release of kinins and lytic enzymes. The growth of new capillaries and fibroblastic activity at the site is inhibited, and **healing is delayed.** Corticosteroids inhibit the hypothalamio-pituitary-adrenal axis (HPA axis).

The **immunosuppressive action** is due to the cytolytic action of glucocorticoids on the **lymphocytes** and **thymocytes**. The corticosteroids **inhibit homograft rejection reactions.**

THERAPEUTIC USES

Their uses can be subdivided into two main heads: (A) **Endocrinal disorders**; and (B) **Non-endocrinal disorders.**

A. **Endocrinal disorders**

1. **Primary adrenocortical insufficiency (Addison's disease).** Hydrocortisone 20 to 30 mg daily orally may be administered.
2. **Acute adrenocortical insufficiency (Addisonian crisis):** It is an emergency and treated by **hydrocortisone hemisuccinate** 100 mg IV rapidly, followed by **hydrocortisone hemisuccinate** 100 mg IV infusion slowly in 1000 ml of 0.9 percent sodium chloride solution every 8 hourly.
3. **Adrenocortical hyperfunction:** In conditions like Cushing's syndrome. The aim of therapy is to suppress pituitary ACTH production. **Prednisone** and **fludrocortisone** have been tried.
4. **Diagnostic use:** Glucocorticoids (dexamethasone or betamethasone) are employed to test the integrity of the hypothalamo-pituitary-adrenal system.

B. **Non-endocrinal disorders**

1. **Rheumatic and other joint disorders:** Patients who require corticosteroids are started on small daily doses of **prednisone** or **prednisolone,** e.g., 5, 7.5, or 10 mg in addition to salicylates or other NSAIDs. Some times corticosteroids may have to be injected **intra-articularly,** i.e., directly into the involved joints. Sterile aqueous suspensions of **triamcinolone** often provide relief for 2-4 weeks after each injection. Corticosteroids are used in **acute** and **chronic gout**, and gouty arthritis.
2. **Collagen diseases:** In addition to rheumatoid arthritis, they include disseminated lupus erythematosus, acute rheumatic fever and carditis, periarteritis nodosa, scleroderma, and pemphigus vulgaris.
3. **Allergic disorders:** Used in the emergency management of anaphylactic shock, blood transfusion reactions, Stevens-Johnson syndrome, atopic and contact dermatitis, allergic rhinitis, allergic conjunctivitis, hay fever and angioneurotic oedema. Corticosteroids are employed as immunosuppressants to avoid and control **homograft rejection reactions.**
4. **Dermatologic disorders:** Corticosteroids are effective in psoriasis, seborrheic dermatitis, pruritus vulvi or ani, and dermatitis herpetiformis.
5. **Ophthalmic disease:** These include irtis, iridocyclitis, choroiditis, keratitis, uveitis, and corneal ulcers.
6. **Respiratory diseases:** These include bronchial asthma and status asthmatics.
7. **Haematologic disorders:** Used in the management of blood dyscrasias including acquired or autoimmune haemolytic anaemia, and idiopathic thrombocytopenia.
8. **Neoplastic disease:** Employed as part of the multiple drug regime for acute lympathic leukaemia in children, chronic lympathic leukaemia in adults, and to control hypercalcaemia in cancer. Also used in Hodgkin's disease and other lymphomatous neoplasms.
9. **Gastrointestinal diseases:** Employed in cases of ulcerative colitis, regional enteritis, and intractable sprue.
10. **Acute infectious diseases:** Used in cases of **Gram-negative septicaemia** and **endotoxic shock**, and to control

complications of **tuberculous meningitis, tuberculous laryngitis, acute military tuberculosis, acute caseous pneumonia, viral infection, mumps orchitis, measles, encephalitis** and appropriate anti-infective chemotherapy must be administered together with the corticosteroids.

11. **Miscellaneous disorders :** These disorders include **sarcoidosis, Loeffler's syndrome, myasthenia gravis, infectious mononucleosis, haemorrhagic shock, Bell's palsy, neuritis** and **subacute thyroiditis.**

Contraindications

Corticosteroids must be used with great caution in the following conditions:

1. **Peptic ulcer.**
2. **Infections.**
3. **Hypertension with congestive heart failure.**
4. **Psychosis.**
5. **Diabetes mellitus.**
6. **Osteoporosis.**
7. **Glaucoma.**
8. **Pregnancy.**

Absolute contraindications include psychoses, severe psychoneuroses, active peptic ulcer, herpes simplex keratitis, and infections that cannot be effectively controlled by chemotherapy.

Adverse Reactions

Metabolic toxicity: Most patients receiving glucocorticoids for longer than 2 weeks develop changes termed as **iatrogenic Cushing's syndrome,** and develop 'Cushingoid' features. **Hyperglycaemia, glycosuria** and **diabetes** may be developed or aggravated. There is an increase in appetite and **weight gain. Myopathy** may develop as a result of a negative nitrogen balance. **Osteoporosis** occurs as a result of loss of bony matrix. **Avascular aseptic necrosis of bone** can occur. **Peptic ulcers** develop. **Body growth in children is retarded.** The patients may develop **hypertension, oedema** and **congestive heart failure**. Effect on mineral metabolism may lead to **sodium retention, oedema, hypopotassemia** and **hypochloraemic alkalosis.**

Behavioural toxicity: Patients develop a **euphoria** and on prolonged administration steroids may cause **psychological** and **physical** dependence, leading to a **steroid withdrawal syndrome.**

Ocular toxicity: Corticosteroids may raise the intraocular pressure, and cause a **steroid induced glaucoma**. **Posterior subcapsular cataracts** develop on long-term steroid therapy.

Adrenal suppression: When patients are maintained on long-term corticosteroid therapy there is an appreciable **suppression of the pituitary-adrenal axis** due to the feedback mechanism.

Other complications: Corticosteroids may cause **superinfection, exacerbation of infection, accelerated blood coagulation, delayed wound healing,** and **rarely hypersensitivity reactions.**

Precautions

The two major aspects to be taken care of are *infection, and hypothalamo-pituitary-adrenal (HPA) axis suppression.*

Infection: Glucocorticoids therapy predisposes the patient to infection of all types (bacterial, viral, fungal, parasitic).

Hypothalamo-pituitary-adrenal axis (HPA) suppression: Exogenous glucocorticoid administration due to a negative feedback to the HPA results in suppression of the HPA axis.

Intermittent Dosage Schedules

These dosage schedules are **tuned to the circadian rhythm** followed by the HPA axis and the **single dose** is administered in the morning when the pituitary adrenal axis is least amenable to damage.

Single daily dose schedule: Instead of administration of several small doses during the day, the total daily steroid dose is administered at about 8.00 AM.

Alternate Day Therapy (ADT)

The ADT regimen consist of administration of a 48-hour dose of an intermediate-acting glucocorticoids between 7.00 to 8.00 AM every other morning.

The ADT regimen is useful in the treatment of **asthma, uveitis, nephrotic syndrome,** and **disseminated lupus erythematosus.** Some patients of **rheumatoid arthritis,** and **ulcerative colitis** may develop symptoms on the 'off' day when medication is withheld.

Steroid Withdrawal

Once the patient is put on long-term steroid therapy, withdrawal of the drug becomes difficult on two scores: (i) the withdrawal may set up an **acute exacerbation** of the disorder; and (ii) a **steroid withdrawal syndrome** may develop as the patient craves to take the steroid for the euphoria it produces. Steroids are capable of producing both **psychological** and **physical** dependence.

GUIDELINES FOR CORTICOSTEROID THERAPY

1. **Accurate diagnosis.**
2. Corticosteroid therapy is started only after alternative therapy has failed.
3. The dosage should be determined, and the **smallest dose** should be used.
4. Systemic administration of a **single large dose** is usually without adverse effects.
5. When possible, **administer corticosteroids locally.**
6. Pharmacologic doses of **glucocorticoids should not be abruptly stopped**, as an adrenal crisis is likely to develop.

MINERALOCORTICOIDS

Aldosterone is the major physiological mineralocorticoid in man, but is unsuitable for routine medical use as it is inactivated when given orally. **Fludrocortisone**, a synthetic corticosteroid is the most often used compound when long-term mineralocorticoid treatment is required.

Aldosterone

Aldosterone is synthesized mainly in the **zona glomerulosa** of the adrenal cortex. **The most important stimulus to aldosterone secretion is a reduction in blood volume, leading to a fall in mean renal arterial pressure, which results in the release of renin from the juxtaglomerular apparatus of the kidney.** Released aldosterone induces the **reabsorption of sodium,** and **loss of potassium with hydrogen ions** in the urine.

Hyperaldosteronism is of two types: **Primary hyperaldosteronism** (Conn's disease) is usually due to an adrenal adenoma or sometimes a carcinoma. **Secondary hyperaldosteronism** occurs in disorders like *congestive heart failure, nephrotic syndrome, cirrhosis with ascites, renal artery stenosis, sodium deprivation and potassium excess.*

Deoxycorticosterone (DOC)

DOC is a mineralocorticoid with almost no glucocorticoid activity. It is available for parenteral administration as **replacement therapy in chronic primary adrenocortical insufficiency**, and in certain forms of congenital adrenal hyperplasia. **Subcutaneous pellet** implantation maintains the mineralocorticoid effect for 2 to 3 months. *Adverse reactions* include sodium and water retention, hypokalemia, hypertension, cardiac enlargement, and congestive heart failure.

Fludrocortisone

Fludrocortisone has very high mineralocorticoid and moderate glucocorticoid activity. **It is the most often used mineralocorticoid**, as it is the only compound available for oral use, and is employed for the management of **chronic primary adrenocortical insufficiency. Adverse reactions** include oedema, hypertension and hypokalaemia. It is available as fludrocortisone acetate, and the dose ranges between 0.05 to 0.5 mg daily orally for several months.

ALDOSTERONE ANTAGONISTS

These are steroids which **compete with aldosterone** for the binding site in the distal renal tubule. **Spironolactone** is such an agent used clinically as a potassium-sparing diuretic.

DRUG INTERACTIONS

The metabolism of adrenocorticosteroids in the body is increased by drugs that induce the hepatic microsomal enzymes, e.g., **phenobarbitone, phenytoin and rifampicin.** Corticosteroids have a hyperglycaemic effect, and the dose of **hypoglycaemia agents** in the diabetic patients may require an increase.

7.6 FEMALE SEX HORMONES AND ORAL CONTRACEPTIVES

There are three types of sex hormones, **androgens, oestrogens** and **progestogens.** Both the sexes produce all the three types, but androgens predominate in males, oestrogens and progestogens in females. In the ovaries oestrogens are secreted by the **Graafian follicle,** and progesterone is secreted by the **corpus luteum.**

PHYSIOLOGIC CONSIDERATIONS

The oestrogens and progesterone are responsible for the **cyclic** changes occurring in the endometrium (menstrual cycle). The oestrogens are synthesized in the ovaries, adrenals, placenta and testes. In women the ovaries are the main source of oestrogens. At **puberty** the ovary begins a 30 to 40 years period of cyclic function, under the influence of pituitary gonadotrophins, the most obvious manifestation being **cyclic uterine bleeding.** Ultimately the uterus fails to respond to pituitary gonadotrophins, and there is a cessation of cyclic bleeding termed as **menopause**.

The anterior pituitary stimulates the ovary mainly through two gonadotropic hormones, namely **follicle stimulating (FSH),** and **luteinizing (LH) hormone.** Additionally the LH in precise balance with the FSH causes the maturation of the follicle, ovulation, and formation of the corpus luteum. A third hormone **prolactin** also initiates mammary gland proliferation and secretion of milk. The placenta produces a **chorionic gonadotrophin**, which can be extracted and purified from the urine of pregnant women. Oestrogens and progesterone inhibit the formation of FSH and LH, respectively by a **negative feedback mechanism** and prevent ovulation.

At the beginning of each cycle FSH increases the oestrogen secretion by the ovarian follicle. This causes proliferation of the endometrium (**proliferative phase**). The oestrogen secretion reaches its peak just before midcycle, and synchronized with the brief surge in LH and FSH, precedes ovulation. Thus, under the influence of LH, on about day 14 of the cycle the follicle ruptures and the ovum is released. **Ovulation** is associated with a **rise in basal body temperature** (BBT). After this under the continuing influence of LH, the corpus luteum secretes progesterone (**Fig. 7.3**). Under progesterone effect the uterine glands become coiled and secretory (**secretary phase**). If the ovum is not fertilized the corpus luteum regresses and the endometrium is shed, i.e., **menstruation** occurs. If fertilization occurs, the corpus luteum continues to secrete oestrogen and progesterone during the early weeks of pregnancy.

OESTROGENS

The term 'oestrogen' is used as a **generic** term including all compounds having oestrogenic activity.

Biosynthesis, Metabolism and Excretion

The major natural oestrogens produced by women are **oestradiol, oestrone** and **oestriol.** The follicular synthesis of oestradiol is regulated by the pituitary gonadotrophins (LH and FSH) acting together. In the first trimester of pregnancy, the **human chorionic gonadotrophin** (HCG) promotes the steroidogenic activity of the corpus luteum.

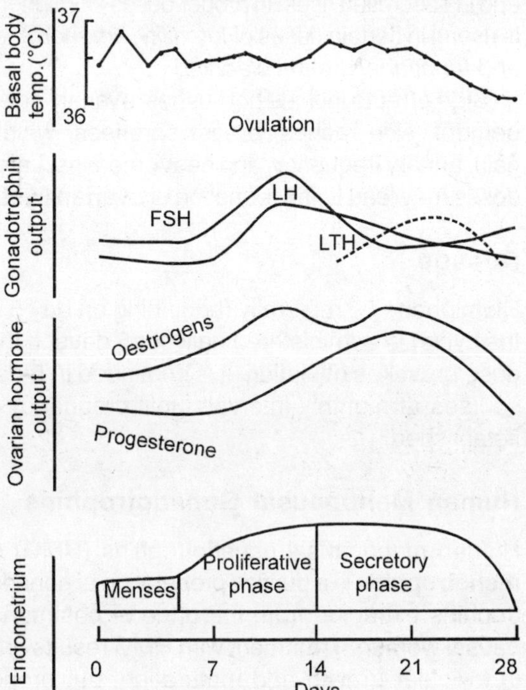

Fig. 7.3: *The menstrual cycle, showing graphically the pituitary and ovarian hormone output, and the basal body temperature record.*

The initial step in the synthesis of oestrogens is the conversion of acetate to cholesterol. Cholesterol is then converted to **pregnenolone** and **progesterone.**

Oestrogens are metabolized by the liver, **conjugated** to glucuronide and sulphate, and excreted in the urine and bile.

Actions

Oestrogens are responsible for the **development of the female sexual organs at puberty, and the development and maintenance of secondary sexual characteristics.** The oestrogenic effect is exerted on the uterus and adnexa, vagina, clitoris and breast. They cause proliferation of the endometrium of the uterus (proliferative phase); and **ductal growth in the breast.** They contribute to the growth of axillary and pubic hair, and alter the distribution of body fat to produce a **female body contour.** They induce the typical feminine psychological get up and voice. They have **anti-androgenic** actions.

Oestrogens promote osteoblastic activity, and **maturation of epiphyses in bones.** Oestrogens have a **hypocholesterolaemic effect**, and promote *salt and water retention* producing oedema.

Mode of Action

Oestrogens are bound in the target organs to a specific macromolecule–the **oestrogen receptor**. This hormone-receptor complex is transferred to the nucleus where it increases RNA synthesis followed by increased protein synthesis. Oestrogens have a **weak anabolic action.**

Therapeutic Uses

Oestrogens are used for r*eplacement therapy* in oestrogen deficient patients.

1. **Menopausal syndrome.**
2. **Ovarian dysgenesis.**
3. **Primary amenorrhoea.**
4. **Carcinoma of the prostate** in the male.
5. **Vulvo-vaginitis** in children.
6. Functional uterine bleeding and **endometriosis.**
7. **Acne** and **hirsutism.**
8. **Dysmenorrhoea.**
9. **Suppression of lactation.**
10. **Postpartum breast engorgement.**
11. For **oral contraception** in combination with progestogens.

Contraindications

Oestrogens are not to be used in **oestrogen-dependent neoplasms** of the endometrium or breast, **premenopausal carcinomas** of the breast or uterus, uterine fibroids, renal and hepatic diseases, **hypertension** and **thromboembolic diseases.**

Toxicity

Anorexia, nausea and **vomiting** is observed frequently specially with the synthetic compounds.

Nausea and **breast tenderness** commonly occur, and can be minimized by using the smallest effective dose of oestrogens. Salt and water retention leads to weight gain, oedema and cardiac failure. There is an **increased frequency of migraine. Hypertension** may develop on prolonged use. Prolonged oestrogen therapy increases the incidence of **thromboembolic disorders** and **hepatic dysfunction.**

Preparation and Dosage

Three types of oestrogens are available: (i) the **naturally** occurring steroid oestrogens; (ii) **semisynthetic steroid oestrogens;** and (iii) the **synthetic non-steroidal oestrogens**. Their specifications are summarized in **Table 7.3.**

OVULATION INDUCING AGENTS

Representative agents are: clomiphene, human menopausal gonadotrophin, urofollitrophin, and human chorionic gonadotrophin.

Clomiphene Citrate

Clomiphene has an **antioestrogenic** action. Thus through the hypothalamic mechanism, it increases pituitary gonadotrophin (FSH and LH) secretion and stimulates ovulation. The ovaries are enlarged, ovulation, and sustained functioning of the corpus luteum are induced. **Clomiphene binds to oestrogen receptors, thereby decreasing the number of receptors available for oestrogen action.** This is sensed by the hypothalamus and pituitary that the oestrogen level is low, and FSH and LH secretion rises. In proper doses clomiphene is useful in certain cases of *infertility, amenorrhoea* and *functional uterine bleeding.*

Side effects include hot flushes, ovarian enlargement, skin rashes, breast soreness, weight gain, urinary frequency, and heavy menses. Large doses may lead to the formation of **ovarian cysts.**

Dosage

Clomiphene 50 mg orally (beginning on day 5 of the cycle) is administered daily for 5 days. If this dose provokes ovulation, it is continued in 5-day courses at monthly intervals until pregnancy is established.

Human Menopausal Gonadotrophins

Human menopausal gonadotrophins (HMG) or **menotrophins** is a purified preparation of gonadotrophins extracted from the urine of postmenopausal women. Treatment with HMG results only in follicular growth and maturation; but proper ovulation is induced by subsequent administration of human chorionic gonadotrophins (HCG).

Menotrophins is used to treat infertility in women with **primary** or **secondary amenorrhoea, polycystic ovary syndrome, anovulatory cycles,** or **irregular menses.** It is used with HCG to stimulate spermatogenesis in men who have **primary** or **secondary hypogonadotrophic hypogonadism.**

Dosage: Menotrophins is available as a powder for injection with 75 U FSH activity, and 75 U LH activity per 2 ml ampoule, or 150 U FSH and 150 U LH activity per 2 ml ampoule. The contents of

Table 7.3 : *The three types of common oestrogen preparations available, and their mode of administration*

Classification	Preparation	Usual route of administration	Dose range (mg)
1. *Naturally-occuring oestrogen*	Oestradiol 17-β	IM	0.22-1.5
2. *Semisynthetic steriodal oestrogens*	Ostradiol benzoate	Oral	0.1-1.0
	Ethinyloestradiol	Oral	0.05-0.1
	Mestranol	Oral	0.1-0.2
3. *Synthetic non-steroidal oestrogen*	Diethylstilboestrol	Oral	0.2-1

the ampoule are dissolved in 2 ml of sterile saline and administered IM. In women usually 1 ampoule per day (75 U each of FSH and LH) is given IM for 9-12 days, followed by HCG 10,000 U IM one day after the last dose of menotrophins.

Adverse effects of menotrophins include ovarian enlargement with or without abdominal pain, *ovarian hyperstimulation syndrome* (abdominal pain, ascites, pleural effusion, ovarian enlargement), haemoperitoneum, ovarian cysts, and rarely arterial thromboembolism. Multiple births occur with HMG/HCG treatment in about 15 percent of pregnancies. In men, gynaecomastia occurs.

Human Chorionic Gonadotrophin

HCG is a purified polypeptide hormone, produced by the human placenta, and extracted from the urine of women during the **first trimester of pregnancy.**

HCG is used for **induction of ovulation** in anovulatory women who have been pretreated with HMG. HCG is also used to treat **cryptorchidism** (undescended testes), and for the treatment of **male hypogonadism** secondary to pituitary hypofunction.

Dosage: HCG is available as a powder for injection containing 200 U/ml, 500 U/ml, 1000 U/ml, and 2000 U/ml after reconstitution. HCG is given IM and the dosage is highly individualized.

Adverse reactions include ovarian hyperstimulation, rupture of ovarian cysts with haemoperitoneum, multiple births, arterial thromboembolism, depression, and gynaecomastia in males.

PROGESTOGENS

Progesterone, a steroid derivative of pregnane, is the main natural progestogen. It is secreted by the **ovary, placenta, testes** and **adrenals.** In addition to its hormonal effects, it serves as a precursor of oestrogens, androgens and adrenocorticosteroids. It is ineffective orally.

Biosynthesis, Metabolism and Excretion

The biosynthesis of progesterone mainly occurs in the **corpus luteum** and the **placenta.** It is synthesized from acetate, cholesterol and pregnenolone. Progesterone is rapidly absorbed following administration by any route. It has a short plasma half-life of 5 minutes. It is **rapidly metabolized in its first passage through the liver,** and excreted in the urine.

Actions

Just prior to ovulation, there is an elevation in FSH and LH levels, and the secretion of progesterone is initiated at this time (**Fig. 7.3**). The LH facilitates the transformation of a follicle to a corpus luteum, which secretes progesterone and oestrogen. **Progesterone is secreted by the corpus luteum mainly in the second half of the menstrual cycle (luteal phase). Progesterone elevates the basal body temperature shortly after ovulation.** This elevation may be used to detect ovulation in women, and is the basis of the 'rhythm method' of birth control.

Progesterone prepares the endometrium for the **implantation of the ovum** (nidation). It promotes **aleveolar (acinar) growth in the oestrogen primed breast. Progesterone renders the uterus less sensitive to oxytocin and ergonovine.**

Mode of Action

Studies support the presence of **progesterone receptors**, which are macromolecules located in the cytoplasm and nucleus of the target organs. Progesterone on entering the target cells binds with the cytoplasmic receptors. As a result of this, progesterone increases the metabolic activity and growth of the female reproductive organs.

Therapeutic Uses

Progestogens are mainly used with oestrogens as **oral contraceptives.** They may be tried in **threatened or habitual abortion.** They are used in cases of **dysmenorrhoea, premenstrual tension, menstrual irregularities, and functional uterine bleeding. Chemical pregnancy tests are based on the detection of "human chorionic gonadotrophins" in urine.**

Toxicity

Sodium and water retention may occur. Progesterone and progestational agents administered early in pregnancy may lead to **masculinization of the external genitalia in the female foetus.**

Dosage

Progesterone (20-60mg IM daily) may be given in an oily solution.

Synthetic Progestational Agents

Synthetic progestogens are mainly of three types: (i) **progesterone derivatives;** (ii) **testosterone derivatives;** and (iii) **19-nortestosterone derivatives.** They possess optimal progestational activity, and are **orally active with a longer duration of action.**

PROGESTERONE INHIBITOR

Mifepristone (RU 486)

Mifepristone is a '19-norsteroid' compound. It binds strongly to the progesterone receptor and inhibits the activity of progesterone. It may be useful in the treatment of *endometriosis, Cushing's syndrome, breast cancer, and other malignancies that contain progesterone or glucocorticoid receptors.*

The major use of *mifepristone* is as an ***abortifacient*** to terminate early pregnancy. A ***single oral dose*** of the 'abortion pill' containing mifepristone 600 mg plus 200 mcg of **misoprostol** (a synthetic analogue of PGE_1) has been found to terminate pregnancy in 95% of patients during the first 7 weeks.

Adverse reactions include vomiting, diarrhoea, flatulence, headache, and sometimes profuse vaginal bleeding.

ORAL CONTRACEPTIVES

There are at least **nine** methods of birth control. They are the **pill** (combined), the **minipills** (progesterone only), **intrauterine devises (IUDs), diaphragms, condoms, condoms plus foam, foam, natural family planning** (basal body temperature method, cervical mucus method), and **sterilization** (tubal ligation for women, or vasectomy for men). The other methods including **calender rhythm, vaginal suppositories** and **tablets** have much lower effectiveness. The comparative estimates of effectiveness reported in literature are shown in **Table 7.4.**

Types of Formulations

Three types of oral contraceptive formulations are available: (i) Oestrogen-progestogen combinations (**combination pills**); (ii) sequential oestrogen-progesterone preparations (**sequential pills**); and (iii) continuous low-dosage progestogen preparations (**minipills**).

Oestrogen-progestogen combinations: The combination pill administered as a single daily dose from day 5 to day 25 of the menstrual cycle (21 days), counting the first day of menses as day 1. Withdrawal bleeding occurs within 3 to 4 days on completion of the course. In between there are *7 pill free days*, and the course is restarted on day 5 of the next cycle. **On repeating this schedule the cycle becomes anovulatory with regular cyclic bleeding.** The combination pills are almost 100 percent effective in preventing conception.

Sequential oestrogen-progestogen preparation: In the sequential regime also pills are administered from day 5 to day 25 of the menstrual cycle (21 days). From day 5 to day 20, a single pill daily containing *oestrogen alone* is administered, followed by single *oestrogen-progestogen combination pill* from day 21 to day 25 (16+5=21). There are *7 pill free days* during which withdrawal bleeding occurs. Serial packs are available, containing 16 oestrogen pills, 5 oestrogen-progestogen pills, and 7 placebo pills. **The woman is just instructed to take one pill a day in serial order.**

Low-dosage progestogen preparations: The minipills are preparations containing a progestogen alone (norethindrone, norgestrel). These progestogens in low dosage are to be taken daily continually to control fertility. **This schedule is less effective than the combination, or sequential contraceptive schedules.**

Table 7.4 : *Comparison of contraceptive efficacy of various contraceptive methods*

Method	Pregnancy rate per year (%)	
	Theoretical effectiveness	Use effectiveness
The pill (combined)	0.1	4-7
The "Minipill" (Progestogen only)	2.5	4
Intrauterine Devices (IUDs)	1-3	4-9
Vaginal spermicides	3	2-30
Foam	3	22
Condom and Foam	1	5
Condoms, Diaphragms	3	3-20
Rhythm	13	25-30
No contraception	Pregnancy would occur in 80 to 85% of women	

Mode of Action

The hypothalamic gonadotrophin releasing hormone (FSH-LH-RH) is inhibited which leads to a **suppression of FSH and LH release** from the anterior pituitary. A direct inhibiting effect on the pituitary secretion of gonadotrophins is also likely. In the **combination pills,** the suppression of FSH and LH caused by the oestrogen is enhanced by the progestogen. In contrast, the **sequential pills** depend on oestrogen alone to suppress FSH and LH release. The **inhibition of ovulation is mainly due to the oestrogenic component of the pill,** and progestogens serve to ensure prompt **withdrawal bleeding.**

In addition, these preparations **increase the viscosity of the cervical mucus,** and the secretion is less copious rendering it hostile to penetration by sperms.

Efficacy

A pill missed early in the cycle is more likely to result in an accidental pregnancy than a pill missed latter on in the cycle. **If there have been many omissions during the cycle, it is advisable to use conventional contraceptive methods in addition, to avoid accidental pregnancy. Combination oral contraceptives are extremely reliable for prevention of pregnancy, and the combination pills are more reliable than the sequential pills.**

Therapeutic Uses

1. **As oral contraceptives:** It is advisable that additional contraceptive means be employed during the first two months of medication, as suppression of ovulation may not be complete. Normal ovulatory cycle follows within 1 to 3 months of stoppage of medication.
2. The combination products have been employed in **endometriosis** when severe dysmenorrhoea is the major symptom. Suppression of ovulation is followed by painless periods. They have been used in certain cases of **premenstrual tension** and **menstrual irregularities**. In cases of **functional sterility** suppression of ovulation for 3 to 6 months may increase the chances of conception (rebound effect).

Contraindications

The **absolute** contracindications are thromboembolic or arterial disease, diabetes mellitus, hyperlipidaemia, liver disease , breast and uterine carcinoma, undiagnosed vaginal bleeding, migraine, and pregnancy. The **relative** contraindications are hypertension, epilepsy and depression.

Special Precautions

Each woman before oral contraceptive medication must be subjected to a **gynaecologic examination, evaluation of the cardiovascular, and liver function.** Care must be observed in women with a history of asthma, diabetes, endocrine disorders, epilepsy and migraine. Discontinuation of medication is advised on the occurrence of migraine-type headaches, and first signs of thrombophlebitis or embolism.

Drug Interactions

In 1971 it was first reported that **rifampicin**, an antituberculous drug, caused a failure of contraception, and pregnancies resulted. Breakthrough bleeding and failure of contraception was noted in patients on anticonvulsant drugs.

Adverse Reactions

Mild side effects include nausea, vomiting, headache, lethargy, breast discomfort (mastalgia), breakthrough bleeding (spotting), oedema and mild depression. Libido is often increased.

More serious side effects may be profuse breakthrough bleeding, oligomenorrhoea or amenorrhoea, weight gain, increased skin pigmentation, acne, hirsutism and vaginal infection.

Very serious side effects include the increased risk of deep vein thrombosis, and pulmonary embolism. There is a 5- to 10- fold increase in the incidence of **thromboembolic disorders.** Cerebral or coronary thrombosis may occur. **Severe hypertension, decreased glucose tolerance,** and **secondary diabetes mellitus** may develop. **Liver damage** and **cholestatic jaundice** have been reported.

Preparations and Dosage

Currently a number of oral contraceptive preparations are available. Some representative agents are listed in **Table 7.5.**

Intrauterine Progesterone Contraceptive System (Progestasert)

This system is a T-shaped intrauterine device (IUD) containing 38 mg of progesterone dispersed in

Table 7.5 : *The composition of some oral contraceptive preparations*

Trade name	Progestogen (mg)	Oestrogen (mg)
The combination pills*		
Bandhan	Levonorgestrel (0.15)	Ethinyloestradiol (0.03)
Duoluton-L	Levonorgestrel (0.25)	Ethinyloestradiol (0.05)
Mala-D	Levonorgestrel (0.30)	Ethinyloestradiol (0.03)
Orgalutin	Lynestrenol (2.5)	Ethinyloestradiol (0.05)
Ovral	Levonorgestrel (0.25)	Ethinyloestradiol (0.05)
Ovral-L	Levonorgestrel (0.15)	Ethinyloestradiol (0.03)
Ovulen	Ethinyloestradiol diacetate (1.0)	Ethinyloestradiol (0.1)
Suvida	Norgestrel (0.30)	Ethinyloestradiol (0.03)
The sequential pills**		
Ortho-novum SQ	Norethindrone (2.0)	Mestranol (0.08)
The minipills***		
Micronor	Norethindrone (0.35)	–

* Combinations : For 21 days, and 7 off days.

** Sequentials : only oestrogen for 14 to 16 days, then combination for 5 or 6 days, and 7 or 8 off days.

*** Minipills : Taken daily continuously.

silicone oil. On its insertion into the uterine cavity, progesterone is continuously released at an average rate of 65 mcg/day. The system suppresses the proliferation of endometrial tissue, creating an environment unfavourable for implantation. It also decreases sperm survival time by altering the cervical mucus, but does not prevent ovulation. After 1 year the system has to be changed.

Adverse reactions include dysmenorrhoea, amenorrhoea, cervical erosion, vaginitis, endometritis, spotting, prolonged menstrual flow, uterine perforation, ectopic pregnancy and pain. The device should be inserted immediately after menstruation to ensure absence of pregnancy.

POSTCOITAL CONTRACEPTION

When coitus has occurred without contraceptive protection, and pregnancy is not desired, large doses of oestrogens may be administered during the preimplantation stage to avoid the unwanted pregnancy. Such interceptive postcoital measures are referred to as 'morning after' contraception. Large doses of the oestrogens (diethylstilboestrol is claimed to be most effective) are administered **within 72 hours after unprotected sexual exposure.** Various regimens may be used (**Table 7.6**).

Table 7.6: *The various postcoital contraceptive oestrogen regimens*

Oestrogen	*Mode of administration (oral)*
Diethylstilboestrol	25 mg twice daily for 5 days
Ethinyloestradiol	2.5 mg twice daily for 5 days
Oestrone	5 mg thrice daily for 5 days

These high doses of oestrogens disturb the passage of the ovum through the fallopian tubes. They also alter the endometrium and interfere with nidation.

Lately, the Drug Controller General of India has approved the e-pill for "Emergency Oral Contraception". The e-pill contains levonorgestrel (0.75 mg/tablet) in packs of 2 tablets (under the brand name EC 2, Pill 72, E-pill, Norlevo). The two tablets have to be taken as soon as possible, within 72 hours of unprotected sex. Effectiveness depends on the time taken after intercourse, i.e., 24 hrs or less (95%); 25-48 hrs (85%); and 48-72 hrs (58%). This measure should not be relied upon routinely.

To **summarize**, the oral contraceptives do provide a reliable means for reversible contraception, but the directions for their use, and precautions must be strictly observed.

7.7 MALE SEX HORMONES, ANABOLIC STEROIDS AND ANTI-IMPOTENCY DRUGS

The male sex hormones or **androgens** are mainly secreted by the **testes,** and to a lesser extent by the **adrenal cortex** and the **ovary.** The most potent natural androgen is **testosterone,** and is secreted by the testicular **interstitial cells of Leydig.**

ANDROGENS

Physiologic Consideration

At puberty there is an increased secretion of pituitary gonadotrophins, follicle-stimulating hormone (FSH), and the luteinizing hormone (LH, same as interstitial cell stimulating hormone, ICSH in males). The FSH stimulates the metabolic activity of the **Sertoli cells** in the seminiferous tubules, and promotes spermatogenesis. The ICSH promotes the development of the **interstitial cells** of Leydig, which synthesize and secrete **testosterone.**

Biosynthesis, Metabolism and Excretion

Testicular steroidogenesis mainly occurs in the interstitial cells (**Leydig cells**), and also in the sustentacular cells (**Sertoli cells**). The interstitial cells contain cholesterol ester from which the natural androgen, testosterone is synthesized.

In man, testosterone is inactivated in the liver to **androsterone, epiandrosterone** and **etiocholanolone**, which are conjugated with sulphate and glucuronic acid. These inactive conjugates are passed in the urine.

Testosterone cannot be given orally as it is rapidly inactivated in the liver. The oral preparation **methyltestosterone** is rapidly absorbed and slowly inactivated by the liver.

Actions

Androgens are responsible for the development of the primary and secondary sex characters in the males at puberty, and are necessary for **spermatogenesis.** At puberty ICSH induces testosterone production and release causing growth of the sex organs, the development of pubic hair and a male hair distribution, rapid growth of the skeleton and musculature, and deepening of the voice. There is an increase in body weight, thickening and increased oiliness of the skin (acne), growth of the beard, fusion of epiphyses, and later on a development of the male pattern of baldness. **Oestrogens have appreciable antiandrogen activity.**

Mode of Action

The active form of testosterone is **5-α dihydrotestosterone**. Androgens bind to a **cytoplasmic receptor**, and increase synthesis of protein and RNA. Androgens promote the development of the male accessory glands (prostate, seminal vesicles) by causing increased protein synthesis.

Therapeutic Uses

Testosterone has a combined androgenic-anabolic pharmacologic profile.

1. In the male androgens are used in **cryptorchidism,** and in **hypogonadism** or castration. Their use in impotency is equivocal. May be used in **male climacteric.**
2. In the female they are used in **inoperable breast cancer.**
3. In both sexes they can be used as **anabolic agents**. May be used in **senile osteoporosis.**
4. Testosterone is capable of stimulating haemopoiesis, and may be used in **refractory** and **aplastic anaemia,** certain **leukaemias,** and in **thrombocytopenia.**

Contraindications

The contraindications are pregnancy and lactation, carcinoma of the prostate and male breast, cardiac and renal disease. Androgens should be used with great caution in infants and young children.

Toxicity

Androgens can lead to **sodium retention, hypertension, oedema** and **congestive heart failure. Hypercalcemia, premature closure of epiphyses** and **stoppage of linear growth** may result. Masculinization or virilization, clitoral enlargement, deepening of voice, baldness and hirsutism may occur in females. **Precocious puberty** (priapism and excessive libido) and acne occur. Hepatic dysfunction and **cholestatic jaundice** has been reported. Large doses in adult males lead to **suppression of spermatogenesis.**

Preparations and Dosage

1. **Testosterone injection:** Usually administered as 50 mg IM three times weekly.
2. **Testosterone pellets:** Pellets of 100 mg are available and are implanted subcutaneously into the medial side of the thigh.
3. **Testosterone propionate:** 5 to 25 mg in oil, given IM two to four times weekly.
4. **Methyltestosterone:** It is a natural androgen which is active when given in a dose of 20 to 50 mg daily sublingually or orally.

ANTIANDROGENS

Cyproterone Acetate

Cyproterone acetate is a synthetic compound with antiandrogenic action. It **possibly acts by preventing the binding of dihydrotestosterone to its receptor in the target cells.** It is a potent **competitive antagonist** of testosterone. **It may be used to decrease sexual drive.**

ANABOLIC STEROIDS

Testosterone has potent anabolic activity, but because of its associated androgenic activity it cannot be used freely, as it causes **virilization.** Steroids have been synthesized with an aim to dissociate the anabolic and androgenic activities. Chemically they are derivatives of testosterone. These drugs are predominantly anabolic but **retain weak androgenic activity.**

Actions

In therapeutic doses the **protein anabolic action is predominant.** These steroids induce a positive **nitrogen balance,** i.e., the nitrogen taken in is greater than the nitrogen lost from the body. This retained N is incorporated into amino acid and protein leading to **growth, regeneration,** and **hypertrophy of body tissue.** This is clinically manifested by **increase in muscle mass, and body weight.** They prevent the resorption of bone.

Preparation and Dosage

The **anabolic: Androgenic** ratio indicates the anabolic potency of these compounds, and for testosterone this ratio 1:1. All agents except nandrolone are active orally **(Table 7.7).**

Therapeutic Uses

These compounds have been used in the treatment of **osteoporosis, chronic renal failure, wasting due to prolonged immobilization, radiotherapy, cancer** (except carcinoma prostate) or **severe illness.** They may be used in high doses in patients with **metastatic carcinoma of the breast.** They have been used in **growth retardation, refractory** and **aplastic anemia,** and to **antagonize glucocorticoid-induced osteoporosis.**

The use of anabolic steroids to promote muscle growth and ***increase performance in athletes*** has attracted much attention. These drugs may be ***abused*** by athletes to improve their performance. Hence their use by athletes is officially banned.

Contraindications

As these agents are related to testosterone they are contraindicated in **prostatic cancer, severe liver insufficiency, severe nephrosis, pregnancy** and **lactation,** and in **male breast cancer.**

Toxicity

Salt and water retention leading to oedema may occur. **Hepatoma** may develop in patients on long-term therapy. If used during pregnancy they may lead to **virilization of the foetus.** They should not be continuously used for periods exceeding 4 weeks. High doses in women may produce **menstrual disorders, deepening of the voice, and hirsutism.** In children they may lead to **premature closure of epiphyses** and **virilization.**

DANAZOL

Danazol inhibits the release of FSH and LH from the anterior pituitary (**antigonadotrophic action**). It also has a **weak androgenic effect.** It **competitively** interferes with the binding of sex steroids to the cytoplasmic receptors.

Danazol is used to treat **endometriosis, fibro-**

Table 7.7 : *Pharmacologic profile and dosage of anabolic steroids*

Compound	Anabolic : Androgenic ratio*	Usual dosage
Nandrolone phenylpropionate	6:1	25-50 mg IM every week
Nandrolone decanoate	4:1	25-50 mg IM every 3 weeks
Stanozolol	6:1	6 mg orally/day

*the ratio for testosterone propionate is 1:1

cystic breast disease, hereditary angioedema, gynaecomastia, infertility and **menorrhagia.** Danazol is used as 50,100,200 mg capsules. Therapy is started during menstruation to rule out pregnancy. The usual dosage ranges between 100 to 400 mg/day in 2 to 3 divided doses for 3 to 9 months, depending on the disease. **Adverse reactions** include flushing, sweating, vaginitis, oedema, hirsutism, acne, oily skin, weight gain, voice deepening, decreased breast size, and clitoral hypertrophy. Vaginal bleeding, nervousness, and hepatic dysfunction have also been reported.

ANTI-IMPOTENCY DRUGS

Impotence or *erectile dysfunction* (ED) is the inability of a male to achieve satisfactory erection of the penis for sexual intercourse. Normally, erection is induced by parasympathetic stimulation initiated by the CNS, and facilitated by sensory stimuli from the penis. This dilates penile arteries and relaxes trabecular smooth muscle through a second messenger, probably ***nitric oxide***. This favours flow of blood into the ***corpora cavernosa*** leading to tumescence. The increased pressure compresses the venules against the fibrous tissue layer called the ***tunica albuginea***, which prevents the outflow of blood from the penis causing an erection. The causes of impotence may be ***psychological***; or ***organic***; or *drug induced* or a mixture of the above factors.

Phentolamine and Papaverine

The combination of the alpha-adrenoceptor blocker ***phentolamine*** (2 mg) with the nonspecific vasodilator ***papaverine*** (12-40 mg) when injected into the corpora cavenosa of the penis causes erection in man suffering from ***erectile dysfunction.*** The long-term efficacy of this therapy is not known. There is a risk of local fibrotic reactions on prolonged use. *Priapism* may occur.

Alprostadil (PGE_1)

Intracavernosal injection of the vasodilator ***alprostadil*** (PGE_1) is used to produce penile erection in men with ED. Doses of 0.2 to 140 mcg are used. Penile pain occurs frequently. Prolonged erection and *priapism* may occur in some patients.

Lately, ***triple therapy*** combining papaverine, phentolamine and alprostadil has been reported to be effective with a lower incidence of adverse effects.

Sildenafil Citrate

Sildenafil is the first oral pill to treat erectile dysfunction (ED). It is popularly known as the 'little blue pill' or 'the virility pill'. ***Sildenafil citrate*** was licensed by the FDA, USA in 1998.

Mode of Action

Sildenafil enhances the smooth muscle relaxant effect of ***nitric oxide*** (NO), a critical **second messenger** released in the corpora cavernosa in response to sexual stimulation. Sildenafil is a phosphodiesterase (PDE) inhibitor, and conserves cyclic GMP. Thus cyclic GMP is conserved, and sexual stimulation gives a more "natural" erectile response. Viagra has no effect on libido (sexual desire). *Dosage*: One Viagra pill is best taken about an hour before sexual activity. *Adverse reactions*: Viagra is generally well tolerated, but side effects include **headache, flushing, GI disturbances,** and **urinary tract infection.** The 'pill' may cause serious side effects or even death among users suffering from **diabetes mellitus** or **cardiac problems.** The elderly are at a greater risk.

Lately, **tadalafil** and **vardenafil**, both phosphodiesterase (PDE) inhibitors, have been introduced for the treatment of erectile dysfunction.

The Vitamins

8

The vitamins are essential microconstituents of diet, which do not give energy, but are necessary for the normal metabolism of the body. Adequate amounts reach the body via a well balanced diet. The toxic effects of vitamin A and D, specially in infants and children must always be kept in mind.

CLASSIFICATION

The vitamins may be categorized into two: (i) the **fat-soluble vitamins;** and (ii) the **water-soluble vitamins.** They are further detailed in **Table 8.1.**

FAT-SOLUBLE VITAMINS

Vitamin A

Mode of action: Vitamin A plays many essential roles in the body. It maintains the **functional** and **structural integrity of epithelial cells** throughout the body.

Toxicity: Prolonged overdosage leads to **hypervitaminosis A.** The children are more liable to this syndrome although it has been detected in adults also. Hypervitaminosis A is characterized by *anorexia, irritability, periosteal thickening, dry skin, pruritus with desquamation, fatigue, myalgia, nystagmus,* and *hepatosplenomegaly*. The intracranial pressure may be increased.

Vitamin D

Mode of action: Vitamin D itself is inactive. In the body it is converted by hydroxylation to **calcifediol** and **1, 25-dihydroxycholecalciferol** (Calcitriol). These two products are the active forms of vitamin D.

The **primary action** of vitamin D is to increase the absorption of calcium and phosphorus from the intestines, and also to reciprocally increase the renal excretion of phosphorus.

Toxicity: Acute or chronic administration of large amounts of Vitamin D leads to ***hypervitaminosis D.*** Initially there is hypercalcaemia, fatigue, vomiting and diarrhoea. With prolonged hypercalcaemia there is ***metastatic calcification,*** i.e., deposition of calcium in soft tissues.

Vitamin E

Vitamin E is supposed to maintain the germinal epithelium. Based on this feature vitamin E therapy is tried in cases of **infertility in women, habitual abortion, progressive muscular dystrophy, peripheral vascular disease, refractory anaemias** and **haemolytic anaemias.**

Vitamin K

Mode of action: Vitamin K promotes the hepatic synthesis of prothrombin, factors II, VII, IX and X.

Toxicity: In man menadione is irritating to the skin and respiratory tract. It may lead to vesication. Menadione can induce **haemolytic anaemia, hyperbilirubinaemia** and **kernicterus** in the newborn.

Table 8.1 : *The vitamins, their dietary allowances (RDAs), and therapeutic doses*

Vitamin	Major dietary sources	Recommended Dietary Allowances (RDA)			Main dificiency disorder	Therapeutic Doses	
		Children	Adults			Oral	Parenteral
			Males	Females			
1. Fat-soluble vitamins							
Vitamin A	Fish liver oils, egg yolk, milk, butter, green and yellow vegetables, tomatoes, yellow fruits	2000-3500 IU	5000 IU	4000IU	Night blindness, xerophthalmia, hyperkeratosis of the skin, increased susceptibility to colds, influenza and infections, keratinization of epithelial tissues	25,000-100,000 IU	50,000 IU IM
Vitamin D	Fish liver oils, egg yolk milk, butter, margarine, salmon, sardines	400 IU	200-400 IU	200-400 IU	Rickets, Osteomalacia, infantile tetany	Ergocalciferol 50,000-500,000 IU Cholicalciferol 400-1000 IU Calcitrol 0.5-1.0 mcg/day Calcifediol 300-350 mcg/week Dihydrotachysterol 0.8-2.4 mg/day	 50,000-200,000 IU IM – 1-2 mcg IM – – –
Vitamin E	Wheat germ, vegetable oils, green leafy vegetables, nuts, cereals, eggs, dairy products	7-10 IU	12-15 IU	12 IU	Deficiency in animals produces sterility, loss of embryo, muscular dystrophy, paralysis, Deficiency state not established in humans, possibly haemolytic anaemia, muscular lesions, creatinuria	d-alpha-Tocopherol 10-200 mg d-alpha-Tocopheryl acetate 10-200 mg d-alpha-Tocopheryl acid succinate 10-200 mg	Tocopherols, mixed concentrates 10-200 mg IM –
Vitamin K	Green leafy vegetales liver, cheese, egg yolk, tomotoes, meats, cereals	Extremely small	–	–	Hypoprothrombinaemia, haemorrhage	Menadiol sodium diphospht (K4) 5 mg Menadione 1 mg Menadione sodium bisulfite 2-5 mg	 5-75 MG im or SC – 2-5 mg IM or SC

Vitamin	Major dietary sources	Recommended Dietary Allowances (RDA)			Maindificiency disorder	Therapeutic Doses	
		Children	Adults			Oral	Parenteral
			Males	Females			
II. Water soluble vitamins							
Vitamin B complex							
Thiamine (B_1)	Liver, whole grain, enriched bread, cereals, pork, egg yolk, rice polishings	0.7-1.2 mg	1.2-1.4 mg	1.0-1.1 mg	Beriberi, anorexia, peripheral neuritis, constipation	5-100 mg	5-100 mg IM, IV
Riboflavine (B_2)	Organ meats, milk, eggs, green vegetables, enriched bread	0.8-1.4 mg	1.4-1.7 mg	1.2-1.3 mg	Stomatitis, glossitis, facial dermatitis, photophobia, cheilosis, corneal vascularization	1-5 mg	1-10 mg parenteral
Nicotinic acid (B_3) (Niacin)	Liver, fish, poultry, red meat, enriched bread and cereals, rice polishings, bran	9-16 mg	16-19 mg	13-15 mg	Pellagra (nervousness insomnia, dermatitits, diarrhoea dementia, delusions, confusion)	20-50 mg	20-50 mg parenteral
Pantothenic acid (B_5)	Organ meats, egg yolk, peanuts, whole grains Cauliflower, rice polishings	*	*	*	"Burning foot" syndrome weakness, fatigue, mood changes, dizziness	20-100 mg	250-500 mg, IM every 6 hrs for 2-3 days for postoperative abdominal distension and paralytic ileus
Pyridoxine (B_6)	Yeast, red meat, liver, whole grains, soya beans, green vegetables	0.9-1.6 mg	1.8-2.2 mg	1.8-2.0 mg	Anaemia, CNS lesions, epileptiform convulsions in children, glossitis, stomatitis, cheilosis	5-100 mg	5-100 mg parenteral
Cyanocobalamin (B_{12})	Liver, red meat, milk, egg yolk, oysters, clams	2-3 mcg	3 mcg	3 mcg	Pernicious anaemia, glossitis, confusion, muscle incoordination, paresthesias	10 mcg-1 mg	10 mcg-1 mg parenteral
Vitamin C Ascorbic acid	Citrus fruits (oranges, lemons, limes), tomatoes green vegetables, potatoes, onion, turnips, grapefruits, green peppers, strawberries	45 mg	50-60 mg	50-60 mg	Scurvy (petichiae, bleeding gums, bruising, impaired wound healing, loosened teeth)	100 mg-1 g	100 mg-1 g parenteral

* RDA not established

WATER-SOLUBLE VITAMINS

Vitamin B Complex

Thiamine (Vitamin B_1)

Mode of action: In the body thiamine functions in the form of the coenzyme thiamine pyrophosphate in which adenosine triphosphate (ATP) acts as the pyrophosphate donor.

Thiamine + ATP→Thiamine pyrophosphate + AMP

The body requirement of thiamine is related to the metabolic rate, and is highest when carbohydrate is the main source of energy.

Toxicity: Thiamine can lead to toxic reactions on parenteral administrations. *Hypersensitivity reactions* can occur rarely.

Riboflavine (Vitamin B_2)

Mode of action: Riboflavine is a component of **flavoprotein enzymes**, which are necessary for the oxidation of carbohydrates and amino acids.

Nicotinic Acid (Niacin)

Mode of action: Nicotinic acid functions in the body as its amide. Nicotinic acid has a **vasodilator activity**, which is lacked by nicotinamide. Nicotinic acid has a **cholesterol-lowering effect.**

Toxicity: Nicotinic acid may produce flushing, pruritus, gastrointestinal distress, activation of peptic ulcer and hepatotoxicity.

Pyridoxine (Vitamin B_6)

Mode of action: The name pyridoxine (vitamin B_6) is given to three closely related substances **pyridoxol, pyridoxal** and **pyridoxamine.** The antitubercular drug, **isoniazid**, inhibits the enzyme pyridoxal kinase, and thus acts as **anti-vitamin B_6**. Pyridoxal phosphate is involved in the metabolic transformation of amino acids.

Toxicity: No definite toxic manifestations are described.

Folic Acid and Cyanocobalamin (Vitamin B_{12}) see Table 8.1 and Chapter 5.1.

Pantothenic Acid

There is no definite evidence of a disease entity developing from the lack of pantothenic acid in man.

Biotin

There is no established therapeutic indication for biotin in man.

Choline and Inositol

These two agents have a **lipotropic action**, i.e., they decrease the fat content of the liver. Choline has been employed in man to **prevent fatty infiltration** and **cirrhosis of the liver.** Inositol does not produce any convincing therapeutic effects.

Para-aminobenzoic Aid

Para-aminobenzoic acid (PABA) has been included in the vitamin B complex group. PABA is an essential metabolite for the growth of certain bacteria, but there is no evidence that PABA is a dietary essential for man.

Ascorbic Acid (Vitamin C)

Lind in 1757 wrote an exhaustive treatise on **scurvy**, which is the first scientifically described deficiency disease. He further showed that when oranges and lemons were included in the diet, scurvy could be prevented.

Mode of action: Vitamin C is a **strong-reducing agent**, and probably helps in **oxidation-reduction reactions** induced by various enzymes in the body. It is involved in the maintenance of the **integrity of collagen in mesenchymal tissues,** specially in the blood vessels. Ascorbic acid is involved in the **carbohydrate metabolism.** It also occurs in high concentrations in the adrenal cortex and medulla. In the cortex it is possibly concerned intimately with the **synthesis of adrenocorticosteroids**, and in the medulla it prevents the oxidation of adrenaline. Vitamin C promotes the process of **healing of wounds.**

Toxicity: Serious toxicity due to Vitamin C is uncommon, but **diarrhoea** may occur with high dosage. On prolonged therapy **acidification of urine** is likely to lead to the **formation of oxalate stones in the urinary tract.**

MULTIVITAMIN PREPARATIONS

Oral dosage forms (usually capsules) containing varying quantities of many vitamins are available in the market, and are in wide use. Now it is generally agreed that in most cases such a multivitamin therapy is **irrational and is a waste of expensive drugs.**

Systemic Anti-Infective Agents

9

9.1 DEVELOPMENT OF CHEMOTHERAPY

Anti-infective drug treatment of systemic infections was put on a rational basis only with the work of the famous German chemist, **Paul Ehrlich** (1854-1915). He was acknowledged as the 'Father of Chemotherapy'.

The modern era of chemotherapy began with sulphanilamide in 1936. The 'golden age' of anti-microbial therapy started with the production of the antibiotic **penicillin** in 1941.

TERMS AND CONCEPTS

Chemotherapy applies to the use of both **natural** and **synthetic chemicals** to interfere with the functioning of foreign cell populations. This term also includes **antineoplastic drugs** used to treat cancer.

Antibiotics are chemical compounds produced by living microorganisms (bacteria, fungi, actinomycetes) which at high dilutions are capable of **inhibiting** or **killing** bacteria and other microorganisms.

Synthetic anti-infective drugs differ only in their origin, in that they are synthetic. The term **antimicrobial agent** includes both types (antibiotics and synthetic chemotherapeutic agents).

Selective toxicity refers to the ability of chemicals to strike selectively at foreign cells in ways that harm them, without causing significant damage to the host cells, ideally speaking.

Potency or activity per milligram of a chemotherapeutic agent is usually expressed on the basis of **'minimum inhibitory concentration'** (MIC) at which it is capable of inhibiting the multiplication of one of the susceptible microorganisms.

Bacteriostatic activity refers to the ability of a compound to inhibit the growth and multiplication of microorganisms, i.e., inhibited growth in time results in death of the organism. **Bactericidal activity** means an actual lethal effect on the microorganisms. Both these terms are based on the *in vitro* testing of antimicrobial drugs.

Antibacterial spectrum, also known as antimicrobial spectrum refers to the range of activity of the compound. Antibiotics are often classified as **broad** or **narrow-spectrum** depending upon the range of activity.

MODE OF ACTION OF ANTI-INFECTIVE AGENTS

Most of the commonly used chemotherapeutic agents act by one of the following basic mechanisms:

i. *Inhibition of bacterial cell wall synthesis*;
ii *Inhibition of cytoplasmic membrane function*;
iii. *Inhibition of nucleic acid synthesis;*
iv. *Inhibition of protein synthesis;*
v. *Control of microbial enzymes;* and
vi. *Substrate competition with an essential metabolite.*

CLASSIFICATION OF ANTIMICROBIAL DRUGS

The antimicrobials may be classified according to their activity:

1. **Narrow-spectrum drugs** (effective against gram-positive cocci and bacilli). Penicillin G, the semisynthetic penicillinase-resistant penicillins, the macrolides, the lincomycins, vancomycin and bacitracin.
2. **Narrow-spectrum drugs** (primarily effective against the aerobic gram-negative bacilli). The aminoglycosides and polymyxins.
3. **Broad-spectrum drugs** (effective against both gram-positive and gram-negative bacteria and chlamydiae and rickettsiae). The broad spectrum penicillins (ampicillin and carbenicillin), the cephalosporins, the tetracyclines, chloramphenicol, trimethoprim, and the fluorquinolones.

BACTERIAL SENSITIVITY TESTING

Sensitivity testing *in vitro* is the most certain way to select the right drug against the organism responsible for the infection. Sensitivity and resistance (S and R) studies are desirable, if facilities exist.

BACTERIAL RESISTANCE TO ANTIMICROBIAL DRUGS

Considered by species, bacteria are **susceptible** to some antibacterial drugs and **resistant** to others. But strains may develop that are resistant to drugs which are supposed to be normally effective against that species. Such a change is particularly true in **staphylococci, gram-negative bacilli** and ***Mycobacterium tuberculosis.*** Bacterial resistance is a major medical problem.

TYPES OF BACTERIAL RESISTANCE

Bacterial resistance to antimicrobial drugs is either **natural** or **acquired.** A related phenomenon is **dependence** which occurs rarely.

PREVENTION OF RESISTANCE

Unnecessary exposure to antimicrobial drugs tends to favour the development of resistance. They should not be used for treating colds, or other trivial infections caused by viruses. Instead they should be reserved for treating patients whose illnesses have proved to be caused by a specific microorganism which is susceptible to the drug. Once the drug has been selected it should be used in **high enough doses**, for **long enough periods** to eradicate the infection.

ADVERSE REACTIONS TO ANTI-INFECTIVE AGENTS

1. **Direct toxic effects** upon such organs as the gastrointestinal tract, liver, kidneys or the auditory, optic and other peripheral nerves.
2. **Allergic reactions** and other types of hypersensitivity reactions affecting the skin, bone marrow, circulating blood and other structures.
3. **Superinfections** are a result of drug induced overgrowth by resistant bacterial strains or fungal organisms.

PROPHYLACTIC USE OF ANTIMICROBIAL DRUGS

Antimicrobial drugs are often used to **prevent** infections in people who have been exposed to pathogens, or who are thought to need special protection against disease. In some situations ***chemoprophylaxis*** is recommended as a rational procedure (**Table 9.1**).

COMBINATION OF ANTIMICROBIAL DRUGS

The combined use of two or more antimicrobial agents is sometimes superior to treatment with a single drug. On the other hand, two drugs given together may not be more effective than one drug alone, particularly when the drugs are combined in a fixed-dosage mixture. Thus, the use of antibiotics in fixed-dosage combinations is to be avoided. The interactions of two antimicrobial drugs may result in **addition, synergism,** or **antagonism.**

Table 9.1: *Some indications for chemoprophylaxis with antimicrobial drugs*

Antimicrobial drugs	Indication
Pencillin G	Prior to oral surgery to prevent the development of subacute bacterial endocarditis in patients with rheumatic endocarditis; congenital heart disease.
Chloroquine	Prevention of malaria
Co-trimoxazole	Prophylaxis of recurrent urinary tract infections
Isoniazid	Prevention of tuberculosis in susceptible close contacts
Doxycycline	Prevention of "traveller's diarrhoea"
Rifampicin	Prophylaxis of meningococcal meningitis

CAUSES OF FAILURE OF CHEMOTHERAPY

Usually a 5 to 7 day treatment is sufficient to cause a resolution of a susceptible infection. If the patient's condition does not improve the following should be considered:

1. Failure due to a wrong diagnosis, wrong choice of drug, and wrong dose, and inadequate duration of therapy.
2. Failure due to development of antimicrobial resistance.
3. Failure due to superinfection.
4. Failure of the patient to comply with the thorapoutic rogimon.

ANTIBIOTIC MISUSE

Antibiotic misuse is a consequence of three main factors: (i) the **availability** of a wide selection of drugs; (ii) the **limitation on physician's time;** and (iii) the **demand from the patient** who cannot fully appreciate the dangerous consequences of antibiotic use.

9.2 SYNTHETIC ANTIMICROBIALS (SULPHONAMIDES, CO-TRIMOXAZOLE AND QUINOLONES)

The sulphonamides were the first effective chemotherapeutic agents employed systemically for the prevention and cure of bacterial infections in man. In 1935 **Gerhard Domagk** reported that the red dye **prontosil** protected mice from streptococcal infection, a discovery for which he was awarded the Nobel prize in medicine for 1938.

SULPHONAMIDES

The sulphonamides as a class of **bacteriostatic** agents, had a short period of clinical use, because of the introduction of antibiotics with a broader and more certain action against microorganisms.

Classification

The available sulphonamides can be grouped as under:

I. **Systemic use**
   1. ***Short-acting agents***
      Sulphadiazine
      Sulfisoxazole
      Sulphamethizole
      Sulphasalazine
   2. ***Intermediate-acting agents***
      Sulphamethoxazole
   3. ***Long-acting agent***
      Sulphadoxine

II. **Local use**
   1. ***Ophthalmic***
      Sulphacetamide
   2. ***Topical***
      Silver sulphadiazine

Antibacterial Spectrum

Sulphonamides are effective against many *gram-*

positive organisms, some gram-negative diplococci and bacilli, actinomyces, nocardia, chlamydia and *some protozoa*. The sulphonamides are an effective adjunct to pyrimethamine in treating *toxoplasmosis*, and to quinine and other antimalarials to treat *chloroquine-resistant malaria*.

Mechanism of Action

The sulphonamides are **antimetabolites** of para-amino benzoic acid (PABA). They inhibit the synthesis of DNA and therefore prevent certain bacteria from replicating. The sulphonamides are primarily **bacteriostatic** agents. The action of sulphonamides is by **competitive antagonism.**

Acquired Resistance to Sulphonamides

Resistance to sulphonamides originates from **random mutation**. Once such resistance is developed, it is usually **persistent** and **irreversible.**

Pharmacokinetics

The sulphonamides are well absorbed from the gut. Approximately 70 to 100 percent of an oral dose is ***rapidly absorbed***, and appears in the urine within 30 minutes of ingestion. After absorption the sulphonamides become **bound to protein**, and to some extent are **acetylated** and are excreted by the kidneys.

Mode of Administration and Dosage

The doses of currently used agents are summarized in **Table 9.2.**

Therapeutic Uses

The sulphonamides have remained first choice drugs in very few conditions.

1. **Urinary tract infections (UTI):** In infections caused by susceptible **gram-negative uropathogens**. The preferred agents are sulfisoxazole and sulphamethizole.
2. **Ulcerative colitis:** Patients of ulcerative colitis are benefited by oral administration of **sulphasalazine.**
3. **Respiratory tract infections:** For the treatment of **pneumococcal pneumonia**, and **lower respiratory tract bacterial infections.**

Table 9.2: *The recommended dosage schedule of some sulphonamides*

Non-proprietary Name	Usual dosage: Initial	Usual dosage: Maintenance
1. Sulphadiazine	4 g orally	1 g 4 hourly
Sulphadiazine sodium	100mg / kg IV or SC upto a total dose of 5 g	30-40 mg/kg IV or SC every 6-8 hours
2. Sulfisoxazole	4 g orally	1 g 4 to 6 times daily
Sulfisoxazole diolamide	IV or SC 100 mg/kg initially and same for 24 hours maintenance	
3. Sulphamethizole	2-3 g orally	0.5 g 4 to 6 times daily
4. Sulphasalazine	4 g orally	1 g 4 times daily
5. Sulphamethoxazole	2 g orally	1 g bid or tid
6. Sulfadoxine	Available as 0.5 g tablets, and also as a solution for injection (1 g / 4 ml); Adult dose is 1-2 g once weekly	
7. Sulphacetamide sodium	Ophthalmic solution available in 10, 20 and 30% strengths	
8. Silver sulphadiazine	0.1% ointment for topical application	

4. **Other chlamydial infections:** Eye diseases like **trachoma** and **inclusion conjunctivitis** respond to sulphonamide therapy. Sulphacetamide sodium is effective when applied topically in these infections.
5. **Systemic mycoses:** The sulphonamides even now are often life saving in **nocardiosis.** Treatment requires administration of very high doses of sulfisoxazole or sulphadiazine for many months.
6. **Protozoal infections: Malaria** caused by *P.falciparum* strains resistant to chloroquine may be controlled with quinine and pyrimethamine combined with sulphadiazine or sulfadoxine. **Combination of sulphadoxine with pyrimethamine may be used for prophylaxis of pneumocystis carinii pneumonia in patients of AIDS.**
7. **Burns and skin disorders: Silver sulphadiazine** is the preferred sulphonamide.

Adverse Reactions

1. **Hypersensitivity reactions: Exfoliative dermatitis** or rarely **Stevens-Johnson syndrome** may occur.
2. **Renal damage:** Crystalluria can occur causing blockade in the kidney, tubules, ureters or bladder. Crystalluria can be avoided by high fluid intake, and maintaining an ***alkaline reaction*** in the urine.
3. **Blood dyscrasias: Agranulocytosis, thrombocytopenia** or **aplastic anaemia** may occur.
4. **Effects on the foetus and neonate:** The sulphonamides may produce **kernicterus** in the foetus and neonate.
5. **Miscellaneous reactions:** Other adverse reactions include goitre and hypothyroidism, arthritis, cardiomyopathy, psychiatric disturbances, insomnia and nightmares.

Caution and Contraindications

Sulpha hypersensitivity and **advanced kidney disease** with an elevated blood urea nitrogen. Caution is required in patients with **liver disease, blood dyscrasias,** and **impaired kidney function.**

Drug Interactions

Sulphonamides increase the effect of **oral anticoagulants** and **methotrexate**. They also potentiate the action of **oral sulphonylurea hypoglycaemic agents, thiazides** and the **uricosuric agents.**

TRIMETHOPRIM: SULPHAMETHOXAZOLE (CO-TRIMOXAZOLE)

Trimethoprim was marketed in combination with sulphamethoxazole as **co-trimoxazole.** Trimethoprim is chemically related to pyrimethamine. The introduction of the combination of trimethoprim with sulphamethoxazole is an important advance, as the two drugs act on **sequential steps** leading to a folate deficiency in the susceptible organism, thereby having a **synergistic** effect.

Antibacterial Spectrum

The antibacterial spectrum of trimethoprim is similar to that of sulphamethoxazole, although the former is 20 to 100 times more potent than the latter. The spectrum includes gram-negative species like *E.coli*, salmonellae, *Haemophilis influenzae* and proteus species. Malarial parasites are sensitive to trimethoprim.

Mechanism of Action

The *sequential action* of sulphonamides and trimethoprim explains the **synergistic action** of this combination (**Fig. 9.1**).

Pharmacokinetics

Absorption of co-trimoxazole by the oral route is rapid, peak plasma levels occur between 2 to 4 hours after administration, persists upto 7 hours, and detectable amounts have been found after 24 hours. Both agents are mainly excreted in the urine, in the free and metabolized form.

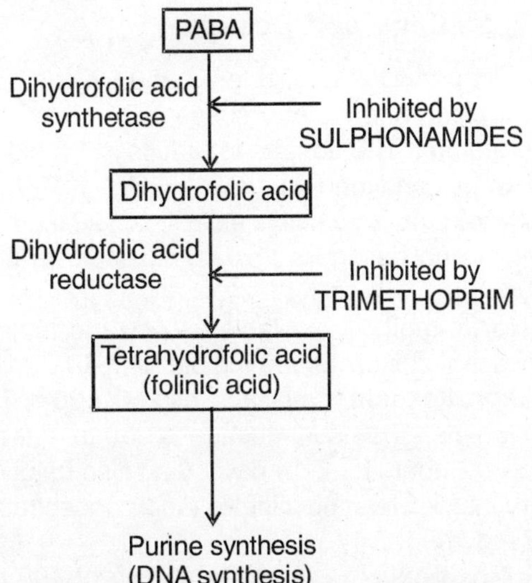

Fig. 9.1: *Sequential blockade of folinic acid production by sulphonamides and trimethoprim.*

Adverse Reactions

Adverse reactions include *headache, tinnitus, vertigo, peripheral neuritis, glossitis and stomatitis.* Allergic reactions like *pruritus , urticaria , periorbital oedema, generalized skin eruptions, anaphylactic reactions, serum sickness, and Stevens-Johnson syndrome* can occur. Blood dyscrasias, *purpura, haemolytic anaemia, hypoprothrombinaemia,* and *methaemoglobinaemia* have been reported.

Therapeutic Uses

1. **Urinary tract infections:** Used in **acute, chronic** or **recurrent** urinary tract infections.
2. **Respiratory tract infections:** *It has been used as long-term treatment in the prophylaxis of episodes of bronchitis.*
3. **Gastrointestinal infections:** Co-trimoxazole is useful in the treatment of **shigellosis,** and **typhoid fever.**
4. **Septicaemia:** Useful for the treatment of septicaemias and serious infections due to gram-negative bacilli.
5. **Plague:** Effective in the treatment of bubonic plague.
6. **Venereal disease:** Gonorrhoea in both men and women may be treated with co-trimoxazole.
7. **Meningitis:** Co-trimoxazole has been used in cases of neonatal meningitis due to *E.coli.*
8. **Miscellaneous infections:** Co-trimoxazole has been used in the treatment of **cholera, brucellosis** and **melioidosis.** Used to treat **nocardiosis, histoplasmosis, chloroquine-resistant falciparum malaria**, and prophylaxis of traveller's diarrhoea.

Preparations and Dosage

Tablets each containing 80 mg trimethoprim and 400 mg sulphamethoxazole are available. The usual dosage of this combination is 1 to 2 tablets twice daily. Double strength tablets containing double amounts of each ingredient are also available. For intravenous use 5 ml ampoules containing trimethoprim 80 mg and sulphamethoxazole 40 mg in a vehicle with 40 percent propylene glycol is available.

QUINOLONES AND FLUOROQUINOLONES

Nalidixic, a 4-quinolone, synthesized in 1962, and other chemically related compounds exert antimicrobial action by inhibiting DNA synthesis. Fluoroquinolones like **enoxacin, norfloxacin** and **ciprofloxacin** have an extended spectrum of action including *gram-positive organisms*, and the more serious gram-negative organisms such as **Pseudomonas aeruginosa** and *gram-negative aerobic bacteria*. The antimicrobial action is accomplished by a specific action on **DNA gyrase**, the enzyme responsible for the unwinding and supercoiling of bacterial DNA prior to its replication.

Antibacterial Spectrum

The quinolones exert a **bactericidal** action against susceptible organisms. The fluoroquinolones, enoxacin, norfloxacin, ciprofloxacin and others are potent against gram-negative bacteria and also active against staphylococci and *Pseudomonas aeruginosa.*

Ciprofloxacin is the prototype member. Its oral absorption is rapid and complete, first-pass metabolism is minimal, food delays rate of absorption but not total amount absorbed, peak serum levels attained within 1 to 2 hours, and urinary excretion is complete within 24 hours. It is also effective against *respiratory, skin, soft tissue, bone and joint infections due to organisms resistant to most other broad-spectrum antibiotics.*

The basic pharmacokinetics of the newer fluoroquinolones is presented in **Table 9.3.**

Table 9.3: Pharmacokinetics of the newer fluoroquinolones

Fluoroquinolone	*Plasma Half-life (hrs)*	*Oral Bio-availability (%)*	*Peak serum concentration (mcg/ml)*
Levofloxacin	5-7	95	8
Lomefloxacin	8	95	3
Ofloxacin	5-7	95	8
Pefloxacin	10	90	6
Sparfloxacin	16-22	90	0.1-1.5

Therapeutic Uses

Ciprofloxacin has potent activity against gram negative bacteria including *P. aeruginosa.* It is effective in resistant **urinary tract infections, prostatitis, biliary infections, osteomyelitis, cystic fibrosis** complicated by **P. aeroginosa,** lung infection, all forms of **gonorrhoea** and against bacterial bowel infections caused by **Shigella and Salmonella.** Ciprofloxacin may be combined with rifampicin for treatment of **serious staphylococcal infection.**

Norfloxacin is used to treat uncomplicated urinary tract infections including those caused by gram-negative rods and gram-positive cocci, urethral and cervical gonorrhoea.

Adverse Reactions

Quinolones and fluoroquinolones are well tolerated drugs. Common adverse reactions are nausea, headache, dizziness, abdominal discomfort, photosensitivity and skin rash. Hypersensitivity reactions can occur.

Preparations and Dosage

Nalidixic acid is available as 250,500 or 1000 mg tablets, and an oral suspension containing 250 mg/5ml. The dosage for adults is 1 g qid for 1-2 weeks and then 2 g/day.

Cinoxacin is available as 250 or 500 mg capsules. Usual dosage is 1 g daily bid or qid for 7-14 days.

Norfloxacin is available as 400 mg tablets. The usual dosage is 400 mg bid for 7-10 days.

Ciprofloxacin is available as 250, 500 or 750 mg tablets. The usual dosage is 250 to 750 mg every 12 hours for 7-14 days. Can also be given by IV infusion over 60 minutes (final concentration 1-2 mg /ml).

Moxifloxacin is used in a dose of 400 mg daily in tablet form.

9.3 ANTIBIOTICS

Microorganisms are subject to either favourable or antagonistic reactions owing to the presence of other living organisms. If the association is **unfavourable (antagonistic)**, the process is designated as **antibiosis.** A substance elaborated by a growing microorganism which exhibits such an antagonistic influence is termed as an **antibiotic** (life against life).

DEFINITION

An antibiotic is a chemical substance produced by a microorganism which at a **high dilution** can **inhibit the growth** and/or **multiplication** or **kill** another microorganism.

CLASSIFICATION

Antibiotics may be classified according to their *mode of action.*

According to the mode of action

i. **Inhibitors of bacterial cell wall synthesis:** Penicillin, cephalosporins, bacitracin, cycloserine and others.
ii. **Inhibitors of protein synthesis:** Amino-

glycosides, tetracyclines, chloramphenicol, macrolides, lincosamides.

iii. **Inhibitors of bacterial cell membrane function:** Polymyxins, nystatin, amphotericin B.

iv. **Inhibitors of nucleic acid metabolism:** Griseofulvin, actinomycin.

The above listing of agents is *not* complete, and is only representative of the particular class.

INHIBITORS OF BACTERIAL CELL WALL SYNTHESIS

The most important members are the **penicillins** and the **cephalosporins,** designated as the **beta-lactam antibiotics.** They have a bactericidal action.

Penicillins

Introduction of 'Penicillin G'

In 1928, **Alexander Fleming** (later Sir Alexander Fleming), while working in St. Mary Hospital, London, noted that some colonies of staphylococci were lysed when the medium was contaminated by a mould later classified as ***Penicillium notatum***.

Chemistry

The first compound in general use was penicillin G, which has a **benzyl** side chain, and subsequently it was found that substituting **phenoxy-methyl** or **phenoxyethyl** groups greatly increased acid stability and the first 'oral' penicillins came into use.

Mode of Action

In **gram-positive organisms** the cell wall consists of a **mucopeptide layer** known as **peptido-glycan** which supports the lipoprotein cell membrane. **Gram-negative bacteria** have a complex cell wall structure.

The **beta-lactum antibiotics** (penicillins, cephalosporins) prevent the normal synthesis of the bacterial cell wall by **selectively inhibiting the synthesis of mucopeptide in the bacterial wall** of susceptible multiplying bacteria. The progeny have **defective cell walls** which are subject to **lysis.** The bacterial cell swells and bursts open due to a hypotonic environment.

Antibacterial Spectrum

Apart from the "broad-spectrum" penicillins, penicillin has a r**elatively narrow spectrum of activity.** It is highly effective against such gram-positive cocci like the *streptococcus* and the *pneumococcus*. Penicillin is effective against the gram-negative cocci that cause *meningitis* and *gonorrhoea*. It is effective against gonococci, pneumococci and meningococci.

Bacterial Resistance

Bacterial resistance to penicillin is usually due to the elaboration of *beta-lectamases* (penicillinases) by the bacteria, *which split the beta-lactam ring*, rendering penicillin inactive.

Penicillin Preparations

Penicillin G as such is rather unstable and currently relatively stable **sodium** and **potassium salts** are used cllinically. Due to the limitations of penicillin G a range of *semisynthetic penicillins* is available for clinical use as listed below:

A. **Natural Products:** Penicillin G potassium or sodium, Penicillin G benzathine, Penicillin G procaine, Penicillin G benzathine and procaine penicillin combined.

B. **Semisynthetic derivatives:** *Acid- Resistant*, Penicillin V; *Penicillinase- Resistant*, Cloxacillin, Dicloxacillin, Methicillin, Nafcillin, Oxacillin; *Broad-Spectrum Penicillins*, Amoxycillin, Ampicillin, Bacampicillin, Cyclacillin; *Antipseudomonal Penicillin* (Extended Spectrum) Azlocillin, Carbenecillin, Mezlocillin, Piparacillin, Ticarcillin.

Pharmacokinetics

Three main types of penicillin G are available: (i) penicillin G for oral use; (ii) aqueous penicillin

G for parenteral use; and (iii) depot preparations as suspensions for parenteral use, also known as 'respository' or 'long acting' preparations of pencillin G.

As penicillin G is absorbed into the blood, a large part of it is *bound to plasma proteins*. It is distributed widely in the body, and tissue concentrations usually are about 20 percent of simultaneous plasma levels.

Probenecid is a drug which was developed to delay the rapid renal excretion of penicillin, when administered with it. Probenecid **competes** with penicillin for the tubular transport system that transfers the antibiotic from the blood to the tubular fluid. **As a result penicillin remains in the blood and tissues at a higher level for longer periods.**

Therapeutic Uses of Penicillin G and Phenoxypenicillins

1. **Pneumococcal infections:** Penicillin G remains the drug of choice for the treatment of infections of all types caused by *Strep. penumoniae*. For *uncomplicated cases* penicillin G or procaine penicillin G (300,000 to 600,000 unit IM 12 hourly) are employed.
2. **Streptococcal infections.** Streptococcal pharyngitis responds well to oral therapy with penicillin V, 500 mg every 6 hours for 10 days, or procaine penicillin G 600,000 units IM daily for 10 days, or by a single injection of benzathine penicillin G 1.2 million units IM.
3. **Staphylococcal infections: Nafcillin, oxacillin** or **methicillin** may be used.
4. **Meningococcal infection.**
5. **Clostridial infections.**
6. **Gram-negative infections:** The newly introduced **antipseudomonal penicillins** (carbenicillin, ticarcillin, carfecillin, mezlocillin) are effective.
7. **Venereal disease (gonorrhoea and syphilis). Gonorrhoea:** Benzylpenicillin is the most active drug against sensitive strains of ***Neisseria gonorrhoeae.*** Penicillin is still the drug of choice for the treatment of syphilis.

Guidelines for Penicillin G Administration

Intramuscular injection: This is the most commonly employed route of administration for penicillin G. For an adult 0.5 to 1 mega unit 6 hourly is sufficient to cure most infections, caused by sensitive organisms.

Intravenous injection: This route may be justified when a very high concentration in the blood is desired. An injection of 10 mega units diluted in 10 to 20 ml of physiological saline may be administered intravenously.

Intravenous infusion: For the treatment of serious invasive infections like **meningitis, septicaemia**, occasionally **pneumonia** or **endocarditis,** intravenous infusion may be justified.

Toxicity

The untoward effects are chiefly of three kinds: (i) **hypersensitivity reactions;** (ii) **direct toxicity;** and (iii) **miscellaneous reactions.**

i. **Hypersensitivity reactions:** Its practical significance is that it causes *potentially fatal reactions.*
ii. **Direct toxicity: Pain** and **sterile inflammation** may occur at the site of intramuscular injection. **Thrombophlebitis** sometimes occurs on intravenous administration of penicillin.
iii. **Miscellaneous reactions: Superinfections** occur rarely.

Several semisynthetic penicillins (**carbenicillin, methicillin, ticarcillin**) and even penicillin itself may induce platelet dysfunction leading to bleeding. With excessive doses of semisynthetic penicillins, particularly **ampicillin** and **methicillin**, bone marrow depression and agranulocytosis may occur. **Cloxacillin, oxacillin, nafcillin, methicillin and carbenicillin** have been reported to occasionally cause liver damage.

Semisynthetic Penicillins

The compounds included are the **acid-resistant penicillins**, **penicillinase-resistant penicillin, broad-spectrum penicillins,** and **antipseudomonal penicillins.**

Acid-resistant Penicillins

Phenoxymethylpenicillin (Penicillin V): It produces 2 to 5 times the blood levels compared to similar doses of penicillin G. ***Penicillin V*** 125 mg is approximately equal to 250,000 units of penicillin G.

Penicillinase-Resistant Penicillin (Anti-staphylococcal Penicillin)

Cloxacillin: It is ***acid-stable*** and is effectively absorbed after oral administration but can also be given parenterally. Absorption from the gut is incomplete (30-50%). When given orally on an empty stomach 1 g of cloxacillin produces a peak plasma level of 5-10 mcg/ml in 1 hour.

Broad-spectrum Penicillins

The broad-spectrum penicillins include ***ampicillin*** and ***amoxycillin, carbenicillin*** and ***ticarcillin***. Broad-spectrum penicillins are mainly used for treating *Pseudomonas aeruginosa* and *proteus* infections.

1. **Ampicillin:** Ampicillin was the first broad-spectrum penicillin. Ampicillin diffuses into gram-negative bacteria more readily than penicillin G.
   Therapeutic uses: Ampicillin is mainly indicated in the treatment of exacerbations of ***chronic bronchitis, otitis media*** and ***meningitis.*** It has second place in the treatment of ***acute typhoid*** but may ***eradicate the carrier-state*** because of high drug levels in the bile.
   Toxicity: Rashes with ampicillin are common and often develop later than with penicillin G. Gastrointestinal disturbances (usually diarrhoea) occur.
2. **Amoxycillin:** Amoxycillin is a derivative of ampicillin. On an oral dose of 250 mg, the average peak levels of 4 mcg/ml plasma are reached in 2 hours. *The drug also penetrates purulent and mucold bronchial secretions more effectively than ampicillin.*
   Adverse effects of amoxycillin are similar to those of ampicillin.

Extended-spectrum Penicillins (Antipseudomonal Penicillins)

1. **Carbenicillin:** Carbenicillin is active against *Ps. aeruginosa* and *Proteus* species, and also against certain gram-negative organisms. *It is not absorbed when given by mouth and has to be administered parenterally.* The drug is given intravenously in amounts of 25-30 g/day when such levels are needed. **Side effects** of intravenous carbenicillin include ***hypokalaemia*** and alteration in platelet function with spontaneous bleeding.
2. **Ticarcillin:** This semisynthetic penicillin is 2-4 times more active than carbenicillin against ***Ps. aeruginosa*** and is also active against anaerobic organisms.

Cephalosporins

Cephalosporins are structurally and pharmacologically related to penicillins. They are **water soluble, broad-spectrum, semisynthetic, bactericidal** antibiotics derived from **7-aminocephalosporanic acid (7-ACA)**.

Antibacterial Spectrum

Cephalosporins and related compounds are divided into **first, second,** and **third generation** agents.

Mode of Action

Cephalosporins and cephamycins have a penicillin-like action. **They inhibit mucopeptide synthesis in the bacterial cell wall**, rendering it defective and osmotically unstable. These drugs are **bactericidal.**

Pharmacokinetics: *Cephalexin, cephradine, cefadroxil* and *cefaclor* are well absorbed from the gut. Pharmacokinetic data about these agents are summarized in **Table 9.4.**

Cephalosporins are widely distributed in most tissues and fluids, with maximum concentrations in liver and kidneys. Most cephalosporins and their metabolites are mainly excreted via the kidneys.

Table 9.4: *Pharmacokinetic data of some cephalosporins and related compounds*

Compound	Protein binding (%)	Half-life (min)	Peak-serum level (Ig IV dose) (mcg/ml)	Routes	Dose (Adults)
First generation					
Cephalexin	5-15	30-70	–	Oral	1.0 g 6 hourly
Cefadroxil	20	70-80	–	Oral	1.0 g 12 hourly
Cephradine	8-17	45-120	86	Oral IM/IV	Oral:1 g 6 hourly 1: 2 g 6 hourly
Cephalothin	65-80	25-60	30-64	IM/IV	1: 1-2 g 4 hourly
Cephapirin	40-54	20-40	40-73	IM/IV	1: 1-2 g 4 hourly
Cefazolin	70-86	90-130	185-189	IM/IV	1: 1-1.5 g 6 hourly
Second generation					
Cefaclor	22-25	36-54	–	Oral	0.25 g 8 hourly
Cefamandole	56-78	30-60	88-139	IM/IV	1: 2 g 4 hourly
Cefoxitin*	65-79	40-60	56-110	IM/IV	1: 2 g 4 hourly or 3 g 6 hourly
Cefuroxime	33-50	60-114	43-98	IM/IV	1: 3 g 8 hourly
Cefonicid	98	210-294	221.3	IM/IV	1: 2 g 24 hourly
Ceforanide	80	150-210	125	IM/IV	1: 1 g 12 hourly
Third generation					
Cefotaxime	30-51	60	81-102	IM/IV	1: 2 g 4 hourly
Moxalactam**	40-57	114-210	71-94	IM/IV	1: 4 g 8 hourly
Ceftizoxime	30	66-133	46-136	IM/IV	1: 3-4 g 8 hourly
Ceftriaxone	85-95	348-522	151	IM/IV	1: 2 g 12 to 24 hourly
Cefoperazone	82-93	102-156	73-153	IM/IV	1:1.5-4 g 6, 8 or 12 hourly
Cefotetan*	78-91	180-276	158	IM/IV	1: 1 or 2 g 12 hourly
Ceftazidime	10-17	114-120	69-90	IM/IV	1: 1 g 8 hourly

I = Injection, IM = Intramuscular, IV = Intravenous, *Cephamycin, **beta-lactum

Therapeutic Uses

The majority of **gram-positive cocci** and **gram-negative bacteria** are susceptible. Cephalosporins are indicated for **preoperative, intra-operative** and **postoperative prophylaxis** to reduce the incidence of infection in patients undergoing surgery which is likely to be contaminated, e.g., *gastrointestinal surgery, cesarean section, vaginal hysterectomy* or *cholecystectomy*.

Nosocomial infections (hospital infections) are usually caused by organisms which are resistant to many commonly used antimicrobials. Third generation cephalosporins are helpful in such situations.

Adverse reactions: Gastrointestinal disturbances and **hypersensitivity** can occur. Cephalosporins should be administered cautiously to *penicillin-sensitive patients*, as there is evidence of **partial-cross sensitivity** between the two groups.

Eosinopenia, transient neutropenia, leucopenia, thrombocytopenia, agranulocytosis and **haemolytic anaemia** may occur. Cephalosporins are **nephrotoxic** and may cause acute tubular necrosis. **Pseudomembranous colitis** has been reported. **Superinfection** may occur.

Drug interactions: Probenecid administered concurrently with cephalosporins increases and prolongs plasma levels by competitively inhibiting renal tubular secretion. **Alcoholic beverages** may produce acute alcohol intolerance. Concomitant use of **loop diuretics and aminoglycosides** increases nephrotoxicity.

Other Beta-lactam Antibiotics

Aztreonam

Aztreonam is monocyclic beta-lactam compound (a monobactam) isolated from ***Chromobacterium violaceum***. It has wide-spectrum of action against **gram-negative aerobic pathogens** but is inactive against gram-positive organisms or anaerobes. Aztreonam *inhibits cell wall synthesis*.

Dosage: For urinary tract infection: 500 to 1 g IV or IM every 8 to 12 hours. Other infections: 1 g to 2 g IV or IM every 6 to 12 hours.

Adverse reactions include vomiting, confusion, insomnia, hypotension, tinnitus, altered taste, breast tenderness, blood dyscrasias, jaundice and hepatitis.

OTHER INHIBITORS OF BACTERIAL CELL WALL SYNTHESIS

Bacitracin

It is **bactericidal** against gram-positive organisms, specially common skin pathogens like staphylococci, streptococci and Neisseria.

Parenteral use of bacitracin has been stopped because of its **nephrotoxicity.**

For topical use, combination of **bacitracin** with **neomycin** or **polymyxin B** widens the spectrum of activity. Such combinations are effective in the treatment of **ulcers, sycosis, external otitis, pyodermas, infected traumatic and surgical wounds,** and **impetigo.**

Cycloserine

Cycloserine is a broad-spectrum **bactericidal** antibiotic produced by ***streptomyces orchidaceous.*** Its use should ordinarily be restricted to the treatment of **tuberculosis** provided it is tolerated. **Cycloserine** (Seromycin) is initially given in doses of 15 mg/kg body weight orally, increased by increments of 250 mg every few days (if tolerated).

Vancomycin

Vancomycin is a **bactericidal** glycopeptide antibiotic obtained from ***Streptomyces orientalis***, primarily effective against gram-positive organisms. It is possibly the *most potent antibiotic against staphylococci*, but because of its toxicity, its use should be reserved for cases where less toxic antibiotics have failed to control infection. Most serious reactions involve the kidney and the eight cranial nerve (cochlea). It may cause **fatal uraemia** and **permanent deafness.**

Vancomycin is administered in dose of 1 g IV, to adults twice daily. *Oral vancomycin* 3-4 g daily may be of value in the treatment of staphylococcal enterocolitis and pseudomembranous colitis.

Beta-lactamase Inhibitors

Some molecules can bind to beta-lactamases and inactivate them, preventing the destruction of beta-lactams which are substrates for these enzymes. Two such compounds are *clavulanic acid* and *sulbactam*.

Clavulanic acid is produced by **Streptomyces clavuligerus.** It is well absorbed orally and can also be given parenterally. It has been combined with **amoxycillin** for oral administration and with **ticarcillin** for parenteral administration.

Sulbactam is another beta-lactamase inhibitor structurally resembling clavulanic acid. It is used orally or parenterally along with *ampicillin*. It is available for IM or IV use combined with *ampicillin*. The usual dose is 1 to 2 g of ampicillin with 0.5 to 1 g sulbactam every 6 hours. This combination is used for the treatment of *mixed intra- abdominal and pelvic infections*.

INHIBITORS OF PROTEIN SYNTHESIS

The antibiotics which inhibit bacterial protein synthesis are a heterogenous group and include the **aminoglycosides, tetracyclines**, **chloramphenicol, macrolides** and the **lincosamides.**

Aminoglycosides

Most aminoglycosides are prepared by natural fermentation from various species of *Streptomyces*. The aminoglycosides include *streptomycin, kanamycin, gentamicin, tobramycin, sisomicin, paromomycin, netilmicin* and *framycetin*.

Antibacterial Spectrum

All the aminoglycosides are **bactericidal** and active against gram-positive and mainly gram-negative organisms. **Streptomycin** and **kanamycin** are also active against **Mycobacterium tuberculosis**, while **amikacin, gentamicin** and **tobramycin** have activity against **Streptococcus faecalis** and **Ps. aeruginosa.**

Bacterial Resistance

Bacteria frequently develop permanent resistance to aminoglycosides. Bacterial resistance can be rapidly acquired, and is partly mediated by the **R-factors** transmitted between bacteria. **Cross-resistance** is usually complete within the group.

Mode of Action

The aminoglycosides ***inhibit bacterial protein synthesis*** and are **bactericidal.** They enter bacteria by transport on the carrier system naturally utilized by spermine.

It has been observed *in vitro* studies that there is 10 to 80 fold increase in potency going from pH 5.5 to 8.0. Hence in the treatment of **urinary tract infections** simultaneous administration of urinary alkalinizers is advisable.

Pharmacokinetics

The aminoglycosides are poorly absorbed following oral administration. They are concentrated in the kidney, and are excreted unchanged by glomerular filtration. *Thus in the presence of renal insufficiency they must be given in reduced dosage to avoid toxicity.*

Toxicity

The adverse reactions to aminoglycosides are **ototoxicity, nephrotoxicity** and **neuromuscular blockade.**

i. **Ototoxicity:** Both auditory and vestibular divisions of the 8th cranial nerve are involved. The ototoxic effects are often **reversible.**
ii. **Nephrotoxicity:** The nephrotoxicity is usually **mild** and **reversible.** It is dose related and tends to develop after the first week of therapy.
iii. **Neuromuscular blockade:** The aminoglycosides have a **curare-like action** and may sometimes cause neuromuscular blockade that can lead to paralysis and fatal respiratory arrest.

Allergic and local **hypersensitivity reactions, superinfection** and **granulocytopenia** have been reported with the aminoglycosides.

Streptomycin

Streptomycin was the first aminoglycoside, isolated from ***Streptomyces griseus*** by Waksman and others in 1944. It is active against most strains of human and bovine **Mycobacterium tuberculosis** and a number of **gram-positive** and **gram-negative** organisms.

Mode of Action

Streptomycin may be **bactericidal** or **bacteriostatic** depending on the organism involved, the concentration of the drug, and the period of contact between the antibiotic and the organism. It acts by **inhibition of protein synthesis.**

Bacterial resistance and dependence: A high degree of resistance to streptomycin can be developed rapidly. This abrupt 'one step' resistance was first demonstrated when streptomycin was used to treat urinary tract infections.

Pharmacokinetics

Streptomycin is usually injected intramuscularly. In patients over 40 years the dose of 0.75 g is recommended. Penetration of the blood-brain barrier is poor, some drug may enter the CSF if the meninges are inflamed.

Therapeutic uses: The major indication of streptomycin is in the **multidrug treatment of tuberculosis,** in combination with isoniazid, ethambutol, or rifampicin. To treat mixed urinary tract infections streptomycin may be advantageously combined with *nitrofurantoin.*

Toxicity: Severe vertigo frequently results. **Deafness** can also occur in babies born of mothers given streptomycin during pregnancy. Streptomycin may rarely cause **peripheral neuritis, facial** and **peripheral paraesthesias,** and **optic neuritis** with **scotomas.**

Streptomycin may induce **curare-like neuromuscular blockade. Hypersensitivity** to streptomycin is common and handling of the drug can cause contact dermatitis in nurses, pharmacists or physicians. **Exfoliative dermatitis, stomatitis, eosinophilia, serum sickness** and **anaphylactic shock** may occur. **Superinfection** mainly due to staphylococci and fungi may occur.

Kanamycin

Kanamycin is obtained from ***Streptomyces kanamyceticus***. Many strains of **Escherichia coli, Enterobacter, Klebsiella, Proteus, salmonella, shigellae** and **Mycobacterium tuberculosis** are susceptible.

Pharmacokinetics: Kanamycin is poorly absorbed on oral administration. On IM injection it is readily distributed to most of tissues and tissue fluid compartments, except the CSF. Excretion is primarily through renal *glomerular filtration.*

Therapeutic Uses

Kanamycin is useful in the treatment of serious ***gram-negative infections*** originating in the ***urinary or biliary tracts,*** or found in patients postoperatively. It is ineffective against *Ps. Aeruginosa* infections.

Toxicity: As with other aminoglycosides parenteral use of kanamycin causes *ototoxicity*, mainly causing *cochlear damage*, which is usually bilateral and irreversible. It may induce **neuromuscular blockade,** leading to respiratory paralysis. Acute tubular necrosis may occur. **Hypersensitivity reactions** and paraesthesias have been reported.

Gentamicin

Gentamicin is the *most important* of the aminoglycosides, and is used widely for the treatment of serious infections.

Gentamicin is a **broad-spectrum bactericidal** antibiotic chemically related to streptomycin isolated from ***Micromonospora purpurea.***

It is effective against most strains of ***Pseudomonas aeruginosa***. It is also effective against **E. coli, Klebsiella, Enterobacter, Serratia,** Indole negative **Proteus, Shigella, Salmonella, Hemophilus influenzae** and **Neisseria.**

Mode of Action

Gentamicin like other aminoglycosides, causes inhibition of bacterial protein synthesis and invariably produces a *bactericidal effect.*

Pharmacokinetics: *Gentamicin is usually given IM or IV.* From the IM site absorption is rapid and peak levels are attained in less than 1 hour. It is excreted via the kidneys.

Therapeutic Uses

The main indications of gentamicin remain serious **gram-negative septicaemia** and **neonatal sepsis; meningitis** and **other CNS infections, biliary tract infections, acute pyelonephritis or prostatitis,** and occasionally in **severe staphylococcal infections** when other drugs have failed.

Toxicity: The main side effects of gentamicin are **vestibular damage** and **reversible nephrotoxicity.**

Gentamicin may rarely cause **neuromuscular blockade,** and **gastrointestinal superinfection.**

Hypersensitivity, granulocytopenia and disordered liver function have been reported.

Dose: Gentamicin is available in vials of 2 ml containing 80 mg gentamicin sulphate. For local application a cream or ointment is available, for use in the eye or ear infection gentamicin drops (gentamicin base 0.3%) may be applied.

Gentamicin is usually administered **intramuscularly** but may be given **intravenously.** The adult dose is 80 mg 8 hourly IM, and for children the dose is 4 mg/kg/day in three divided doses.

Tobramycin

Tobramycin is derived from **Streptomyces tenebrarius.** It is similar to gentamicin in its antibacterial spectrum, degree of effectiveness and toxicity.

Tobramycin alone or in combination with the penicillins or cephalosporins is used to treat **septicaemias** and susceptible infections of the soft tissue, bone, lung and urinary tract.

Toxic effects are similar to those of gentamicin e.g. ototoxicity in particular.

Amikacin

Amikacin is active against a wide variety of **gram-negative organisms,** including some species that are resistant to gentamicin and tobramycin. It is principally used for the treatment of **serious infections caused by gram-negative bacilli resistant of gentamicin.**

Ototoxicity and **nephrotoxicity** occur as with other aminoglycosides.

Neomycin: Framycetin: Paromomycin

These three aminoglycosides are similar and they have an *antibacterial spectrum like kanamycin*, and are considered too toxic for systemic administration. Their use is limited to oral and *topical administration.* All the three drugs are capable of causing **irreversible deafness.**

Tetracyclines

The first member of this family was *chlortetracycline* derived from the soil organism ***Streptomyces aureofaciens***. This was followed by *oxytetracycline* produced from the ***Streptomyces rimosus***. Molecular modification by removing the chlorine atom from chlortetracycline produced *tetracycline*. Today they are known as the 'older' tetracyclines.

Investigation of the mutant strains of *Streptomyces aureofaciens* led to the discovery of **demethyl-chlortetracycline**. A number of other tetracyclines, including **rolitetracycline, lymecycline, metha-cycline, clomocycline, doxycycline** and **minocycline** have become available, and are labelled as 'newer' tetracyclines.

Antibacterial Spectrum

The tetracyclines have a broad antibacterial spectrum which covers **gram-positive** and **gram-negative bacteria, Rickettsiae, Treponema pallidum, mycoplasma** and the **Chlamydiae** e.g., the psittacosis and **lymphogranuloma venereum** organisms.

Mode of Action

Tetracyclines enter bacterial cells by either passive diffusion through 'pores' on by an active transport system. Inside the bacterial cells, they *bind specifically to 30S ribosomes*, thereby *inhibiting protein synthesis*.

Bacterial Resistance

An increasing proportion of pathogens is developing resistance to the tetracyclines which results from diminished permeability to the drugs. **Cross resistance** develops within the group.

Pharmacokinetics

The tetracyclines are usually given orally, but can be given intravenously, intramuscularly and by local application (to the eye and ear). Absorption from the stomach and intestines is variable and incomplete. Hence absorption is depressed by food (*except for doxycycline*). After absorption there is a varying degree of plasma protein binding.

Therapeutic Uses

The main clinical indications are:

1. Acute exacerbation of chronic bronchitis.
2. Non-specific urethritis.
3. Primary atypical pneumonia (Mycoplasma pneumonia).
4. Rickettsial infections (e.g. typhus).
5. Brucellosis.
6. Lymphogranuloma venereum.
7. Pustular acne (prolonged treatment).
8. Trachoma and inclusion body conjunctivitis.
9. Cholera.
10. Syphilis (in penicillin allergic patient it is the first choice).
11. Actinomycosis.
12. Meningococcal carriers.

The tetracyclines are usually **contraindicated** during pregnancy, lactation, peptic ulcer and hepatic disease.

Toxicity

Gastrointestinal upset: Anorexia, heartburn, nausea, vomiting, flatulence and most often diarrhoea occur. **Cheilosis, black hairy tongue, glossitis,** and **tenesmus** occur.

Superinfection: The tetracyclines rapidly depress the normal body flora which makes superinfection likely. **Necrotizing (pseudo-membranous) entercolitis** may also develop.

Hypersensitivity reactions may occur. **Photo-sensitivity reactions** are common with demethyl-chlortetracycline and doxycycline.

Deposition in tissues: Children may show **brown staining of teeth** if tetracyclines are administered before the appearance of first teeth, and pigmentation of permanent teeth can result.

Renal damage: In patients even with normal renal function the tetracyclines may impair the urinary concentrating ability.

Administration and Dosage

The usual dose of chlortetracycline, tetracycline and oxytetracycline is 250 mg 6 hourly. In severe infections this dose may be doubled. The comparable doses for demethylchlortetracycline, methacycline or lymecycline are 150-300 mg 6 hourly. Doxycycline is given in a dose of 200 mg on the first day follow by 100 mg daily for 5-7 days.

Chloramphenicol

Chloramphenicol was isolated from ***Streptomyces venezuelae*** (a soil organism) in 1947. Now chloramphenicol is manufactured synthetically.

Antibacterial spectrum: It is effective against many **gram-positive** and **gram-negative** organisms, and exhibits activity against the **Chlamydiae** and **Rickettsiae.** Because of its toxicity on the bone marrow, the use of chloramphenicol is ***restricted to salmonelloses,*** and infections due to rickettsiae.

Mode of Action

Chloramphenicol is primarily **bacteriostatic** and inhibits bacterial protein synthesis in susceptible organisms.

Pharmacokinetics: The drug is well absorbed from the intestine but large particle size may impair absorption. Fine suspension of chloramphenicol can be given intramuscularly, and the sodium succinate salt can be injected subcutaneously, IM or IV. Chloramphenicol penetrates tissues better than any other antibiotic.

Therapeutic uses: Because of a small but definite incidence of **serious bone marrow depression,** chloramphenicol therapy is restricted to those infections only in which other drugs are not as effective. The accepted indications are **enteric fever** and **H. influenzae meningitis.**

A convenient regimen in adults is to give 1g on the first day, 1.5 g on the second day, 2.0 g on the third day, and 3.0 g thereafter to a total of about 35.0 g. Some authorities believe that the dose rarely needs to exceed 2 g per day.

Toxicity

Haematological abnormalities: The **first** is a true toxic reaction as a result of direct haemotoxicity, manifested by bone marrow depression, is dose related, progressive and **reversible** upon stoppage of therapy.

The **second** more serious type of bone marrow depression which may occur after a single dose or following prolonged therapy, is **aplastic anaemia.**

Hypersensitivity reactions: Rarely anaphylactic and Jarish- Herxheimer-like reactions have been reported.

Gastrointestinal disturbances: Nausea, vomiting, glossitis, enterocolitis and diarrhoea may occur. **Superinfection** may occur.

The grey (gray) syndrome: The **neonates** and **premature infants** on large doses of chloramphenicol may readily develop the 'grey syndrome' characterized by progressive abdominal distension, vomiting, refusal to suck, dyspnoea, cyanosis and loose greenish stools.

Preparations and Dosage

Chloramphenicol (250 mg) capsules are available for oral use. The daily adult dose varies between 1.5 to 3.0 g in divided doses every 6 to 8 hourly.

Chloramphenicol palmitate is a less bitter form of the drug and as a suspension is available for paediatric use containing 125 mg/ 5ml. The dose ranges from 50-100 mg/kg/day.

Chloramphenicol sodium succinate is provided in 1g vials for parenteral use. The usual dose is 50 mg/kg/day in divided doses.

Ophthalmic preparations are available as drops (0.5%), ointment (1.0%) and aplicaps (1.0%).

Macrolides

The macrolides include **erythromycin, oleandomycin, triacetyloeandomycin (troleandomycin)**. Amongst these members only erythromycin maintains a regular place in therapeutics. Newer macrolides are **azithromycin, clarithromycin** and **spiramycin.**

Erythromycin

Erythromycin was isolated from **Streptomyces erythreus** in 1952. Its effectiveness has diminished due to the development of bacterial resistance.

Antibacterial Spectrum

Erythromycin has an antibacterial spectrum between that of penicillin G and the tetracyclines. Bacterial resistance to erythromycin develops rapidly.

Mode of Action

Erythromycin is bound to the 50S subunit of the ribosome, and blocks the execution of instructions coded by mRNA. The macrolides do not attach to human ribosomes.

Therapeutic uses: Erythromycin is used as *an alternative in the penicillin allergic patient*, or in the treatment of penicillin-resistant gram-positive organisms. It is also useful in primary atypical pneumonia caused by **Mycoplasma pneumoniae,** and in syphilis or infections with **Haemophilus influenzae.**

Toxicity: Erythromycin is one of the safer antibiotics. Gastrointestinal disturbances and allergy being the commonest adverse reactions. Occasionally **superinfection** with **Candida albicans** may develop.

Hypersensitivity reactions with fever, eosinophilia, lymphocytosis, headache and skin rashes are sometimes seen.

Preparations and Storage

Erythromycin stearate: The usual dose for erythromycin stearate is between 250-500 mg every 6 hourly.

Erythromycin ethyl succinate is available dissolved in polyethylene glycol base for IM use. Dose: 100 mg every 4-8 hourly.

Erythromycin lactobionate is a soluble salt suitable for slow IV injection or infusion. Dose:- 300 mg every 6 hourly or 600 mg every 8 hourly.

Oleandomycins

Oleandomycin and the related compound *triacetyloeleandomycin (troleandomycin)* are similar to erythromycin. The use of oleandomycins is limited to the treatment of very severe susceptible infections.

Azithromycin

Azithromycin is a macrolide as active as erythromycin against *gram-positive organisms*, but more active against *gram-negative organisms* like *H. influenzae*. It is more acid-stable than erythromycin and is well tolerated. It is inactive against *Pseudomonas*. Its *mode of action* is through inhibition of protein synthesis.

Azithromycin is indicated in *upper* and *lower respiratory tract infections, skin* and *soft tissue infections, urogenital infections* including *gonorrhoea,* and *uncomplicated genital chlamydial infections.*

Dosage: 500 mg OD for 3 days, or 500 mg once on day 1, and 250 mg OD on the next 4 days. Doses should be preferably taken 1 hour before or 2 hours after a meal.

Adverse reactions include anorexia, dyspepsia, constipation, headache, photosensitivity, hepatitis and mild neutropenia, and rarely tinnitus and taste disturbances.

Clarithromycin

Clarithromycin is a macrolide with a spectrum of activity similar to that of erythromycin. It is *inactive against Pseudomonas* and *Enterobacteriaceae.* Its indications are similar to those of erythromycin. It is also used for the eradication of *H. pylori* infection. *Dosage:* 200-500 mg bid for 7-14 days. For *H. pylori* infection 1.0 to 1.5 g daily in divided doses as part of the multidrug regimen is given.

Spiramycin

Spiramycin is effective not only in infections of the ***upper*** and ***lower respiratory tract,*** but also in some *protozoal infections* like ***toxoplasmosis*** and ***cryptosporidiosis.*** Other indications include *skin infections, gonococcal and chlamydial urethritis, prostatitis, trachoma,* and *prophylaxis of meningococcal meningitis.*

Dosage: Usual dose is 6-9 million IU/day orally in 2 or 3 divided doses for 5 days.

Adverse reactions: It is one of the best tolerated antibiotics. GI side defects are less frequent than with erythromycin.

Lincosamides (Lincomycins)

The lincosamide antibiotics, **lincomycin** and **clindamycin** are similar to the macrolides regarding their antibacterial spectrum, mode of action and therapeutic applications. These antibiotics have a very *limited use because of their serious side effects.*

INHIBITORS OF BACTERIAL CELL MEMBRANE FUNCTION

The 'surface active' antibiotics like the **polymyxins** and some **antifungal drugs** (e.g. nystatin, amphotericin B) damage the bacterial cell membrane by increasing the permeability. The antifungal antibiotics are considered in **Chapter 9.13.**

Polymyxins

Polymyxin B

Polymyxin B has a molecular weight of about 1000, and readily forms water soluble salts with mineral acids. The usual preparation is polymyxin B sulphate.

Antibacterial spectrum: Polymyxin B has a narrow spectrum limited to action against gram negative organisms (excluding Proteus and Neisseria). It is particularly active against *Ps. aeruginosa.* Other susceptible organisms are *Enterobacter aerogenes, E. coli, H influenzae, Bordetella pertusis, Klebsiella pneumoniae, salmonella* and *shigella.*

Mode of action: It *impairs the bacterial cell membrane function* and causes leakage of small molecules (e.g. phosphate, nucleosides) from the bacteria. This increased membrane permeability is the reason for their lethal effect.

Therapeutic uses: The polymyxins are second-choice agents in the treatment of **Pseudomonas aeruginosa** infections, particularly those of the urinary tract, external ear, conjunctiva and meninges, and in **septicaemia** when other drugs like carbenicillin and gentamicin are ineffective.

Toxicity: Adverse effects are minimal on topical application. Nausea, vomiting and diarrhoea, and superinfections with gram-positive bacteria, proteus or fungi may follow oral therapy. Kidney damage, with development of proteinuria and haematuria is the most dreaded adverse reaction in patients on systemic therapy.

Preparations and Dosage

Polymyxin B sulphate is available for local, oral or systemic administration. The average oral dose is 4.0 mg/kg daily. Intramuscularly or preferably IV the daily dose is 1.5-2.5 mg/kg in 3 or 4 divided doses.

Colistin

Colistin, a **bactericidal polypeptide antibiotic**, obtained from **Bacillus colistinus,** is identical with polymyxin E. It is available as colistin sulphate for oral use, and colistin sulphomethate sodium (sodium colistimethate) for parenteral use.

Colisitin has an antibacterial spectrum and mode of action similar to that of polymyxin B, but is less potent.

It has been suggested that colistin and polymyxin B be reserved for the treatment of systemic **Pseudomonas aeruginosa** infections, when less toxic antibiotics have failed.

The pattern of toxicity with colistin is similar to that of polymyxin. In addition **peripheral neuritis, nystagmus, amblyopia, transient deafness** and **leucopenia** may occur on systemic use.

Preparation and Dosage

Colisitin sulphate: It is suspended in distilled water (5 mg/ml) immediately before use. The recommended dose is 5-15 mg /kg/day in divided doses. The usual dose for children is 3-5 mg /kg/ day in divided doses.

Colistimethate sodium: It is available for IM administration in doses of 150 mg with the local anaesthetic dibucaine, 8mg. The usual IM dose is 2.5-5.0 mg/kg/day in divided doses.

MISCELLANEOUS ANTIBIOTICS

Spectinomycin

Spectinomycin is an ***aminocyclitol*** produced by **Streptomyces spectabilis.** It is active against a number of gram-negative bacterial species, and it readily inhibits most strains of **Neisseria gonorrhoeae** (gonococci). It inhibits protein synthesis in the bacteria. There are ***similarities in its action and that of the aminoglycosides.*** Spectinomycin is rapidly absorbed after IM injection and a single 2 g dose produces peak plasma levels of about 100 mcg/ml by 1 hour. It is not significantlly bound to the proteins, and is excreted in a biologically active form in the urine within 48 hours.

Spectinomycin is used to treat **acute genital** and **rectal gonorrhoea.**

Adverse effects occur infrequently and include pain at the site of injection, nausea, chills, fever, urticaria, insomnia and oliguria. Rarely **haematologic, renal** and **hepatic damage** may occur.

The recommended dose of spectinomycin dihydrochloride is 2 g/day in men and 4 g/day in women as a single deep IM injection.

The antibiotics **rifampicin, capreomycin, cycloserine** and **viomycin** have been discussed in **Chapter 9.4** dealing with chemotherapy of tuberculosis; cytotoxic antibiotics in **Chapter 9.10;** and the antifungal antibiotics nystatin, amphotericin B, griseofulvin and hamycin are discussed in **Chapter 9.13.**

9.4 CHEMOTHERAPY OF TUBERCULOSIS (ANTITUBERCULOUS DRUGS)

As recently as 60 years ago, tuberculosis was considered a serious health hazard. Chemotherapy has radically changed the outlook of this disease. The significance of the year 1948 is that it marks the introduction of **streptomycin**. Now hospitalization is necessary only for the seriously ill, and most patients are now treated in ***ambulatory-care clinics*** of general hospitals.

TUBERCULOUS INFECTIONS

Tuberculosis is a chronic infection caused by ***Mycobacterium tuberculosis*** and occasionally ***Mycobacterium bovis.*** Infection of the upper lung is the most common form of tuberculosis.

CLASSIFICATION

Antituberculous drugs are divided into *two* groups: (i) the primary drugs or the '*first line*' drugs which are used in standard therapeutic regimens, due to their **high level of efficacy,** and **acceptable degree of toxicity**; and (ii) the secondary drugs or the '*second line*' drugs which are used occasionally because of **bacterial resistance** or certain **patient-related factors.** The individual members are listed below:

i. **Primary drugs:** Isoniazid (INH), Rifampicin, Ethambutol, Pyrazinamide, Streptomycin.
ii. **Secondary drugs:** Ethionamide, Para-aminosalicylic acid (PAS), Cycloserine, Viomycin, Kanamycin, Amikacin, Capreomycin, Thiacetazone, Ciprofloxacin, Ofloxacin, Moxifloxacin.

PRIMARY DRUGS

Isoniazid (INH)

Isoniazid (isonicotinic acid hydrazide) introduced in 1952, is even now the most effective drug for the treatment of tuberculosis. It is very close to being an **ideal** drug as it is least toxic, most efficacious, and the least expensive of the available primary drugs.

Antibacterial spectrum: Isoniazid is both *tuberculostatic* and *tuberculocidal in vitro*. Some **atypical mycobacteria** are also susceptible to isoniazid action.

Mode of action: The main action being the ***inhibition of the biosynthesis of mycolic acids,*** which are important constituents of the mycobacterial cell wall. Only isoniazid-sensitive tubercle bacilli take up the drug, where it combines with certain ***intracellular mycobacterial enzymes,*** and interferes with the bacterial cell metabolism.

There is no cross-resistance between isoniazid and other anti tuberculous drugs.

Pharmacokinetics: Isoniazid is readily absorbed from the gut, diffuses well into the body tissues, including the CNS. It also ***penetrates into macrophages so that it is effective against intracellular tubercle bacilli.*** It is partly metabolized by acetylation in the liver. People are divided genetically into 'slow' and 'rapid' acetylators of isoniazid, which depends upon the group's ethnic make up. Slow acetylating patients should be treated with lower doses, and fast acetylators on the contrary require more frequent administration of isoniazid.

Therapeutic uses: Isoniazid is used for the treatment of tuberculosis, in combination with other drugs. It may be used alone for **prophylaxis.**

Toxicity: Toxic effects are more frequent in slow acetylators. The commonest effects are restlessness, insomnia, nausea, vomiting and muscle twitching. **Peripheral neuritis** may occur with higher doses which can be reversed or prevented by the use of pyridoxine 10-20 mg daily.

Dosage: For **pulmonary tuberculosis** upto 300 mg daily or upto 1 g (14 mg/kg) twice weekly is given orally. For **tuberculous meningitis** it is given in a dose of 10 mg/kg daily orally. For oral use 50 and 100 mg tablets are available.

Rifampicin

The rifamycins are complex antibiotics obtained from ***Streptomyces mediterranei.*** **Rifampicin** (rifampin) is a *semisynthetic derivative of rifamycin B*, and is well absorbed on oral administration.

Antibacterial spectrum: Rifampicin has a *broad-spectrum* of activity and inhibits the growth of many gram-positive cocci (e.g. gonococci and meningococci), and gram-negative bacteria such as *Escherichia coli, Pseudomonas,* indole positive and negative proteus and *klebsiella*.

Rifampicin is highly effective against most strains of ***Mycobactrium tuberculosis,*** and many atypical mycobacteria. Rifampicin is also active against ***Mycobacterium leprae*** **(Chap. 9.8).**

Mode of action: It has a high lipid solubility and ***diffuses easily through cell membranes to kill intracellular bacteria.*** Resistance by mycobacteria and other microorganism may develop rapidly.

Pharmacokinetics: Absorption of rifampicin from the gut is almost complete, but is impaired by food. The t½ is 2 to 5 hours, and renal insufficiency does not significantly raise the plasma levels. It is metabolized by **deacetylation** and is excreted mainly in the bile.

Therapeutic uses: The usual dose is 600 mg orally, given once daily, either 1 hour before or 2 hours after a meal. The dose for children is 10-20 mg/kg with a daily maximum of 600 mg. Combined with vancomycin or a beta-lactam antibiotic, rifampicin may be useful in cases of **osteomyelitis** or **staphylococcal endocarditis.**

Toxicity: On daily treatment regimens, signs of **hepatic toxicity** may appear but are usually transient. The drug should be used with caution in alcoholics and patients with hepatic disease.

Rifampicin markedly **induces hepatic microsomal activity,** and can accelerate the metabolism of several drugs like oestrogens, corticosteroids, sulphonylureas and anticoagulants. **The effectiveness of oral contraceptives is reduced, and where appropriate the method of contraception should be changed.** The urine saliva and other **body secretions are coloured orange-red (pink).**

Ethambutol

Ethambutol is used as a **first-line drug** in the treatment of tuberculosis. It is a *bacteriostatic* agent. Mycobacterial resistance develops slowly, and no cross resistance has been described. *It effectively inhibits strains which are resistant to INH or streptomycin.*

Ethambutol is well absorbed from the gut, and the absorption is not affected by the presence of food in the stomach. The plasma t½ is 5-6 hours. About 80 percent of the drug is excreted unchanged in the urine.

Ethambutol is used in the treatment of **tuberculosis** in combination with other drugs, usually rifampicin and isoniazid. The usual adult dose is 15 mg/kg given once a day.

Ethambutol produces very few **adverse reactions**. In high doses it may cause **loss of visual acuity due to retrobulbar neuritis** and **loss of colour vision.** Ethambutol today has virtually replaced PAS.

Pyrazinamide

It is chemically related to nicotinamide and is a **bactericidal** drug active against **M. tuberculosis.** It is particularly useful in ***tuberculous meningitis*** because of good meningeal penetration. **Hepatotoxicity** is the most common untoward effect. Other adverse effects are **arthralgias, anorexia, vomiting, fever, urticaria,** and **diabetes mellitus**. Dose is 20-30 mg/kg/day orally with a maximum of 3 g daily.

Streptomycin

The pharmacology of streptomycin has been discussed in detail in **Chapter 9.3.** Streptomycin is used in combination with other primary drugs in the treatment of tuberculosis. The *use of streptomycin for the treatment of pulmonary tuberculosis has sharply declined.* The usual dose is 1 g IM daily.

SECONDARY DRUGS

Alternative or second-line drugs discussed below are **less effective** and **more toxic** than the primary drugs. These drugs are used under the following circumstances: (i) in the treatment of patients when the **conventional primary therapy has failed;** and (ii) when the **organism is resistant** to the primary drugs, or in **infection with atypical mycobacteria.**

Ethionamide

It suppresses the multiplication of human strains

of **M. tuberculosis,** and is used for the treatment of tuberculosis resistant to first-line drugs. **Adverse reactions** are gastrointestinal disturbances including anorexia, salivation, metallic taste, nausea, vomiting and diarrhoea. **Peripheral neuropathy, optic neuritis, and hypothyroidism** may occur. The **usual dose** is 0.5-1 g orally daily, in divided doses or as a single dose at night.

Para-aminosalicylic acid (PAS): PAS is an analogue of p-aminobenzoic acid and acts in a similar way as the sulphonamides. It is bacteriostatic to most strains of **M. tuberculosis.** It is readily absorbed from the gut, and distributed in tissues and body fluids, with the exception of CSF. At present PAS is infrequently used. The average daily dose is 8-10 g orally in divided doses.

Cycloserine (Seromycin): It is a broad-spectrum antibiotic isolated from **Streptomyces orchidaceus.** The *inhibition of cell wall synthesis* is responsible for its inhibitory effect on *M. tuberculosis*.

Cycloserine is used in combination with other effective drugs to treat tuberculosis resistant to first-line drugs. The untoward reactions commonly involve the CNS manifesting as tremors, vertigo, confusion, psychotic states with suicidal tendencies, and grand mal seizures. Pyridoxine 100 mg/day may minimize the CNS effects. **Cycloserine is the most toxic of the second-line drugs.** The usual dose is 0.5-1 g/day orally in divided doses.

Viomycin: Viomycin is an ***aminglycoside***, and is most active *in vitro* against *M. tuberculosis*. Almost all strains of the tubercle bacillus are inhibited. Viomycin inhibits protein synthesis in *M. tuberculosis*. **Some cross-resistance to streptomycin, kanamycin and capreomycin exists. Toxic effects** are much more severe than streptomycin and include eighth nerve damage, and kidney damage. The usual dose is 1g IM daily.

Kanamycin (Kantrex)

Kanamycin is an ***aminoglycoside*** **(Chap 9.3).** It inhibits the growth of *M. tuberculosis*. It is sometimes incorporated into the multiple drug regimens. The usual dose is 1 g IM daily.

Amikacin (Amikin): Amikacin is also an ***aminoglycoside.*** It is very active against several mycobacterial species. It is given IM or IV in a dose of 15 mg/kg in 2 divided doses.

Capreomycin: Capreomycin is a polypeptide antibiotic isolated from **Streptomyces capreolus.** It has marked suppressive effect against *M. tuberculosis* and *M. bovis. Capreomycin approaches streptomycin in therapeutic efficacy, and there is no cross resistance between the two.* Capreomycin is toxic to the ***eighth cranial nerve leading to hearing loss,*** tinnitus and vertigo. The usual dose is 1 g IM daily.

Thiacetazone: Thiacetazone (same as amithiozone) is *bacteriostatic*, and is effective against **M. tuberculosis, M. bovis** and **M. leprae.** It can be used as a tuberculostatic or antileprotic agent. The usual dose is 150 mg/day orally in divided doses.

Ciprofloxacin and Ofloxacin

These fluoroquinolones are detailed in **Chapter 9.2.** Both **ciprofloxacin** and **ofloxacin** are active against *M. tuberculosis*. They are also active against *atypical mycobacteria*. The fluoroquinolones are important drugs against tuberculosis specially for ***strains that are resistant to first line drugs.*** *Dosage*: *Ciprofloxacin* 750 mg orally bid, *Ofloxacin* 600-800 mg orally as a single dose. Inclusion of **moxifloxacin** 400 mg daily as a single dose in the drug-combination therapy of **multidrug resistant** (MDR) tuberculosis is likely to shorten the duration of the course from 6 to 4 months.

CORTICOSTEROIDS AND TUBERCULOSIS

Corticosteroids are often useful adjuncts to the primary antituberculosis drugs in **fulminating pulmonary tuberculosis (tuberculous pneumonitis), tuberculous meningitis** and **pericarditis.** In these conditions corticosteroids may be life-saving. Corticosteroids decrease interstitial pulmonary inflammation, improve gas exchange, and decrease pleural, pericardial and meningeal fibrosis. They also offer benefit by their **antitoxic,**

antipyretic and **antianorectic** properties in the treatment of moribund tuberculous patients. In the unconscious patient large IV doses of **methylprednisolone** (80 to 120 mg/day) may be given initially, followed by 40 mg daily for a short period of time. In conscious patients **prednisone** 30-40 mg/day may be given orally. The treatment should be limited to a maximum of 6 weeks.

Chemotherapeutic Regimens

Except for prophylaxis and some cases of primary tuberculosis in which a single drug may be used (usually isoniazid), both pulmonary and extrapulmonary disease must always be treated with multiple drugs. Pleurisy with effusion is a fairly common form of tuberculosis in young adults, and should be treated with **standard triple-drug therapy,** or by one of the **short-treatment regimens.**

The treatment of tuberculosis may be divided into two phases an **initial phase** using at least three drugs, and a **continuation phase** with two drugs.

Initial phase: Treatment of choice for the initial phase is the daily use of **isoniazid** and **rifampicin** with **ethambutol** or **streptomycin.** These drugs should be continued for 8 weeks.

Continuous phase: After the initial phase, treatment is continued with only 2 drugs, one of which should be **isoniazid** provided it is not contraindicated. The second drug may be **rifampicin, ethambutol** or **streptomycin.**

Duration of treatment: Sufficient data are now available on the outcome of treatment in the initial phase (3 drugs) followed by continuation phase with 2 drugs (isoniazid and rifampicin) which confirm that a course of **9 months duration** gives satisfactory results in **pulmonary tuberculosis.** For **extrapulmonary tuberculosis** a total treatment period of **12 months** is recommended.

More recently it has been found that constant inhibitory concentrations of drugs are not essential. Such an **intermittent schedule** may be employed in stabilized patients during the continuous phase of treatment, and the **twice weekly regimens** may be used. Details of regimens are beyond the scope of this text.

Failure of chemotherapy may be due to: (i) **poor patient compliance;** (ii) **interruption in therapy;** (iii) **inadequate initial triple-drug therapy;** and (iv) **primary mycobacterial resistance** to the drugs in use.

Tuberculous Meningitis

Although there is no consensus on an optimal regimen, the following is considered satisfactory. **Isoniazid** 400mg, plus **pyridoxine** 10 mg daily; **streptomycin** 1 g IM daily; and rifampicin 10 mg/kg daily. Ethambutol 25mg/kg may be substituted for streptomycin. *This treatment is continued for 2 months. Isoniazid and rifampicin are then continued for a further period of 6 months and lastly isoniazid alone for another 6 months. The total duration of chemotherapy comes to 14 months.* **Corticosteroids** are sometimes used in the initial stages of treatment as discussed earlier.

Short-course therapy: The most effective experimental short treatment regimen is an initial intensive phase of 4 drugs: **streptomycin, INH, rifampicin** and **pyrazinamide** for about 8 weeks, followed by twice-weekly **streptomycin, INH** and **rifampicin** for the continuation phase till a total treatment time of 6 months.

Extrapulmonary tuberculosis: Once the diagnosis is established, treatment is generally similar to that of pulmonary disease.

NATIONAL TUBERCULOSIS CONTROL PROGRAMME (NTCP) GUIDELINES

National tuberculosis control programme (NTCP) has provided detailed guidelines for the treatment of various categories of tuberculous patients. Details are beyond the scope of this text.

In 1993 the Revised National Tuberculosis Control Programme (RNTCP) applied the principles of Directly Observed Therapy Shortcourse (DOTS) in the Indian context. It has resulted in the early diagnosis; successful treatment; and prevention of emergence of Multidrug Resistant Tuberculosis

(MDR-TB) in the country. DOTS offers the best means for TB control.

CHEMOPROPHYLAXIS OF TUBERCULOSIS

Prophylactic therapy may be employed effectively to prevent the development of active tuberculosis in certain circumstances. **Isoniazid,** 300 mg daily is very useful for prophylaxis. Its prophylactic use is reserved for household contacts of patients with proven tuberculosis.

9.5 CHEMOTHERAPY OF MALARIA (ANTIMALARIAL DRUGS)

Malaria is a parasitic disease caused by the proto zoan of the genus **Plasmodium.** The continued prevalence of malaria warrants a vigorous attack on the malarial parasite, and on its insect vector, the **female anopheles mosquito.**

TYPES OF MALARIA

Four species of the genus Plasmodium cause human malaria: (i) **Plasmodium falciparum,** causes **malignant tertian** (MT) malaria; (ii) **Plasmodium vivax,** causes benign tertian (BT) malaria, and relapses are common. The term **tertian** indicates that the attacks of chills and fever typically tend to recur every third day; (iii) **Plasmodium malariae,** causes **quartan** (Q) malaria. The term **quartan** indicates that the spikes of fever come every fourth day; and (iv) **Plasmodium ovale,** causes a rare form of relapsing malaria. It is tertian in nature. Infections caused by *P. vivax, P. malariae* and *P. ovale* are classified as **'relapsing malarias'** because they have a secondary exoerythrocytic stage of development. In contrast, *P. falciparum* has no exoerythrocytic stage in its life cycle.

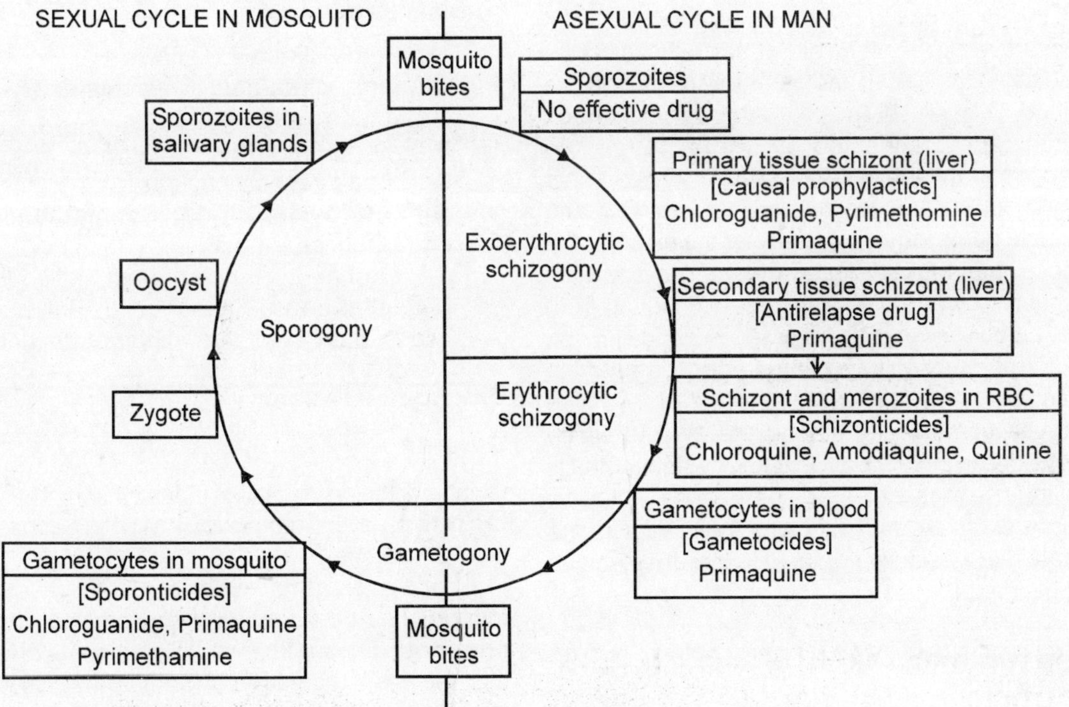

Fig. 9.2: *The life cycle of the malarial parasite, and the points of action of various categories of antimalarial drugs (diagrammatic).*

LIFE CYCLE OF THE MALARIAL PARASITE

Broadly speaking the parasite runs its **asexual cycle** in man, and the **sexual cycle** in the mosquito (**Fig. 9.2**). The human phase begins when an infected **female Anopheles mosquito** bites man and injects **sporozoites** from her salivary glands. The injected sporozoites localize in the liver parenchyma cells, develop into **primary tissue schizonts** and mature within 8-21 days to form **merozoites.** This constitutes the **preerythrocytic stage** during which the subject remains symptom-free. On maturity the merozoites of all four species are liberated from the liver cells and invade the erythrocytes and begin the **erythrocytic cycle** of asexual development. In all except falciparum malaria, a proportion of merozoites infect more tissue cells, forming **secondary tissue schizonts** and this constitutes the **exoerythrocytic cycle** which may continue for several years and accounts for the **relapse** of infection (secondary exoerythrocytic forms do not occur with *P. falciparum*, hence no relapse). At the end of the erythrocytic cycle the infected red cells rupture releasing merozoites (they reinvade other red cells), pigments and other products in to the blood. This point of time marks the **clinical attack** of malaria manifested by **chills, fever** and **profound sweating.** After several cycles some erythrocytic parasites differentiate into male and female **gametocytes.** No further development of these forms takes place in man. They may be ingested by a female Anopheles mosquito from the blood stream of the infected individual. In the gut of the mosquito, **exflagellation** of the male gametocyte is followed by **fertilization** of the female gametocyte forming the **zygote** which develops in the gut wall as an **oocyst,** eventually giving rise to the infective sporozoites, which on rupture of the oocyst make their way to the *mosquito's salivary glands*. Hence, the cycle is completed.

CATEGORIES OF ANTIMALARIAL DRUG ACTION

1. **Causal prophylaxis:** A casual prophylactic agent prevents infection by its lethal effect on the plasmodia during their **preerythrocytic stages**, e.g., **Primaquine.**
2. **Suppressive treatment:** A suppressive drug causes inhibition of the **erythrocytic stage** of development of the parasite, e.g., **chloroquine.**
3. **Clinical cure:** Drugs in this category interrupt **erythrocytic schizogony** of the plasmodia, and terminate the clinical attack, e.g., **chloroquine** and **amodiaquine.**
4. **Radical cure:** This refers to the eradication of both **exoerythrocytic** and **erythrocytic** phases of the infection, e.g., **primaquine**.
5. **Suppressive cure:** This refers to the complete elimination of the malarial parasite from the body by continued suppressive therapy, e.g., of **pyrimethamine** for 10 weeks.
6. **Gametocytocidal therapy:** This category of drugs destroys the sexual forms of the malarial parasites in human blood, e.g., **primaquine.**

CLASSIFICATION

i. **Cinchona alkaloid:** Quinine.
ii. **4-Aminoquinolines:** Chloroquine, Hydroxychloroquine, Amodiaquine.
iii. **8-Aminoquinolines:** Primaquine.
iv. **Acridine dyes:** Quinacrine.
v. **Diaminopyrimidines:** Pyrimethamine, Trimethoprim.
vi. **4-Quinoline-carbinolamines:** Mefloquine.
vii. **Miscellaneous:** Quinghaosu, Sulphonamides, Sulphones, Artemether, Artesunate.

Cinchona Alkaloid

Quinine

Quinine is the chief alkaloid obtained from the bark of cinchona tree. Commercially it is produced from natural sources.

Pharmacological actions: On the skeletal muscle it has a **curare-like** effect. It induces **bronchoconstriction.** It has an **oxytoxic** effect. Quinine has a **local anaesthetic action**. Its very bitter taste is the basis for its use as a **stomachic bitter** to increase gastric juice secretion.

Antimalarial action: Quinine has been used for **suppressive prophylaxis** and **clinical cure** in all types of malaria, since it is actively **schizonticidal.** With the advent of the synthetic antimalarials, the use of quinine has declined.

Mode of action: Quinine forms a hydrogen bonded complex with double standard DNA causing inhibition of protein synthesis, DNA replication, and transcription to RNA.

Pharmacokinetics: On oral administration, quinine is rapidly and effectively absorbed, mainly from the upper small intestine. Peak levels develop within 1-3 hours, and about 70-80 percent is protein bound. It is degraded in the liver and only 5-10 percent of the active drug is recoverable in the urine.

Therapeutic uses: The valid use of quinine today is in the treatment of **relapsing vivax malaria** in combination with primaquine, and in the treatment of **malignant tertian malaria** due to strains of *P. falciparum* resistant to chloroquine.

Toxicity: Adverse effects due to quinine include: (i) **Cinchonism** which is a mild toxic state with flushed and wet skin, tinnitus, blurred vision, impaired hearing, dizziness, nausea, vomiting and diarrhoea. In severe cinchonism there may be urticarial skin rashes, deafness, diminished vision or even blindness (**quinine amblyopia**), abdominal pain and cardiac arrhythmias; (ii) **Local irritation** is responsible for gastrointestinal discomfort, and thrombophlebitis on IV injection of quinine; (iii) **Bone-marrow depression** may occur; (iv) **Black water fever** due to massive intravascular haemolysis; and (v) **Hypersensitivity reactions** may occur.

Preparation and dosage: Quinine sulphate for oral use, and **quinine dihydrochloride** for IV use. The usual oral dose of quinine sulphate (as base) is 650 mg every 8-hourly for 10 or 14 days for treatment of malaria.

Chloroquine-Resistant Malaria

It is recommended that all falciparum infections should be assumed to be resistant, and treated as:

1. **Quinine sulphate** 650 mg 3 times a day for 3 days, plus **Bactrim Double Strength** (160 mg trimethoprim and 800 mg sulphamethoxazole) 2 tablets 2 times a day for 5 days administered concurrently.
2. Following a course of quinine the patient should be given a dose of 2 tablets of **Fansidar** (50 mg pyrimethamine and 1 g sulfadoxine).

4- Aminoquinolines

Chloroquine

Chloroquine is the most widely used antimalarial.

Pharmacological actions: Chloroquine was primarily developed as an antimalarial, but in addition it is active against **extraintestinal amoebiasis.**

Antimalarial actions: Chloroquine is an excellent blood schizonticidal drug for all 4 types of malaria.

Mode of action: Chloroquine and its congeners block the enzymatic synthesis of DNA and RNA. Chloroquine has a number of other actions like **stabilization of lysosomes,** some **anti-inflammatory** and **antihistaminic** activity.

Therapeutic uses:

1. **Acute malarial attacks:** For *P. vivax* infection the recommended total dose of chloroquine (base) is 1.5 g over a 3-day period (600 mg initial dose, 300 mg after 6 hours and then 300mg for 2 days).
2. **Suppression of malaria.**
3. **Hepatic amoebiasis.**
4. **Rheumatoid arthritis, discoid lupus erythematosus,** and in **acute disseminated lupus erythematosus.**

Toxicity: Occasionally there may be **vertigo, malaise, diarrhoea, blurring of vision** and **urticaria.** After high doses **maculopapular eruptions, exfoliative lesions of the skin, alopecia** and **graying of the hair** may develop. **Hallucinations, agitation** and **peripheral neuropathies** may occur.

Ocular toxicity: Corneal deposits and **retinal retinopathy** may occur.

8- Aminoquinolines

Primaquine Phosphate

Primaquine is the most effective and least toxic of the 8-aminoquinoline.

Antimalarial actions: Primaquine is a **'tissue schizonticide'.**

Therapeutic uses: It is used to induce **'radical cures'** of relapsing malarias.

Toxicity: Side effects seen with larger doses include nausea, headache, disturbances of visual accommodation, pruritus and abdominal cramps. Severe reactions with high dose therapy include **leucopenia** and **methaemoglobinaemia**.

Acridine Dyes

Quinacrine

Quinacrine is **obsolete** as an antimalarial drug, but is used in the management of **giardiasis.**

Diaminopyrimidines

Pyrimethamine

Suppressive cure of some vivax infections may be achieved with pyrimethamine administration in prophylactic doses for 10 weeks after leaving a malarious region.

Mode of action: Both the **antifols** or **dihydrofolate reductase inhibitors,** namely pyrimethamine and trimethoprim, exert a plasmodicidal action by causing a deficiency of tetrahydrofolate which results in the **inhibition of cell division** and **schizogony**.

Therapeutic uses

Pyrimethamine is effective as a **prophylactic** and **suppressive** agent, and has proved useful if given once weekly.

Toxicity: With recommended dosage no significant toxic manifestations are seen. Excessive doses may produce a **megaloblastic anaemia** resembling that of folic acid deficiency.

Preparations and dosage: Pyrimethamine is marketed in scored tablets containing 25 mg (base). The drug is also available in combination with **dapsone** (Maloprim) which is meant for use as a prophylactic. Pyrimethamine in combination with **sulfadoxine** (Fansidar) is available for use in the treatment of multiresistant infections **(Table 9.5)**. **Sulfadoxine** is a sulphonamide with a long t½ of 7 to 9 days.

Trimethoprim

Trimethoprim is mainly used as an antibacterial agent in combination with sulphamethoxazole (co-trimoxazole). It is used for the treatment of multiresistant strains of plasmodia.

4- Quinoline Carbinolamines

Mefloquine

Mefloquine is used in the prophylaxis and treatment of ***chloroquine-resistant*** and ***multidrug-resistant falciparum malaria.***

Adverse effects include vomiting, abdominal pain, disorientation, hallucinations, and depression.

Miscellaneous

Quinghaosu (Artemisinin)

Quinghaosu is effective against asexual blood forms of the parasite. It lacks activity against tissue stages.

Artemisinin Derivatives

Artemisinin is a herbal product traditionally used in China for the treatment of malaria. It is active against *P. vivax* and against both chloroquine sensitive and chloroquine-resistant strains of *P. falciparum*. The two commonly used derivatives are **artemether** and **artesunate.**

Artemether: It is a potent and rapidly acting ***blood schizonticide,*** and is highly efficacious in treating ***chloroquine-resistant falciparum malaria,*** and ***complicated falciparum malaria*** including ***cerebral malaria.***

Dosage: A 5-day dose scheme is followed – 80 mg (one ampoule) IM bid on day 1, followed by 80 mg IM OD for the following 4 days. **Adverse reactions** include nausea, vomiting, abdominal pain, bradycardia, first degree heart block, and transient increase in transaminases.

Table 9.5: *Drugs used for the prophylaxis and treatment of malaria*

Drug	Prophylaxis*	Treatment*	Comments
Quinine sulphate	–	650 mg orally 8-hourly for 10-14 days	Given with primaquine it produces a radical cure in vivax malaria.
Quinine dihydro-chloride	–	600 mg IV slowly, repeated 6-8 hours, maximum dose 1.8 g per day	Drug of choice for *cerebral malaria*, but oral therapy should be started as soon as possible
Chloroquine** phosphate	300 mg orally weekly	600 mg initially, then 300 mg at 6. 24 and 48 hours (1.5 g in 3 days)	Drug of choice for treating acute attacks of malaria (clinical cure) Other uses : Amoebiasis, giardiasis, rheumatoid arthritis and other collagen diseases
Chloroquine hydrochloride	–	3 mg/kg initially IM or IV, then 3 mg/kg every 6 hours. Max. dose 900 mg/24 hours	Acute attacks of malaria
Primaquine phosphate	15 mg orally daily for 14 days after leaving endemic area, or 45 mg weekly for 8 weeks	15 mg orally daily for 14 days	Radical cure for vivax malaria expected in 95% cases treated with primaquine plus chloroquine
Pyrimethamine	25 mg orally weekly	–	For prophylaxis and suppressive cure
Pyrimethamine-sulfadoxine	50 mg pyrimethamine and 1 g sulfadoxine every other week for 6 weeks		For prophylaxis of chloroquine-resistant falciparum malaria
Mefloquine	250 mg weekly for 4 weeks, then 124 mg weekly	1250 mg once, or 750 mg followed after 6-8 hours by 500 mg	Reserved for prophylaxis and treatment of chloroquine-resistant and multidrug-resistant falciparum malaria

* Slight variations in dosage may exist between this Table and the text.

** Doses of chloroquine are in terms of base : chloroquine base 100 mg = chloroquine phosphate 160 mg = chloroquine hydrochloride 125 mg = chloroquine sulphate 137 mg.

Artesunate: It also is a potent ***blood schizonticide*** and is available for oral use in cases of **chloroquine-resistant falciparum malaria** (Dose: 100 mg bid orally on day 1, followed by 50 mg bid for 4 days); and for IM/IV use (Dose: 120 mg IM/IV on day 1, followed by 60 mg IM/IV daily for 4 days). **Adverse reactions** include rash, drug fever, transient first degree heart block, reversible reticulocytopenia and transient elevation of transaminases.

Sulphonamides and Sulphones

The sulphonamides are active against the asexual blood forms of human malarial parasites. **Sulfadoxine** and **sulfalene** have been used for suppression of infection caused by sensitive strains of *P. falciparum*.

Tetracyclines: Tetracyclines in a dose of 250 mg 6-hourly for 7 days can clear asexual forms of **chloroquine-resistant falciparum infections.**

Proguanil

It is active against *pre-erythrocytic forms* of the parasite, but is a *slow and weak blood schizonticide.* Proguanil is mainly used for *causal prophylaxis of falciparum malaria* in doses of 200 mg orally daily starting 1 week before entering, and for 4 weeks after leaving a malarious region. ***Adverse effects*** include GI disturbances, headache, vertigo, rash and hair loss.

9.6 CHEMOTHERAPY OF AMOEBIASIS (AMOEBICIDAL DRUGS)

Amoebiasis is an infection caused by **Entamoeba histolytica.** It is an invasion of the gastrointestinal mucosa, liver and other tissues by the **vegetative trophozoite forms** of the protozoan.

AMOEBIC DISEASE STATES

Amoebiasis in man presents as: (i) asymptomatic intestinal infection; (ii) mild to moderate intestinal infection; (iii) severe intestinal infection (dysentery); (iv) amoebic liver abscess; and (v) amoeboma or extraintestinal infection.

LIFE CYCLE OF THE AMOEBA

Entamoeba histolytica has a two stage life cycle: (i) the **cystic** stage in which the organism can live for long periods both outside the body and within the human intestine; and (ii) the **trophozoite** (vegetative) stage, which is motile, and occurs under suitable environmental conditions in the intestine (colon). It invades the intestinal mucosa forming multiple ulcers (amoebic dysentery). The trophozoites finally find their way to the mesenteric veins to be carried to the liver (amoebic hepatitis and liver abscess). Thus, the trophozoite form is responsible for both the **intestinal** and **extra-intestinal** symptoms of amoebiasis.

The disease is transmitted when mature cysts are ingested. Each cyst develops into 8 trophozoites. A colony is established in the caecum which extends throughout the colon. The trophozoites penetrate the mucosa causing *ulceration, diarrhoea* and *abdominal pain.*

CLASSIFICATION

The amoebicidal drugs may be classified according to their site of antiamoebic action:

I. **Tissue amoebicides**
   a. Dehydroemetine, Emetine.
   b. Chloroquine (mainly active in the liver).
II. **Luminal amoebicides**
   a. **Halogenated hydroxyquinolines.** Iodoquinol, Clioquinol.
   b. **Alkaloid.** Emetine Bismuth Iodide (EBI).
   c. **Amides.** Diloxanide furoate, Teclozan, Etofamide.
   d. **Antibiotics.** Tetracyclines, Erythromycin.
III. **Tissue and luminal amoebicides**
   a. **Nitroimidazoles.** Metronidazole, Tinidazole.

Treatment of amoebiasis may require the **concomitant** or **sequential** use of several drugs. A brief mention of the available drugs follows:

Ipecacuanha Alkaloids

Emetine Hydrochloride

Ipecacuanha is obtained from the dried rhizomes or roots of **Cephaelis ipecacuanha.** Its amoebicidal activity is due to its alkaloid content, mainly **emetine**. Emetine is seldom used today.

Amoebicidal action: Emetine has a **direct** lethal action on *E.histolytica*. Emetine in therapeutic doses only acts against trophozoites.

Emetine given parenterally in toxic doses causes cellular damage in the **liver, kidneys, skeletal** and **cardiac muscle.**

Therapeutic uses: Emetine has a **restricted** use due to its toxicity and availability of safer drugs. However, it may be cautiously employed in extraintestinal amoebiasis.

Toxicity

Gastrointestinal toxicity includes **diarrhoea, nausea** and **vomiting.** Neuromuscular manifestations of toxicity are **muscle weakness,** specially those of the neck and extremities. It is **cardiotoxic** and serious manifestations include **hypotension, cardiac arrhythmias, congestive heart failure** and **death.**

Preparations and dosage: Emetine hydrochloride is administered by deep SC or IM injection. A dose of 65 mg/day for upto 5 days is recommended.

Dehydroemetine

It **retains the amoebicidal property of emetine but is less toxic.** The clinical uses of dehydroemetine are similar to those of emetine.

Its dosage for **severe intestinal amoebiasis** is 1 mg/kg IM or SC for 3-5 days. The maximum daily dose is 0.1 g.

Emetine Bismuth Iodide (EBI)

EBI contains about 25 percent emetine and about 20 percent bismuth. It is an orally administered compound. **Side effects** are similar to emetine. It is seldom used today.

4-Aminoquinolines

Chloroquine Phosphate

Chloroquine is **amoebicidal** and is useful in treating **hepatic amoebic infections.**

Chloroquine is actively amoebicidal for **extraintestinal** parasites.

Adverse reactions: In amoebiasis the longer period of administration increases the frequency of gastrointestinal disturbances. Chloroquine phosphate (in terms of salt) is usually given in a dose of 1g/day orally for 2 days, followed by 0.5 g/day for 2 to 3 weeks to effectively treat hepatic amoebiasis.

Halogenated Hydroxyquinolines

The currently used members of this group are **iodoquinol** and **clioquinol.**

Amoebicidal action: Iodoquinol exerts a **direct amoebicidal action** against trophozoites and cysts of *E.histolytica* in the intestines. It is ineffective in extraintestinal amoebiasis.

Therapeutic uses: Iodoquinol is particularly useful for the treatment of **asymptomatic cyst passers.**

Iodoquinol and **clioquinol** (iodochlorohydroxyquin) are used to treat superficial fungal infections like **athlete's foot,** and **trichomonal vaginitis** for which vaginal inserts are used topically.

Iodoquinol is occasionally used in the treatment of **giardiasis.**

Toxicity: There is increasing evidence that certain 8-hydroxyquinolines can produce *neurotoxicity*. The main findings were *optic atrophy, visual loss, and peripheral neuropathy*.

The most important neurologic toxic reaction, particularly due to iodochlorhydroxyquin (clioquinol) is **subacute myelooptic neuropathy (SMON),** the incidence of which has a peculiar geographic distribution. It was first reported in Japan, where it occurred in epidemic form. This resulted in the cessation of sale of this drug in Japan, and restriction on sale in other countries the world over.

Table 9.6 : *Drug regimens for the treatment of amoebiasis*

Pattern of infection	Drugs of choice	Alternative drugs
1. Asymptomatic intestinal infection	Diloxanide furoate(1)*	Diiodohydroxyquin(2) or Metronidozole (3)
2. Mild to moderate intestinal infection	Diloxanide(1) or Diiodohydroxyquin(2) plus A tetracycline(4) followed by Chloroquine(5)	Metronidazole(3) plus Diloxanide(1) or Paromomycin(6) followed by Chloroquine(5)
3. Severe intestinal infection (dysentery)	Metronidazole(3) plus Diloxanide(1) Diiodohydroxyquin(2)	A tetracycline(4) plus Diloxanide(1) or Diiodohydroxyquin(2) or Dehydroemetine(6) followed by Chloroquine(5)
4. Hepatic abscess	Metronidazole(3) followed by Diloxanide(1) or Diiodohydroxyquin(2) plus Chloroquine(5)	Dehydroemetine(6) plus Chloroquine(5) or Emetine(7) plus Chloroquine(5)
5. Amoeboma or extraintestinal infection	Same as for hepatic abscess, but excluding chloroquine	Same as for hepatic abscess, but excluding chloroquine

* The numerals in parentheses indicate the dosage mentioned below :
(1) Diloxanide furoate, 500 mg tid for 10 days.
(2) Diiodohydroxyquin (iodoquinol) 650 mg tid for 21 days.
(3) Metronidazole, 750 mg tid for 10 days.
(4) A tetracycline, 250 mg qid for 10 days.
(5) Chloroquine phosphate, 1.0 g (500 mg base) daily for 2 days, then 0.5 g (250 mg base) daily for 2-3 weeks.
(6) Dehydroemetine, 1 mg/kg/day IM or SC for 10 days (max. dose 90 mg/day).
(7) Emetine, 1 mg/kg/day IM or SC for upto 5 days (max. dose 65 mg/day).

Preparations: *Iodoquinol* is administered in a dose of 650 mg orally 3 times daily for 21 days. *Clioquinol* is available in the form of an ointment or powder for topical use as an antifungal agent.

Amides

Diloxanide Furoate

Diloxanide is **directly amoebicidal,** and primarily acts against the trophozoite forms of the parasite. It is less effective in acute amoebic dysentery.

Diloxanide furoate is free form serious side effects. Flatulence is common. Nausea, abdominal cramps, dry mouth, pruritus, urticaria and albuminuria may occur rarely.

Antibiotics

A number of antibiotics are of value in the treatment of intestinal amoebiasis, specially **paromomycin, tetracyclines** and **erythromycin.** The *older tetracyclines mainly tetracycline itself is more effective as it remains unabsorbed in the bowel* in relatively larger proportions.

Nitroimidazoles

Metronidazole

Metronidazole is **amoebicidal** at both intestinal and extraintestinal sites, and is currently the preferred drug for all amoebic infections. Metronidazole can be used alone or with other drugs (**Table 9.6**). It was originally introduced as a **trichomonacidal** agent, effective orally.

Toxicity: Frequent reactions are nausea and diarrhoea. Other side effects include unpleasant taste, furry tongue, glossitis, stomatitis, anorexia, abdominal cramps and darkening in the colour of urine.

When taken with alcoholic beverages, metronidazole may produce a **disulfiram-type reaction** (abdominal distress, nausea, vomiting and headache) caused by accumulation of acetaldehyde in the body.

As it is a nitroimidazole, *its potential for depressing the bone marrow* must be kept in mind.

Therapeutic uses: Metronidazole is employed in the treatment of **amoebic dysentery, amoebic liver abscess, amoeboma** and **extra-intestinal amoebiasis.** A course of metronidazole may be *repeated after 2 weeks*, if necessary. Metronidazole is also effective against **giardiasis** and **dracunculiasis,** and **anaerobic** bacteria, specially *B.fragilis.*

Tinidazole is a newer nitromidazole, and is effectively used in the treatment of **amoebiasis, trichomoniasis** and **giardiasis.** Dose: 2 g single daily dose for 3 days in intestinal amoebiasis. Other nitroimidazoles include secnidazole, and niridazole.

GUIDELINES FOR AMOEBICIDAL THERAPY

Success of drug therapy depends upon concomitant or sequential treatment with at least two drugs (**Table 9.6**). The ideal treatment is summarized below:

Table 9.7: *Drugs of choice and alternative drugs for some protozoal infections in man*

Infecting organism	Drug of choice	Alternative drug
Leishmaniasis		
Leishmania donovani (Kala-azar)	Sodium stibogluconate	Pentamidine
L. tropica (Oriental sore)	Sodium stibogluconate	–
L. braziliensis (mucocutaneous leishmaniasis)	Sodium stibogluconate	Amphotericin B
Trypanosomiasis		
Trypanosoma gambiense	Pentamidine	Suramin
T. rhodesiense	Suramin	Pentamidine
T. cruzi (Chaga's disease)	Nifurtimox	Primaquine
Trichomoniasis		
Trichomonas vaginalis	Metronidazole	Topical drugs
Giardiasis		
Giardia lambia	Quinacrine	Metronidazole
Balantidiasis		
Balantidium coli	Oxytetracycline	Iodoquinol
Toxoplasmosis		
Toxoplasma gondii	Pyrimethamine+ trisulfapyrimidines	–

1. **Acute amoebic dysentery:** The drug of choice is metronidazole with or without an antibiotic.
2. **Chronic amoebic colitis:** It is best treated with a 3-week course of **diloxanide** plus **chloroquine.**
3. **Asymptomatic carrier state:** The asymptomatic carrier (cyst passer) is best treated with **diloxanide furoate.**
4. **Extraintestinal amoebiasis: Chloroquine** and **emetine** are the drugs of choice for either acute or chronic extraintestinal infection. **Metronidazole** is also recommended.

OTHER PROTOZOAL INFECTIONS

Apart from malaria and amoebiasis other important protozoal infections in man are **leishmaniasis, trypanosomiasis, trichomoniasis, giardiasis,** and **toxoplasmosis**. The drugs of choice and alternative drugs are listed in **Table 9.7.**

9.7 CHEMOTHERAPY OF HELMINTHIASIS (ANTHELMINTIC DRUGS)

Anthelmintics are drugs used to eradicate parasitic worms (known as helminths) from the human body.

HELMINTHS INFECTING MAN

Three categories of worms, namely **nematodes** (roundworms), **cestodes** (tapeworms), and **trematodes** (flukes) parasitize man.

ANTHELMINTICS

Albendazole (Zentel)

Albendazole is a broad-spectrum oral anthelmintic.

Mode of action: Albendazole blocks glucose uptake by larval and adult stages of susceptible parasites, depleting their glycogen stores. This results in immobilization of the parasite and its death.

Therapeutic Uses and Dosage

1. **Ascariasis, trichuriasis, hookworm and pinworm infections:** A single dose of 400 mg orally is administered with a meal.
2. **Strongyloidiasis:** A dose of 400 mg twice daily for 3-7 days.
3. **Hydatid disease:** A dose of 800 mg /day for 30 days is given.
4. **Neurocysticercosis:** The treatment schedule is 15 mg/kg/day for 30 days.

Adverse reactions: Headache, diarrhoea, epigastric distress, dizziness and insomnia have been reported. When used for 1-3 days, albendazole is almost free of adverse effects.

Diethylcarbamazine Citrate

Diethylcarbamazine is the *drug of choice* for the treatment of **filariasis.** It causes rapid disappearance of microfilariae of **Wuchereria bancrofti, W. malayi** and **Loa loa** from the blood of man. Diethylcarbamazine also kills adult worms of *W. bancrofti*, *W. malayi* and *Loa loa*.

Therapeutic uses and dosage: Diethylcarbamazine is used to treat infections with **W. bancrofti, W. malayi, Loa loa** and **O. volvulus.** In the treatment of **tropical eosinophilia** it causes a rapid disappearance of symptoms in a dose of 2 mg/kg tid for 7 days. For treatment of *W. bancrofti* and *W. malayi* infections the usual dose is 2 mg/kg three times daily after meals for 7 days.

Adverse effects are mild and include dizziness, headache, weakness, nausea and vomiting.

Emetine Hydrochloride

Emetine is an alternative drug for the treatment of **Fasciola hepatica** infection. It is administered by deep intramuscular injection in doses of 1 mg/kg (maximum 65 mg daily) for 10 days.

Ivermectin

It is the drug of choice for **onchocerciasis.** It acts by increasing the release and binding of gamma-aminobutyric acid (GABA), thereby producing paralysis. Thus it also appears to be highly effective in **strongyloidiasis, ascariasis, trichuriasis** and **enterobiasis.** The dosage ranges between 120-230 mcg/kg.

Mebendazole

It is the primary drug of choice for **enterobiasis** and **trichuriasis**. It is particularly useful in the treatment of mixed infections with **whipworms** (trichuriasis), **roundworms** (ascariasis), **hookworms** (ancylostomiasis), and **pinworms** (enterobiasis).

Dosage: Mebendazole is available as 100 mg chewable tablets. For the treatment of **ascariasis, trichuriasis** and **hookworm** infections, 100 mg twice daily for 3 days is given. No pretreatment or post treatment purging is required.

Niclosamide

Niclosamide is the drug of choice for treating tapeworm infections. This agent is administered orally and the concomitant use of a laxative is not required, except for *T.solium*. Niclosamide may destroy *T.solium* segments, thereby releasing viable eggs. The laxative administered 1 to 2 hours after the anthelmintic avoids the possibility of cysticercosis. No serious side effects have been reported.

Adverse reactions include gastrointestinal disturbances, vomiting and diarrhoea. Headache, dizziness and occasionally ECG changes, neuropsychiatric disturbances, insomnia, hallucinations, and seizures may develop. Haemolytic anemia may occur in patients of G-6-PD deficiency. The **usual dose** is 25 mg/kg body weight daily orally in two divided doses, for 5-7 days in schistosomiasis, and for 7 to 10 days in dracunculiasis.

Piperazine

Currently piperazine is an alternative drug for the treatment of ascariasis. The main effect of piperazine on *Ascaris* is to cause **flaccid paralysis** of the worm, which is expelled by peristalsis. After therapy ascaris worms are passed out paralysed and alive, usually 1 to 3 days after treatment. A **laxative** is needed to expel the worms from the intestine.

Piperazine salts are available as tablets, each containing 500 mg, and as syrups and suspensions containing 100 mg/ml. All preparations are equally effective. **Piperazine citrate** and **piperazine phosphate** are official preparations. In **ascariasis** the usual dose is 3.5 g once daily for 2 consecutive days.

Adverse reactions include nausea, vomiting, diarrhoea and allergic reactions. With larger doses muscular incoordination, vertigo, speech difficulty, confusion and **myoclonic contractions** have been reported.

Praziquantel

Praziquantel is effective against **schistosome infections** of all species, and most other **trematode** and **cestode infections.**

Therapeutic uses and dosage: Praziquantel is an extremely active, well tolerated, **broad-spectrum anthelmintic,** and is the drug of choice for treating schistosomiasis. Both **S. mansoni** and **S. haematobium** infections respond well to a single oral dose of 40 mg/kg. **S. japonicum** is treated with half this dose, with administration repeated on 3 occasions within a 12 hour period. For **neurocysticercosis** the dosage is 50 mg/kg/day orally in 3 divided doses for 14 to 30 days.

Adverse reactions occur in some patients within a few hours of administration and include gastrointestinal intolerance with nausea, vomiting and abdominal discomfort.

Pyrantel Pamoate

Pyrantel pamoate is highly effective for the treatment of **oxyuriasis, ascariasis** and **Trichostrongylus orientalis** infections.

The anthelmintic action of pyrantel is due to the inhibition of neuromuscular transmission. It causes a spastic neuromuscular paralysis in the worm, which is subsequently expelled from the hosts intestines.

For **roundworms** and **pinworms** pyrantel is administered orally as a single dose of 11 mg/kg (pyrantel base) body weight to a maximum of 1 g. For **hookworms** this dose is given for 3 consecutive days. Fasting before treatment is not necessary. **Adverse reactions** include anorexia, nausea, headache, drowsiness, rashes and elevated SGOT levels.

During the past three decades many older anthelmintics have been replaced by safer and more effective drugs.

9.8 CHEMOTHERAPY OF LEPROSY (ANTILEPROTIC DRUGS)

The WHO has estimated that 12 to 20 million people worldwide have leprosy (Hansen's disease). The majority are in India, China and Africa. *India alone has about 4 million leprosy patients.*

Leprosy is a chronic infectious disease caused by an acid-fast bacillus, **Mycobacterium leprae,** related to the tubercle bacillus. This bacillus multiples very slowly in the body. It is essentially a disease of **peripheral nerves,** but it also affects the **skin** and the **eyes,** the **mucosa of the upper respiratory tract, muscle, bone** and **testes.**

FORMS OF LEPROSY

Leprosy is classified into four forms: (i) **indeterminate**; (ii) **tuberculoid**; (iii) **lepromatous**; and (iv) **dimorphous** (border-line). Indeterminate leprosy is manifested by some localized hypopigmentation of the skin and sensory loss. When treatment is not given or healing does not occur the condition may progress to **tuberculoid leprosy** in those with high degree of resistance (Lepromin test positive) to the infection, or to **lepromatous leprosy** with low degree of resistance (Lepromin test negative) to the infection. **Dimorphous** form of the disease has some features of both the tuberculoid and the lepromatous types.

CLASSIFICATION OF LEPROSTATIC DRUGS

The available drugs may be classed into the *sulphones* and the *nonsulphones* as under:

1. **Sulphones:** Dapsone, sulfoxone sodium.
2. **Nonsulphones:**
   - i. **Antibiotics:** Rifampicin.
   - ii. **Phenazine dye:** Clofazimine.
   - iii. **Thioureas:** Thiacetazone (amithiozone).
   - iv. **Sulphonamides:** Sulfadoxine.
   - v. **Anti-inflammatory drugs:** Aspirin, Chloroquine, Thalidomide, Antimonials, Corticosteroids.

Sulphones

Dapsone (DDS)

Dapsone is the **sulphone of choice** for the treatment of **all forms of leprosy.** The mechanism of action of the sulphones is similar to that of the sulphonamides. Dapsone is primarily **bacteriostatic.** Continuous treatment with this drug assures a negative bacterial state in almost all patients of **lepromatous leprosy,** provided it is administered for 5 years or more. Patients with **tuberculoid leprosy,** should receive dapsone for 2 years, and those with dimorphous form, for 10 years after an 'inactive' state has reached.

Toxicity: Gastrointestinal upsets (nausea, vomiting, anorexia, abdominal cramps and diarrhoea) occur. Headache, excitement, nervousness, insomnia, **cholestatic jaundice,** drug fever, goitre, haematuria and severe renal failure may develop occasionally. **Acute psychosis** is rare. A **reversible peripheral neuropathy** has also been reported.

Dosage: Dapsone 100 mg daily orally is administered to patients with **lepromatous** and **dimorphous** leprosy, and for **tuberculoid** and **indeterminate** cases 50 mg daily.

Sulfoxone Sodium (Diasone Sodium)

Sulfoxone may be substituted for dapsone. It is **hydrolysed in the gut to dapsone.** *Adverse reactions* are similar to those produced by dapsone. Sulfoxone is administered in a daily dose of 330 mg orally, which may be increased to 660 mg daily, if necessary.

Nonsulphones

Rifampicin

Rifampicin appears to be **bactericidal** for *M.leprae*, while other drugs are bacteriostatic. In oral doses of 300 to 600 mg daily rifampicin renders bacilli non-infective. Rifampicin is expensive, and it may induce *haemolytic anaemia, thrombocytopenia, acute renal failure and hepatitis.*

Clofazimine

Clofazimine is used in patients of leprosy infected with sulphone resistant *M.leprae. Clofazimine interferes with bacterial nucleic acid metabolism by binding to DNA.* Many patients of leprosy receiving sulphones develop **erythema nodosum leprosum,** marked by a sudden and acute flare up of the disease, which is thought to be induced by the therapeutic effect of the sulphones. **Clofazimine effectively prevents the development of this reaction.**

Adverse effects of clofazimine include nausea, diarrhoea and abdominal pain, and development of *skin pigmentation.* The dose of clofazimine is 100-300 mg orally daily. When the symptoms have been controlled, 100 mg twice weekly is effective.

Thalidomide

Thalidomide is used to prevent the skin manifestations of erythema nodosum leprosum in doses of 100-300 mg daily till symptoms subside.

Sulfadoxine

The long-acting sulphonamide, sulfadoxine (0.5 g daily) has been tried in patients not tolerating dapsone.

WHO REGIMENS

According to the WHO Study Group, for treatment purposes leprosy patients are divided into: (i) those suffering from **multibacillary leprosy;** and (ii) those suffering from **paucibacillary leprosy.** A 3-drug regimen is recommended for the former, and a 2-drug regimen for the latter as detailed below:

Multibacillary Leprosy (3-drug Regimen)

Rifampicin : 600 mg once monthly , supervised (450 mg for those weighing, less than 35 kg).

Dapsone : 100 mg daily, self administered.

Clofazimine : 300 mg once monthly, supervised and 50 mg daily, self administered (or, if clofazimine is unacceptable, then *ethionamide* 250 mg daily self administered).

Treatment should be given for at least 2 years, and continued when possible, upto smear negatively.

Paucibacillary Leprosy (2-drug Regimen)

Rifampicin : 600 mg once monthly, supervised (450 mg for those weighing, less than 35 kg).

Dapsone : 100 mg daily, self administered.

Treatment should be given for 6 months.

These WHO regimens are applied worldwide, with minor variations in different countries.

PROPHYLAXIS IN LEPROSY

Chemoprophylactic trials with dapsone have provided evidence of its moderate protective value in people with unduly high risk of contracting leprosy.

9.9 CHEMOTHERAPY OF VIRAL DISEASES (ANTIVIRAL DRUGS)

Infections caused by viruses present special and difficult problems in chemotherapy. The agents that **inhibit** or **kill** the viruses are also likely to injure the host cells. This relationship between the viruses and the host cell, makes **selective antiviral action** difficult to achieve.

TYPES OF VIRUSES

Viruses can be divided into: (i) the **large viruses** (chlamydia) responsible for *trachoma, inclusion conjunctivitis,* and the *rickettsial infections;* and (ii) the **true (small) viruses** including the *pox viruses, herpes viruses, adenoviruses* and *picorna viruses*. The large viruses possess both DNA and RNA, and differ from true viruses both in morphology and in their mode of multiplication.

The *true viruses* contain a core of either DNA (smallpox, chickenpox, herpes simplex, herpes zoster) or RNA (poliomyelitis, mumps, measles, rabies). These viruses can replicate only inside host cells using the host enzyme systems.

PHASES OF VIRAL INFECTION AND REPLICATION

The reproductive cycle of a virus can be divided into five phases:

Phase 1: Attachment and penetration.
Phase 2: Uncoating.
Phase 3: Synthesis of viral components.
Phase 4: Assembly of the virus particle.
Phase 5: Release of the virus.

CLASSIFICATION

The antiviral drugs can be classified as under:

I. **Inhibitors of adsorption and penetration:** Gamma globulin.
II. **Inhibitors of intracellular synthesis**
Inhibitors of nucleic acid synthesis
Ribavarin, idoxuridine, foscarnet, acyclovir, ganciclovir, zidovudine, interferons.
III. **Inhibitors of assembly or release of virus particles**
Amantadine, Rifampicin.

ANTIVIRAL DRUGS

Inhibitors of Adsorption and Penetration

Gamma Globulin

Gamma globulin (IgG) is a fraction obtained from the plasma of normal individuals, and is rich in most of the antibodies found in whole blood.

Therapeutic uses: IM injections given during the early infectious stage (incubation period) can partially alleviate the progression of **hepatitis, measles, rabies, poliomyelitis** and other viral infections. This procedure confers only a passive immunity.

Dosage: Human gamma globulin is given in a dose of 0.22 ml/kg IM. *Adverse reactions* include occasional anaphylactoid reactions, and minor allergic manifestations.

Inhibitors of Nucleic Acid Synthesis

Ribavarin

Ribavarin **inhibits the replication in vitro** of a wide range of RNA and DNA viruses. It has antiviral activity against influenza A and B viruses, and herpes simplex virus.

Therapeutic uses: Ribavarin aerosol is used to treat **influenza A and B virus** infection; and oral therapy of *hepatitis virus, herpes genitalis virus, measles and Lassa fever.*

Dosage: Ribavarin is available as powder for reconstitution as aerosol containing 20 mg/ml in 100 ml vials. The dose to be delivered to infants is 1.4 mg/kg per hour. Treatment is carried out for 12-18 hours per day for 3-7 days.

Adverse reactions: Ribavarin aerosols are generally well tolerated. Conjunctival irritation, rash, wheezing and temporary deterioration in pulmonary function may occur.

Idoxuridine

Idoxuridine (IDU) is rapidly inactivated by enzymes, IDU is used only locally in the eye for the treatment of **herpes simplex keratitis.**

Therapeutic uses: IDU is used for treatment of **herpes simplex keratitis.** IDU is used either as a 0.5 percent ophthalmic ointment, or a 0.1 percent ophthalmic solution.

Adverse effects include local irritation, burning, lacrimation, and conjunctival hyperaemia. Idoxuridine is potentially carcinogenic and is not used systemically.

Foscarnet

Foscarnet sodium **inhibits viral DNA polymerase** and **reverse transcriptase.**

Foscarnet is active against **herpes viruses,** including **cytomegalovirus** and **HIV (Human Immunodeficiency Virus).**

Dosage: An initial bolus dose of 20 mg/kg IV is administered over 30 minutes, followed by a continuous infusion of 230 mg/kg per day for 2 to 3 weeks.

Adverse reactions include reduced renal function, malaise, nausea, vomiting, headache and fatigue.

Acyclovir

Acyclovir has potent antiviral activity against the **herpes viruses**, particularly **herpes simplex type I virus.**

Therapeutic uses: Acyclovir is effective in the treatment of **herpes simplex virus-1** and **type 2-infections, genital herpes, neonatal herpes** and **herpes simplex encephalitis.**

Adverse reactions are minimal and include headache, nausea and vomiting, skin rash, increased hair loss, and depression.

Dosage: Acyclovir sodium is available in 200 mg capsules. The usual dose is 200 mg orally every 4 hours for 10 days. Acyclovir ointment 5 percent is available for topical treatment.

Ganciclovir

Ganciclovir is similar to acyclovir. It is active against all herpes viruses, including cytomegalovirus.

Therapeutic uses: The use of ganciclovir is limited to life-threatening infection with cytomegalovirus as it is a toxic agent.

Adverse reactions include headache, psychosis, convulsions and coma. Ganciclovir suppresses the bone marrow.

Dosage: The usual initial daily dose is 10 mg/kg IV in 2 or 3 divided portions.

Zidovudine (Azidothymidine, AZT)

Zidovudine is a synthetic pyrimidine deoxynucleoside. It is commonly referred to as AZT.

Mode of action: AZT inhibits the enzyme **reverse transcriptase** in the virus, whose function is to use the viral RNA template to produce single-standard DNA. Zidovudine is active against **HIV-1** and other mammalian retroviruses.

Therapeutic uses: The efficacy of zidovudine in patients with AIDS, and in symptomatic patients with **AIDS related complex** (ARC) is well established. It is helpful in **reducing the viral load, and the degree of severity of AIDS-related infections.**

Adverse reactions: The major adverse effects are granulocytopenia and anaemia. Other untoward effects include severe headache, nausea, insomnia and myalgias.

Dosage: Zidovudine is available as 100 mg capsules. The usual dose is 200 mg orally every 4 hours continuously.

Lopinavir is an anti-HIV drug belonging to the *protease inhibitor* class. It selectively kills *human papilloma virus* (HPV), the virus that causes *cervical cancer.* It is used in combination with *ritonavir.*

Newer drugs for Antiretroviral Therapy (ART) for AIDS include *lamivudine, stuvadine, zalcitabine and nevirapine.*

Interferons

Interferons possess complex **antiviral, immunomodulating,** and **anti-proliferative** effects.

There are three major types of human interferons, designated as **alpha, beta** and **gamma.** Now exogenous interferons have been produced using recombinant DNA technology.

Mode of action: Interferons bind to specific cell surface receptors inhibiting viral penetration or uncoating, synthesis of messenger RNA, translation or viral assembly and release.

Therapeutic uses: Interferon alpha is currently used for hairly-cell leukaemia, AIDS related Kaposi's sarcoma, and condylorna acuminata (genital warts).

Dosage: *Interferon alpha-2a* is available in solution or as powder for reconstitution, and is administered by the SC or IM route. The usual dose is 36 x 10^6 IU per day for 5 to 7 days.

Adverse reactions include influenza-like illness, headache, myalgia, nausea and diarrhoea. Bone marrow suppression with *granulocytopenia* and *thrombocytopenia* may occur.

Inhibitors of Assembly or Release of Virus Particles

Amantadine

Amantadine appears to **block a late stage in the assembly** of the influenza A virus.

Therapeutic uses: Amantadine is used for the prophylaxis and treatment of infection with **influenza A virus.** Amantadine is also useful in the treatment of **parkinsonism.**

Dosage: Amantadine hydrochloride is available as 100 mg capsules and as a syrup (50 mg/5ml). The usual dose for adults is 200 mg once daily, or 100 mg twice daily.

Adverse reactions include nervousness, hallucinations, confusion, seizures, and coma. Amantadine should not be administered to pregnant women and nursing mothers.

Rifampicin

Rifampicin prevents the assembly of enveloped mature viral particles. It is not useful in the treatment of human poxvirus infections, but topical application can inhibit human vaccinia lesions.

The goal of research in the field of antiviral drugs has been to find drugs capable of destroying the virus invading host cells without damaging the host cells.

9.10 CHEMOTHERAPY OF MALIGNANCY AND IMMUNOSUPPRESSIVE AGENTS (CYTOTOXIC DRUGS)

Next to heart disease, cancer is the major killer of mankind. The main features of cancer are: (i) ***excessive cell growth***; (ii) ***invasiveness,*** i.e., the ability to grow into surrounding tissue; (iii) ***undifferentiated cells*** or ***tissues***; (iv) the ***ability to metastasize*** or spread to new sites and establish new growths; and (v) a ***shift of cellular metabolism*** towards an increased catabolism.

GUIDELINES FOR USE OF CYTOTOXIC DRUGS

The Cell Cycle

The various phases of the cell cycle are:

i. The **presynthesis phase** (G_1);
   the **non-proliferative subphase** (G_0);
ii. the **DNA synthesis** (S);
iii. the **premitotic phase** (G_2);
iv. the **mitotic phase** (M) in which chromosomes separate into two daughter cells through subphases—**prophase, metaphase, anaphase** and **telophase.**

The **phase specific drugs** act chiefly in certain phases of the cell cycle. Whereas, the **phase nonspecific drugs** act on cells in any phase of the cycle.

Combination Chemotherapy

Cytotoxic drug combinations would be **less toxic** and the different mechanisms of action may also produce a **greater tumour cell-kill.** *A common procedure is to first employ phase nonspecific drugs, followed by phase specific agents.*

Adverse Effects of Cancer Chemotherapy

Immediate side effects with cancer chemotherapy are **nausea** and **vomiting.** The delayed adverse effects involve the tissues or systems with a rapid cell turnover rate:

a. **Bone marrow depression.**
b. **Gastrointestinal tract:** Bleeding, ulceration, and diarrhoea may occur.
c. **Neurotoxicity.**
d. **Hepatotoxicity.**
e. **Teratogenecity and fertility:** Cytotoxic drugs impair fertility, and are carcinogenic.
f. **Immunosuppression:** Resistance to microbial infections is lowered.

g. Superinfection: Fungal and other unusual infections may occur.

CLASSIFICATION OF CYTOTOXIC DRUGS

They may be classed into six major groups: (i) **Alkylating agents;** (ii) **Antimetabolites;** (iii) **Natural products;** (iv) **Hormones and antagonists;** (v) **Radioactive isotopes;** and (vi) **Miscellaneous agents.**

INDIVIDUAL CYTOTOXIC DRUGS

1. Alkylating Agents

Chemically they contain a bis (chloroethyl) amine, ethyleneimine or nitrosourea moiety.

Mode of action: Clinically useful alkylating agents react by **cross-linking** DNA, thus preventing it from acting as a template for RNA. Thus, the DNA structure becomes fragmented and disorganized.

Nitrogen Mustards

Mustine hydrochloride: The major indications for this alkylating agent are in the treatment of disseminated **Hodgkin's disease** and other **lymphomas.**

Mustine is administered immediately after preparation of the solution, intravenously via a fast running infusion. Local extravasation causes severe tissue necrosis. **Thrombosis** and **thrombophlebitis** may occur. Severe vomiting is a common side effect. The most serious side effect is **myelosuppression.**

Cyclophosphamide: This is a very commonly used alkylating agent, and does not have a vesicant action. It can be administered **orally** or **intravenously.**

The major indications for cyclophosphamide are in the treatment of **lymphoproliferative** and **myeloproliferative** diseases. It has a marked **immunosuppressive action.**

Adverse reactions include bone marrow depression and gastrointestinal disturbances. **Alopecia** may occur which is reversible. **Bladder fibrosis** and **carcinoma of the bladder** have been reported on long-term use.

Chlorambucil

Chlorambucil is the drug of choice in **chronic lymphatic leukaemia**, and is also effective in **Hodgkin's disease,** and **non Hodgkin's lymphomas**, and **ovarian carcinomas.**

Melphalan

Melphalan is used in the treatment of **myelomatosis**. It has also been used as an adjuvant in the treatment of **stage II breast carcinoma. Ovarian carcinomas** and **testicular seminoma** also respond.

Melphalan produces a dose related depression of bone marrow function resulting in leucopenia, thrombocytopenia and anemia.

Ethyleneimines

Triethylenethiophosphoamide: Thiotepa may be used by intracavitary instillation in the treatment of **malignant effusions.**

Alkylsulphonates

Busulphan: It is used in the treatment of **chronic myeloid leukaemia.** Hyperpigmentation of the skin commonly occurs, and a rare but serious toxic effects is **interstitial pulmonary fibrosis.**

Triazines

Dacarbazine (DTIC): It has an alkylating action. Dacarbazine is mainly used for **melanoma, Hodgkin's disease** and **soft tissue sarcomas.**

Nitrosoureas

Carmustine (BCNU), lomustine (CCNU) and **semustine (methyl CCNU)** have a high lipid solubility, and cross the blood-brain barrier effectively. This property enables their use in **meningeal leukaemias** and **brain tumours.**

2. Antimetabolites

Folic Acid Analogues

Methotrexate: Methotrexate resembles folic acid and competes with it for the active site of the enzyme **dihydrofolate reductase.** The active form of folic acid (tetrahydrofolic acid) is not formed. By blocking this step, methotrexate prevents the synthesis of nuclear material and the cell dies. Administration of **leucovorin** (folinic acid) bypasses this block and reverses the effect of methotrexate.

Methotrexate can be given orally, IM, IV or intrathecally. After IV injection, it distributes in about 75 percent of body weight.

Methotrexate is the drug of choice for **choriocarcinoma,** and for intrathecal therapy of malignancy. It induces complete remission in **acute lymphoblastic leukaemia.** It is also used to treat **osteogenic sarcoma, epidermoid carcinoma of head and neck** and some **bronchial carcinomas.**

Adverse effects include **myelosuppression**, nausea, vomiting, stomatitis and diarrhoea. Prolonged low dose administration may cause **hepatic fibrosis, intestitial pneumonitis** and **osteoporosis**.

Pyrimidine Analogues

Fluorouracil: It is used in the treatment of **colorectal carcinoma.** It is also effective in **gastric** and **pancreatic adnocarcinoma.** Other responsive tumours are **carcinoma of the breast, bladder, ovary, uterine cervix** and **hepatoma.**

Adverse reactions include oral ulceration and diarrhoea, bone marrow suppression and megaloblastic anemia.

Cytarabine: It is mainly used for induction or maintenance of remission in **acute leukaemias.** Toxic manifestations include nausea, vomiting, stomatitis, and bone marrow depression.

Purine Analogues

Mercaptopurine (Purinethol, 6-MP): It interferes with purine synthesis and is a **cell cycle-specific drug** for the S-phase. In addition it has an **immunosuppressant action.** 6-MP is used in the treatment of childhood **acute leukaemia,** and as a remission maintenance agent.

Toxic effects include leucopenia, thrombocytopenia, haemorrhage, nausea, anorexia, stomatitis, and cholestatic jaundice.

Thioguanine: It is **cell-cycle specific** for the S-phase. Thioguanine is used solely in the treatment of **acute leukaemias.**

3. Natural Products

Vinca alkaloids: These are plant alkaloids extracted from *Vinca rosea*, which cause **metaphase arrest** by interfering with the assembly of microtubules.

Vincristine: It is a major drug in the management of the **leukaemias** and **lymphomas,** particularly for the induction of remission. It is very effective in **malignant lymphomas** and the combination of mustine, vincristine, procarbazine and prednisone (MOPP) is considered the treatment of choice in advanced **Hodgkin's disease.**

Vinblastine: It is often substituted for vincristine in the management of **lymphomas.** It is also used in the management of **malignant teratomata.** It is **cell cycle specific** for the M-phase. *Adverse effects* include gastrointestinal disturbances, alopecia and bone marrow depression.

Antibiotics: Many of the antibiotics bind to DNA and block the transcription of new RNA and DNA and cell replication. The cytotoxic antibiotics include **dactinomycin,** the anthracyclines (**daunorubicin** and **doxorubicin**), **bleomycin mithramycin** and **mitomycin.**

Dactinomycin: It is isolated from **Streptomyces parvullus.**

Dactinomycin is used in combination with surgery and vincristine in the adjuvant treatment of **Wilms' tumour,** with or without radiotherapy. It is also used with methotrexate for **gestational choriocarcinoma.** *Adverse reactions* include gastrointestinal upset, bone marrow suppression and alopecia.

Anthracycline Antibiotics

The anthracycline glucoside antibiotics (doxorubicin and daunorubicin) have been isolated from *Streptomyces peucetius var. caesius*.

Doxorubicin: It is one of the most successful antitumor drugs. It has been used to treat **acute leukaemias,** and many **solid tumours.** The combination of cisplatin and doxorubicin is very effective in genitourinary tumours including bladder, prostate, testicular and ovarian carcinoma.

Daunorubicin

Its main use is in **acute myeloid leukaemia,** and the toxic manifestations are similar to those with doxorubicin.

Bleomycin: It is one of the few drugs to show activity in squamous cell carcinoma. *Testicular tumours, malignant lymphomas, uterine cervix carcinoma and squamous cell carcinomas of the head and neck* are most responsive.

Mitomycin: This is a cytotoxic antibiotic isolated from **Steptomyces caespitosus.** It is a cell cycle nonspecific alkylating agent. It has been used predominantly to treat gastrointestinal tumours.

Enzymes

Asparaginase: Asparagine is a non-essential amino acid normally synthesized by the mammalian tissue cells. The asparagine depleting action of asparaginase **interferes with protein, and also DNA and RNA synthesis in tumour cells.**

Asparaginase is effective in **acute lymphocytic leukaemia. Adverse reactions** include immunosuppression, hypersensitivity reactions ranging from urticaria to anaphylactic shock.

Taxanes

Placitaxel: It is an alkaloid ester obtained from the western yew (*Taxus brevifolia*) and the European yew (*Taxus baccata*). It is approved for primary and secondary treatment of ***advanced ovarian cancer,*** and for secondary treatment of ***breast cancer.*** *Adverse reactions* include neutropenia, thrombocytopenia, peripheral neuropathy, cardiac conduction defects, alopecia, muscle pain, and myelosuppression.

4. Hormones and antagonists

The most useful hormones and antagonists are as follows:

i. **Adrenocorticosteroids:** Hydrocortisone acetate, prednisone, dexamethasone.
ii. **Androgens:** Testosterone propionate, fluoxymesterone.
iii. **Antiandrogens:** Flutamide.
iv. **Oestrogens:** Diethystillboestrol, ethinylo-estradiol.
v. **Antioestrogens:** Tamoxifen, nafoxidine, clomiphene.
vi. **Progestogens:** Hydroxyprogesterone caproate, medroxyprogesterone, megesterol acetate.

Mode of action: Highly specific **cytoplasmic receptors** have been identified for **oestradiol, dexamethasone** and **androstenolone.** The steroid hormones form a mobile steroid-receptor complex which binds directly to DNA in the nucleus and **alters the transcription** of structural or regulatory genes (**Fig. 9.3**).

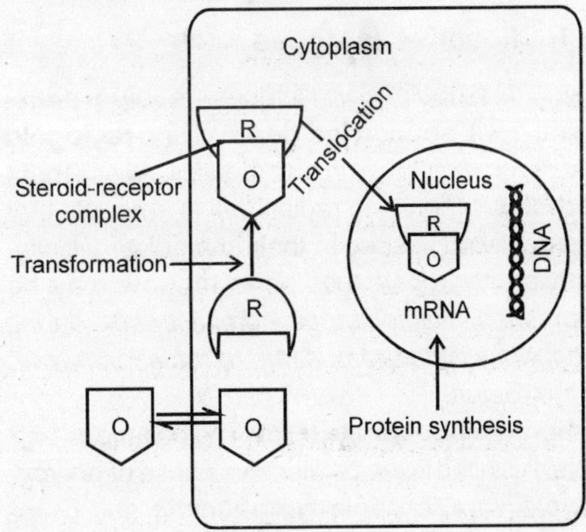

Fig. 9.10-1 : *A model cancer cell which is oestrogen receptor positive. Oestrogen (O) binds to receptor (R). This complex is then bound to chromatin, and RNA synthesis and protein synthesis is initiated. Cells with such steroid hormone receptors respond to hormonal therapy.*

Adrenocorticosteroids: These agents have a ***lympholytic effect;*** and cause regression of lymphatic tissue. The corticosteroids are used for **acute** and **chronic lymphatic leukaemia, Hodgkin's disease, and non-Hodgkin's lymphomas, prostatic carcinoma, and multiple myeloma.**

Androgens: Large doses of androgens induce a regression of **disseminated carcinoma of the breast.**

Antiandrogens: Flutamide is used to treat **cancer prostate.**

Oestrogens: These agents are effective in the treatment of **metastatic breast carcinoma** in postmenopausal patients, and in **carcinoma of the prostate.**

Antioestrogens: Three antioestrogens, namely **tamoxifen, nafoxidine** and **clomiphene** have been useful in the treatment of human **breast cancer.**

Progestogens: The progestogens have been employed in the management of **endometrial carcinoma, breast cancer, refractory prostatic cancer, and rarely carcinoma of the kidney** and **testes.**

5. Radioactive Isotopes

Mainly three radioactive isotopes—**sodium phosphate** (P^{32}), **sodium iodide** (I^{131}), and **radiogold** (**Au^{198}**) are employed in therapeutics. All emit **beta particles** or 'ionizing radiations' in amounts that destroy living tissues in their immediate vicinity. With an overdose the bone marrow may be depressed. *Radioisotope administration during pregnancy is dangerous due to radiation hazard to the foetus.*

Sodium phosphate (P^{32}): The half-life is 14.3 days. It is used in the proliferative phase of **polycythemia vera, chronic lymphocytic** and **granulocytic leukaemia.**

Sodium iodide (I^{131}): I^{131} is used to treat **hyperthyroidism** and inoperable **thyroid carcinoma. I^{131}** has a half-life of 8 days.

Radiogold solution (Au^{198}): This is short-lived radioisotope (t½ 2.7 days) is used to treat **malignant pleural** and **peritoneal effusions,** injected directly into the involved serous cavity.

6. Miscellaneous Agents

Cisplatin: It is mainly used in the treatment of **metastatic testicular and ovarian carcinoma. Adverse effects** include nephrotoxicity, myelosupression, nausea and vomiting.

Hydroxyurea: It is effective in **chronic granulocytic leukaemia** refractory to busulphan an mercaptopurine.

The dosage schedules for the cytotoxic drugs briefed above are complex, and are beyond the scope of this text.

Response to Combination Therapy

Tumours responding to single chemotherapeutic agents often recur, or the drug induced toxicity is intolerable. Regrowth of tumour cells occurs due to incomplete eradication of cancer cells. There are more than 125 different combination regimens in current use.

Cancer and Immunity

Attempts are being made to treat cancer by immunotherapy. Two methods are under trial: (i) **stimulation of nonspecific cellular immunity** by repeated exposure to an antigen. BCG (Bacillus Calmette Guerin) injections are employed; and (ii) **killed tumour cells or extracts** of tumour cells are injected to induce an immune response.

Intermittent high dose chemotherapy now forms the basis of most modern chemotherapeutic regimens. Combination chemotherapy utilizing different drugs is another advancement. **Immunotherapy** of cancer is also being developed to be combined with chemotherapy.

In addition to chemotherapy while treating cancer patients, the following measures have to be adopted: (i) maintenance of nutrition; (ii) treatment of anaemia; (iii) protection against infection; (iv) relief of pain and anxiety; (v) occupational therapy; and (vi) adequate emotional support, particularly in patients with **terminal cancer,** i.e., advanced cancer with poor prognosis.

IMMUNOSUPPRESSION

Drugs that suppress the immune response, play an important role in tissue or **organ transplantation** procedures.

IMMUNOSUPPRESSIVE AGENTS

Azathioprine (Imuran): This drug is a purine analogue (antimetabolite). It is converted in the liver to **mercaptopurine,** which is its active form. It is preferred for immunosuppression in humans, possibly due to its *marginally lower toxicity.* It is the most commonly used cytotoxic immunosuppressant.

Clinically azathioprine is used to prevent **transplant rejection** (in a dose of 1-4.0 mg/kg/day orally), and also in the treatment of **autoimmune** and **collagen disease. Myelosuppression** is its predominant side effect.

Cyclophosphamide: Clinically cyclophosphamide can be used to prevent **graft rejection reactions.** The usual dose is 3.0 mg /kg/day orally for 8 weeks. *Adverse effects* include **myelosuppression, alopecia** and **sterility (azospermia) in the male** as a result of prolonged use.

Glucocorticosteroids: The corticosteroids are the most widely used immunosuppressive agents, and they were the first to be recognized to have **lympholytic** properties.

Corticosteroids are given **prophylactically** to organ transplant recipients where rejection is a problem, e.g., in **renal transplantation.**

Human Rho (D) immune globulin: A major advances in medicine has been the development of a technique of preventing Rh haemolytic disease in the newborn **(erythroblastosis foetalis).**

If an injection of Rho (D) antibody (RhoGAM) is administered (2 ml IM) to the mother within 72 hours after the birth of the baby, the mother's own antibody response to the foreign Rho (D) positive cells is suppressed. When the mother has been treated in this manner, Rh haemolytic disease of the newborn does not occur in the subsequent pregnancy.

Cylosporin: This is an immunosuppressive agent used in **human organ transplantation,** and for the treatment of graft versus host (GVH) syndrome following **bone marrow transplantation.**

Cyclosporin has been used orally in a dose of 10-25 mg/kg daily. **Adverse reactions** include nephrotoxicity, higher incidence of viral infections, transient liver dysfunction, and very little myelosuppression.

To conclude, the immunosuppressive agents currently have three clinical indications: (i) **organ transplantation;** (ii) **autoimmune diseases;** and (iii) **isoimmune disorders** like Rh haemolytic disease of the newborn.

IMMUNOSTIMULATING AGENTS

The major potential uses of these drugs are: (i) **immunodeficiency disorders;** (ii) **chronic infections;** and (iii) **cancer.**

Interferons and interferon-inducers: Their use in infections, certain forms of cancer, is under evaluation.

Immune globulin: An appropriate use of immune globulin is in the treatment of immunodeficiency states due to impaired or absent antibody synthesis.

Levamisole: Studies indicate that both monocyte and T lymphocyte functions are stimulated by levamisole. It has been tried in **rheumatoid arthritis** and **Hodgkin's disease.**

BCG vaccine: It has been employed as a nonspecific immunostimulant (adjuvant) in cancer therapy.

9.11 CHEMOTHERAPY OF URINARY TRACT INFECTIONS (UTI)

Acute urinary tract infections are second in frequency only to respiratory tract infections, and particularly women of child bearing age, are subject to frequent bladder and kidney infections.

DEFINITION

A urinary tract infection is defined as a condition characterized by the persistence of actively multiplying bacteria in bladder urine. When infection is present white blood cells usually accompany the bacteria.

CAUSATIVE ORGANISMS

The majority of urinary tract infections are caused by **Escherichia coli**. Other bowel-derived organisms which cause urinary infections are **Streptococcus faecalis, Proteus mirabilis** and **Klebsiella aerogenes.** In chronic infections **Pseudomonas aeruginosa** and **Staphylococcus aureus** are the causative organisms.

URINARY PH

Deliberate alternation of urinary pH influences the action of some urinary chemotherapeutic agents, which may be taken advantage of clinically.

Urine may be made acidic by the administration of **ammonium chloride** (6-12 g/day orally), **methionine** (3-10 g/day orally), or **ascorbic acid** (4 g/day orally). Alkalinization can be produced by administering **sodium bicarbonate** or **acetazolamide.**

DRUGS FOR URINARY TRACT INFECTIONS

These drugs may be divided into two groups:

1. **Urinary tract antiseptics**
   Methenamine mandelate
   Quinolones: Nalidixic acid, Cinoxacin, Enoxacin, Norfloxacin, Ciprofloxacin, Nitrofurantoin. Co-trimoxazole, Trimethoprim.
2. **Antibiotics**
   Ampicillin
   Carbenicillin
   Cephalosporins
   Aminoglycosides: Kanamycin, Gentamicin.

Urinary Tract Antiseptics

Methenamine Mandelate

Methenamine mandelate is primarily effective against gram-negative bacteria including **Esch. coli.**

Adverse reactions are minimal, excessive formaldehyde liberated by gastric acid can produce gastrointestinal upset.

Methenamine mandelate is available as tablets and oral suspension. The usual dose for adults is 3-6 g orally in divided doses daily.

Quinolones

Nalidixic Acid: Nalidixic acid is active against some strains of **Esch. coli, Enterobacter aerogenes, Klebsiella** species and **Proteus** species.

Adverse reactions are common and serious gastrointestinal upsets may be minimized by administering the drug after meals. Transient fever, myalgia, polyarthritis, eosinophilia, vertigo, sleepiness and amblyopia may occur. **Convulsions** may be precipitated. Superinfection is rare.

Nalidixic acid is available in tablets of 250 and 500 mg. The usual dose is 1 g four times daily for 2 weeks, followed by 1 g twice daily for a further 2 weeks.

Cinoxacin

Cinoxacin is active against most of the **Enterobacteriaceae** which commonly cause UTI. The usual dose is 500 mg every 12 hours.

Enoxacin, Norfloxacin, Ciprofloxacin

These three quinolones are more potent than the older agents (nalidixic acid, cinoxacin). The usual doses are **enoxacin,** 200 mg bid for 3 days, and 400 mg bid for 7-14 days for complicated infections; **norfloxacin,** 400 mg bid for 7-10 days; and **ciprofloxacin,** 250 mg bid orally, or 100 mg twice daily IV over 30-60 minutes for 7 days.

Adverse reactions include nausea, diarrhoea, allergic reactions, headache and dizziness. Convulsions and toxic psychosis has been reported.

Nitrofurantoin

Nitrofurantoin is a urinary antiseptic, and it is effective against most urinary pathogens. It is effective against many gram-positive and gram-negative organisms but many strains of Proteus, *Esch coli, Enterobacter aerogenes*, neisseriae, staphylococci, streptococci and *Pseudomonas aeruginosa* may exhibit resistance. It is primarily a bacteriostatic agent.

Adverse reactions: Apart from **hypersensitivity reactions, polyneuropathy** and allergic pneumonitis may occur. Gastrointestinal upsets are common and predictable. *Haemolytic anaemia* may develop in the G-6-PD deficient patient. A folic acid dependent **megaloblastic anaemia** may develop.

TRIMETHOPRIM-SULPHAMETHOXAZOLE (CO-TRIMOXAZOLE)

Trimethoprim with sulphamethoxazole exert a **synergistic bactericidal action** against a wide range of bacteria. This combination is used in the treatment of **acute, chronic** and **recurrent** UTI, and also in bacteriuria of pregnancy.

Antibiotics

Ampicillin

This agent was the first broad-spectrum penicillin, and is active against many urinary pathogens. It may be administered orally or parenterally. It is often effective but some strains of *Esch. Coli* may be resistant.

Carbenicillin: This agent is a broad-spectrum penicillin with particular activity against **Ps. aeruginosa** and **Proteus species.** Carbenicillin is not absorbed on oral administration, and is given usually by intravenous route. It achieves high concentrations in urine. Infections caused by *Ps. aeruginosa* and *Proteus* species are most difficult to treat, and for this carbenicillin may be combined with gentamicin.

Cephalosporins: Both **cephalothin** (given intravenously), and **cephaloridine** (given intramuscularly) have a place in the treatment of urinary tract infections, specially if accompanied by septicaemia. **Cephalexin** and **cephradine** are two orally absorbed cephalosporins and they have a place in the treatment of UTI due to sensitive strains of *Esch.coli* and *Proteus* species.

Aminoglycosides: Gentamicin and **kanamycin** are two aminoglycosides that are useful in treating acute UTI. Alkalinization of the urine increases the efficacy of the aminoglycosides in UTI.

THERAPEUTIC REGIMEN IN UTI

The treatment of UTI may be considered under the following *four* heads:

1. **Removal of predisposing causes:** The precipitating factors like renal calculi, major anatomical abnormalities must be detected and treated.
2. **Initial therapy:** The patients selected for initial therapy are those with acute symptomatic pyelonephritis, and those with asymptomatic bacteriuria of pregnancy.

   Chemotherapy will be dictated by the results of **urine culture** and **sensitivity tests.** For very seriously ill patients with invasion of the blood stream **ampicillin, kanamycin, gentamicin** or **cephalosporins** should be given parenterally. This treatment should continue for at least 10 days.
3. **Long-term therapy:** A choice of the drug may be made from: **ampicillin** 500 mg/day; ***nitrofurantoin*** 100 mg/day; or ***co-trimoxazole*** 1 tab twice daily. Treatment may continue from 6 weeks to 6 months to eradicate the infection.
4. **Chemoprophylaxis:** An important measure in the prevention of UTI is the avoidance of catheterization and instrumentation. Cultures should be done and sensitivity determined. During prolonged suppressive chemoprophylaxis superinfection may occur.

9.12 CHEMOTHERAPY OF SEXUALLY TRANSMITTED DISEASES (STD)

The STD have increased dramatically over the past 40 years, specially **gonorrhoea** and **non-gonococcal urethritis,** and more recently the two viral conditions **genital herpes** and **genital warts.** Pre- and extramarital sex, a proportion of which is promiscuous, have facilitated the spread of these disease.

The five main venereal diseases are **gonorrhoea, syphilis, chancroid, lymphogranuloma venereum** and **granuloma inguinale. Non-gonococcal urethritis** is also spread by sexual activity. Other diseases in the STD group are the **four** viral infections (**herpes genitalis, genital warts, molluscum contagiosum** and **AIDS**), and two vaginitides (**trichomoniasis** and **candidiasis**).

GONORRHOEA

There has been a gradual increase in the prevalence of strains of **Neisseria gonorrhoea** with mild resistance to the penicillins. However no other antibacterial drug is as active as ***benzylpenicillin*** (penicillin G) against the sensitive strains of gonococci. **Ampicillin** and **amoxycillin** are effective alternatives to penicillin G. Single dose therapy with any of the penicillins is inadequate for ascending genital infection in women (pelvic inflammatory disease); this complication is usually treated with 7-10 day courses of parenteral penicillin G and/or oral ampicillin.

The drug of first choice for penicillinase-producing gonococcal infection is **ceftriaxone**; and for penicillin sensitive infections is **ampicillin plus probenecid,** or **amoxycillin plus probenecid** or **penicillin G plus probenecid.** The aminocyclitol, **spectinomycin dihydrochloride** in a single dose of 2.0 g IM cures 94.8 percent of patients with uncomplicated anogenital infection. In patients allergic to penicillin the newer tetracyclines (*minocycline* or *doxycycline*), or *co-trimoxazole* may be used.

SYPHILIS

Penicillin G is still the drug of choice for the treatment of syphilis, and in contrast to the gonococcus no increased resistance in **Treponema pallidum** has been proved. It must be emphasized that **tetracyclines** and **erythromycin** as alternatives to penicillin, are much less efficient antitreponemal drugs. They should be used only when penicillin is contraindicated. Cephalosporins are promising agents and **ceftriaxone** has shown good results.

NON-GONOCOCCAL URETHRITIS

Non-gonococcal urethritis is almost as frequent as gonococcal urethrirts among the STD. The parasite **Chlamydia trachomatis** is the causative organism in most cases.

The **tetracyclines** are the drugs of choice for the treatment of non-gonococcal urethritis. A minimum course should be 8 to 10 days on full dosage (e.g., **tetracycline** 500 mg 6-hourly), the maximum being 3 weeks therapy. Alternatively **doxycycline** (200 mg initially followed by 100 mg daily); or **minocycline** (200 mg initially followed by 100 mg 12 hourly) may be administered for 8 to 10 days.

VIRAL INFECTIONS

Genital Herpes

Genital ulcers in women and blisters or ulcers in men due to the **Herpes simplex** virus are becoming increasingly common. Genital herpes is a complex infection due to its recurrent nature, and its probable aetiologic association with **squamous cells carcinoma of the cervix.**

Gentamicin or **neomycin** are first choice antibiotics. The antiviral drug, **idoxuridine** may be painted as a 0.5 percent solution at frequent intervals on the part. **Acyclovir** has shown good results. The usual dose is 200 mg orally qid for 5 days, or 5 mg /kg every 8 hourly.

Genital and Anorectal Warts (Condylomata Acuminata)

It is caused by *human papilloma virus* (HPV). It has a long incubation period of about 1 to 3 months. The treatment is best done by chemical destruction of the lesions by the use of 25 percent **podophyllin** in 90 percent alcohol. **Cryotherapy** (application of liquid nitrogen with a swab, or a slush of acetone and carbon dioxide snow) can be successful, specially in the treatment of hard warts.

Mollusca Contagiosa

The pearly papules with an umbilicated centre of molluscum contagiosum on the lower abdomen and thighs can be controlled by application of phenol by a stick, by **cautery** or **cryotherapy** or by **cantharidin.**

Acquired Immunodeficiency Syndrome (AIDS)

AIDS is caused by a retrovirus referred to as the human immunodeficiency virus (HIV). The drugs used are detailed in **Chapter 9.9.**

Vaginitides

A pale, cloudy or mucoid vaginal discharge occurs due to an overproduction of cervical mucus, i.e., mucorrhoea. The contraceptive 'pill' is often the cause. Vaginitis can occasionally be due to a severe cervical erosion.

Trichomoniasis

Vaginitis due to infection with the flagellate protozoan **Trichomonas vaginalis,** is always a sexually transmitted disease by the asymptomatic male sex partner.

The standard treatment is **metronidazole** 200 mg orally 3 times daily for 7 to 10 days for both patient and partner. The treatment of choice is the newer imidazole analogue **tinidazole** in a single 2 g oral dose for both patient and partner. **Alternative regimens** like 3 doses of 1 g **nimorazole** or **tinidazole** 12 hours apart, or a single 1.5 g dose of **ornidazole** orally have been tried.

Candidiasis

The fungus **Candida albicans** is often present in the female genital tract without causing infection. Clinical infection usually occurs when a suitable environment is produced hormonally (in pregnancy, by oral contraceptives, or premenstrually), or in diabetic patients, or following elimination of normal bacterial flora by antibiotic treatment, designated as **superinfection.**

The standard treatment has been **nystatin,** administered vaginally in the form of a cream, pessary or foaming vaginal tablet. The recommended regimen is one applicatorful of cream twice daily, or 2 vaginal tablets (200,000 units) inserted at night for 7 to 14 days.

Miconazole cream (2%) is applied into the vagina at night for 7 days. **Clotrimazole** or **econazole** may be used as pessaries.

CHANCROID

Chancroid is caused by a gram-negative bacillus **Haemophilus ducreyi. Sulfisoxazole,** 1 g qid is the safest drug. Alternatively, **sulphamethoxazole** 800 mg in combination with **trimethoprim** 160 mg may be given 12-hourly for 4 days. **Tetracycline** 500 mg orally qid for 1-2 weeks may be tried.

LYMPHOGRANULOMA VENEREUM

Lymphogranuloma venereum is an acute systemic sexually transmitted disease caused by **Chlamydia trachomatis** types L_1-L_3.

Drug treatment consists of administration of **minocycline** in an initial dose of 200 mg followed by 100 mg twice daily for 21 days. **Trimethoprim-sulphamethoxazole** combination is given as 2 tablets twice daily for 2 to 3 weeks.

GRANULOMA INGUINALE

Granuloma inguinale is caused by **Calymmatobacterium granulomatis.** The lesions occur on the skin or mucous membranes of the genitalia or perineal region.

Drug therapy includes administration of **streptomycin** 1 g IM twice daily for 1 to 3 weeks. **Tetracyclines** are often effective in doses of 500 mg 4 times daily for 3 weeks. **Trimethoprim-sulphaemethoxazole** combination is effective in doses of 2 tablets twice daily for 2 weeks.

Effective control of STD can be accomplished by **contact tracing,** *screening, education* and *social awareness, accurate diagnosis, specific and curative treatment schedules,* and *regular post-treatment surveillance.*

9.13 CHEMOTHERAPY OF FUNGAL DISEASES (ANTIFUNGAL DRUGS)

The fungi, like mammalian cells are **eukaryotic** and posses nuclei, mitochondria and cell membranes containing sterols. The similarity between fungal and mammalian cells works against **selective toxicity,** and the antifungal drugs are in general more toxic than the antibacterial drugs.

MYCOTIC INFECTIONS

Mycotic infections in man can be divided into **two** main groups: (i) **superficial mycoses** confined to the epidermic, the hair and the nails; and (ii) **deep (systemic) mycosis** involving the dermis, bones and viscera.

Superficial Mycoses

Ring worm (e.g., tinea capitis, tinea corporis, tinea cruris, tinea unguium) is caused by the dermatophytes, classified into three genera—**Epidermophyton, Microsporum** and **Tricophyton**—which infect the superficial keratinized tissues chiefly hair, skin, and nails. Other superficial infections include tinea versicolor by **Malassezia furfur; superficial and intestinal candidiasis** by **candida albicans.**

Deep Mycoses

Deep fungal disease can be caused by **Candida albicans** which is normally present in the mouth and the gut.

Other mycoses causing systemic involvement include *Cryptococcus neoformans, Histoplasma capsulatum, Blastomyces dermatitidis, Coccidioides immitis* and *Aspergillus fumigatus.*

CLASSIFICATION OF ANTIFUNGAL AGENTS

1. **Antifungal antibiotics**
   Griseofulvin
   Polyenes: Nystatin, Natamycin, Amphotericin B.
2. **Synthetic antifungal agents**
   Flucytosine
   Co-trimoxazole
   Dapsone
   Imidazoles: Clotrimazole, Miconazole, Econazole
   Triazoles: Fluconazole, Itraconazole.
3. **Miscellaneous antifungal agents**
   Tolnaftate
   Terbinafine
   Ciclopirox olamine
   Benzoic and salicylic acid.

ANTIFUNGAL ANTIBIOTICS

Griseofulvin (Grisovin FP)

Griseofulvin was isolated from *Penicillium griseofulvum.*

Antifungal spectrum: Griseofulvin is effective orally against species of *Epidermophyton, Microsporum* and *Tricophyton* that cause dermatophytic infections.

Pharmacokinetics: Griseofulvin is erratically absorbed on oral administration, mainly because of its poor solubility. Small sized (micronized) particles and a fatty meal facilitate absorption.

Therapeutic uses: Griseofulvin is the treatment of choice for **ringworm** infection of hair, skin and nails.

Toxicity: A minority of patients report headaches, forgetfulness, mental dullness or inattention, which restricts its use in some patients with demanding occupations. **Superinfection** with **candida albicans** has been reported occasionally.

Preparations and Dosage

Griseofulvin (microcrystalline form) 500 mg daily in single or divided doses is administered after meals; 1 g or more daily in divided doses is recommended for obstinate infections.

Polyenes

Nystatin

Nystatin is a polyene antibiotic obtained from *Streptomyces noursei.*

Antifungal spectrum: Nystatin is active against *Candida albicans* infections of the skin and mucous membranes.

Pharmacokinetics: Nystatin is usually applied topically or given orally for its local effect in the bowel lumen.

Therapeutic uses: Nystatin is mainly used in the treatment of **candidiasis of the skin, intestine** and **vagina.**

Toxicity: Nystatin, even in large doses, is relatively non-toxic when applied topically. Contact sensitivity is rare.

Preparations: Nystatin is available in tablets (500,000 units); oral suspension (100,000 units/ml); vaginal cream (100,000 units/4 g); and as pessaries (100,000 units) for insertion into the vagina. The usual oral dose is 500,000 units every 6 hourly, doubled in severe infections; by vagina 100,000-200,000 units for 14 nights or more.

Amphotericin B

Of the two amphotericins, A and B isolated from *Streptomyces nodosus*. Only **amphotericin B** is used in therapeutics.

Antifungal spectrum: The effective antifungal spectrum of amphotericin B is the widest of all antifungal agents. It includes **Histoplasma capslatum** (histoplasmosis); **Cryptococcus neoformans** (cryptococcosis); **Blastomyces dermatitidis** (blastomycosis); **Candida species** (local and systemic candidiasis); **Coccidioides immitis** (coccidioidomycosis); and **Sporatrichum schenckii** (sporotrichosis).

Mode of action: The antifungal activity of amphotericin B is similar to nystatin. It is **fungistatic** or **fungicidal** depending on the concentration and sensitivity of the fungus.

Pharmacokinetics: Amphotercin B is poorly absorbed on oral or IM administration, therefore for systemic mycoses it **must be given intravenously or intrathecally.**

Therapeutic uses: Histoplasmosis, crypttococcosis, coccidioidomycosis, blastomycosis and **systemic candidiasis** are indications for intravenous amphotericin B therapy.

Toxicity: It is a toxic drug and with systemic therapy adverse reactions develop in almost all patients. Common side effects during IV infusions are *fever, chills, headache, nausea, vomiting* and *malaise. Thrombophlebitis* is common, and may be reduced by combining it with hydrocortisone and heparin.

Nephrotoxicity almost invariably occurs. Normochromic normocytic anaemia may develop. Intrathecal administration may cause **chemical meningitis, paraesthesias, radiculitis** and **difficulty in micturition.**

Natamycin

It is related to nystatin and amphotericin B. It is active against most **Candida** species, **Aspergillus fumigatus** and **Trichomonas vaginalis.** Natamycin is poorly absorbed orally, and is usually administered topically. It has been locally used in the treatment of **candidiasis** and **trichomoniasis. Side effects** include nausea, vomiting, diarrhoea on oral administration, and local irritation on topical use. It is available as a 2 percent cream; 1 percent sterile aqueous suspension for oral use and 2.5 percent for inhalation as an aerosol, and *vaginal tablets* containing 25 mg of the drug. The usual dose by mouth is 10 drops of a 1 percent oral suspension after meals; by inhalation 2.5 mg every 8 hourly; and by vagina 25 mg (1 tab) for 21 nights.

SYNTHETIC ANTIFUNGAL AGENTS

Flucytosine

Its antifungal spectrum is restricted to **Crytococcus neoformans, Candida albicans** and some other Candida species, **Torulopsis glabrata** and **Cladosporum** species.

Pharmacokinetics: Unlike amphotericin B flucytosine is well absorbed from the gut. It penetrates adequately into the CSF and lung.

Therapeutic uses: Flucytosine is probably the drug of first choice for **systemic candidiasis** and **cryptococcosis** provided the strains are sensitive. The optimal oral dose is 150 mg/day in 6-hourly divided doses.

Toxicity: The main adverse reactions are gastrointestinal upsets, skin rashes, cosinophilia and **reversible hepatic dysfunction.**

Preparation and dosage: Flucytosine is available as 500 mg scored tablets, and 10 mg/ml in 250 ml infusion bottles. The usual dose by mouth or IV infusion is 150-200 mg/kg/day in divided doses.

Co-trimoxazole and Dapsone

Lately the sulphonamides have been combined with other agents like **tetracycline, chloramphenicol** and **cycloserine.** Recent reports also suggest that **co-trimoxazole** is useful for the treatment of nocardiosis.

Imidazoles

At least three drugs of the imidazole family are useful antifungal agents. **Clotrimazole, miconazole nitrate** and **econazole nitrate** are active against almost all pathogenic fungi and primary resistance is rare.

The antifungal imidazoles have a broad antifungal spectrum which includes **Histoplasma capsulatum, Blastomyces dermatidis, Cryptococcus neoformans, C.immitis** and species of **Aspergillus** and **Candida.** They are also active against the pathogenic dermatophytes.

Triazoles

Fluconazole

Fluconazole is an oral triazole antifungal effective against **local** and **systemic candidiasis,** and **cryptococcosis** (including meningitis).

Fluconazole is available as 50 mg capsules, oral suspension, and intravenous infusion. The usual dose for **mucosal candidiasis** (except vaginal infection) is 50 mg daily for 7-14 days, or longer in cases of **oesophageal candidiasis** or **candiuria.** For acute or recurrent **vaginal candidiasis** a single dose of 150 mg is given.

Adverse reactions include nausea, abdominal discomfort, flatulence, rashes, and elevation of hepatic enzymes in some patients.

Itraconazole

Itraconazole is an orally effective agent, active against **oropharyngeal** and **vulvovaginal candidiasis, pityriasis versicolor,** and other **dermatophyte** infections.

It is available as 100 mg capsules. The usual dose is 100-200 mg daily for 15-30 days. For AIDS associated oropharyngeal candidiasis it is given in a dose of 200 mg daily for 15 days. **Side effects** include dyspepsia, headache, nausea and abdominal discomfort.

MISCELLANEOUS ANTIFUNGAL AGENTS

Tolnaftate

Tolnaftate is effective topically against **dermatophytic infections.** It is also effective in the treatment of **Triochophyton rubrum** infection which is often resistant to griseofulvin. It is available as a 1 percent cream or powder which is to be rubbed into the lesion twice daily for 2 to 3 weeks.

Terbinafine

Terbinafine has been introduced for the oral treatment of **ringworm** infections. The usual dose is 250 mg daily for 2-6 weeks in **tinea pedis;** 2-4 weeks in **tinea cruris;** and 4 weeks in **tinea corporis.** *Side effects* include nausea, anorexia, diarrhoea, rash, urticaria and abdominal discomfort.

Ciclopirox

Ciclopirox olamine is a **broad-spectrum antifungal** used for **tinea pedis, tinea cruris, tinea corporis, candidiasis** and **tinea versicolor** due to **Malassezia furfur.**

Ciclopirox olamine is available as a 1 percent cream to be applied locally twice daily. It has a low incidence of side effects. Also available in solution (10 mg/ml) dosage form.

Benzoic and Salicyclic Acid

Benzoic acid (6%) and salicyclic acid (3%) ointment called **Whitfield's ointment** combines the mild **fungistatic** action of benzoate with the **keratolytic** action of salicylate. It is used mainly in the treatment of **tinea pedis.** *Continuous medication* is needed for several weeks to months.

PHARMACOTHERAPY OF MYCOTIC INFECTIONS

There are many preparations available for topical use in the treatment of **superficial** fungal disease. Chemotherapy of **deep** fungal disease is unsatisfactory, and their use is associated with severe toxicity (**Table 9.8**).

Table 9.8 : *Drugs employed in the treatment of some superficial and deep fungal infections*

Disease	Infecting fungus	Drugs of choice	Alternatives
SUPERFICIAL INFECTIONS			
Dermatomycosis (tinea, ringworm)	*Dermatophytes* Epidermophyton Microsporum Trichophyton	*Topical agents* Miconazole Clotrimazole Ciclopirox	*Topical agents* Tolnaftate Terbenafine *Oral therapy* Griseofulvin, Itraconazole, Terbinafine
Candidiasis	*Candida albicans* Superficial	Miconazole or Clotrimazole (topical)	Nystatin (topical) Itraconazole
	Intestinal	Nystatin (oral)	
DEEP INFECTIONS			
Candidiasis	*Candida albicans*	Amphotericin B with of without Flucytosine	Flucytosine Fluconazole
Cryptococcosis	*Cryptococcus neoforman*		
Aspergillosis	*Aspergillus*		
Histoplasmosis	*Histoplasma* capsulatum	Amphotericin B	Potassium iodide
Coccidioidomycosis	*Coccidioides immitis*		*Sulphonamides*
Phycomycosis	*Mucor*		
Blastomycosis	*Blastomyces dermatitidis*	Amphotericin B	
Maduromycosis	*Madurella mycelomi*	Sulphonamides	Tetracyclines Amphotericin B
Rhinosporidiosis	*Rhinosporidium seeberi*	Amphotericin B	–
Nocardiosis	*Nocardia asteroides**	Sulphonamides Co-trimoxazole	Tetracyclines Erythromycin
Actinomycosis	*Actinomyces israeli**	Pencillin Erythromycin	Sulphonamides Cephalosporins

* Not a true fungus

Local Anti-Infective Agents 10

Antiseptics and **disinfectants** are a widely used group of drugs. Most of these locally effective drugs have a **low therapeutic index** making them unsuitable for systemic use. They are used for various purposes, e.g., sterilization of skin and surgical instruments prior to operations; disinfection of wounds and ulcers; against certain fungal and parasitic infestations of the skin and hair; and for disinfection of rooms and other articles. Collectively the antiseptics and disinfectants may be termed as **local anti-infective agents.**

DEFINITIONS

Antiseptics are drugs that are applied to living tissues for the purpose of killing bacteria, or inhibiting their growth. **Disinfectants** are bactericidal drugs that are applied to inanimate objects (surgical dressings and instruments, dishes, bed pans, rooms, wards, lavatories etc.) to destroy microorganisms, and prevent infection. The term **germicide** is used to cover both antiseptics and disinfectants. **Sterilization** is the process of total destruction of all microbial life, including vegetative bacteria, spores, fungi and viruses. A **sanitizer** is a chemical agent used to reduce the number of bacterial contaminants to a safe level in items like the utensils and cutlery used in cafes, and restaurants, as prescribed by the public health authorities. A **preservative** is an agent that prevents decomposition by either chemical or physical means.

MECHANISMS OF ACTION

Germicidal or local anti-infective activity depends on three basic mechanisms of action: (i) **Coagulation of bacterial proteins;** (ii) **Surface activity** adversely affecting the bacterial metabolism; and (iii) **Poisoning of the enzyme systems** in the bacterial cells is the mode of action of most germicides.

CLASSIFICATION

The local anti-infectives drugs may be subdivided into:

I. **Physical agents:** Heat, ultraviolet light.

II. **Chemical agents:**
   - i. *Acids*: Boric acid, benzoic acid, mandelic acid, salicylic acid.
   - ii. *Oxidizing agents*: Potassium permanganate, hydrogen peroxide.
   - iii. *Phenolic compounds*: Phenol, dettol cresol, hexachlorophene.
   - iv. *Surface-active agents* (Surfactants).
     - a. *Anionic surfactants*: Soaps.
     - b. *Cationic surfactants*: Benzalkonium chloride, benzethonium chloride, cetylpyridinium chloride, cetrimide.
     - c. *Nonionic surfactants*: Nonoxynol-9
   - v. *Alcohols*: Ethyl alcohol, isopropyl alcohol.
   - vi. *Halogens*: Iodine, iodophores, chlorine-releasing preparations (chlorinated lime, Dakin's solution, Eusol, chloramine T, halazone, chloroazodin).

vii. *Aldehydes*:Formaldehyde, glutaraldehyde
viii. *Antiseptic dyes*:
  a. *Acridine dyes*: Acriflavine, proflavine
  b. *Triphenylmethane dyes*: Crystal violet, brilliant green.
ix. *Metals*
  a. *Silver compounds*: Silver nitrate, silver proteinate.
  b. *Zinc salts*: Zinc oxide, zinc sulphate.
x. *Antibiotics*: Bacitracin, neomycin, polymyxin B, framycetin.
xi. *Miscellaneous*: Nitrofurazone, chlorhexidine.

COMMONLY USED LOCAL ANTI-INFECTIVES

Physical Agents

Heat

Saturated steam (120°C) at 2 atmospheres pressure is the most important agent for destroying microorganisms. Both the **vegetative** and **spore forms** of most bacteria are killed after an exposure for 20 minutes. Dry heat is much less efficacious. Simple boiling at normal atmospheric pressure is inadequate to destroy organisms like those for infectious hepatitis. In office practice it is advisable to use disposable syringes and needles.

Ultraviolet Light

The maximum antibacterial effect of light energy is exerted around a wave length of 2700Å. Staphylococci, streptococci and viruses are resistant. This method of disinfection is too expensive for general use. Such techniques have found greatest applicability in burn wards and premature baby units.

Chemical Agents

Acids

Boric acid: It is a weak bacteriostatic agent. Once boric acid was a popular antiseptic agent. But because of its systemic absorption and toxicity, it has been superseded by more efficacious disinfectants.

Benzoic acid: It is a relatively non-toxic agent and can be applied on the skin in a fairly high concentration. It is a **bacteriostatic** agent used extensively as a preservative in foods and drinks. In addition, benzoic acid has **antifungal** action and is used in the treatment of ringworm infection of the skin.

Salicylic acid: It has **weak bacteriostatic** and **antifungal** action. Externally it may be applied as a 1 to 5 percent ointment or dusting powder. In addition 10 percent salicylic acid acts as **keratolytic** agents, and in collodion base (10-12%) it is an effective application for the removal of corns or warts.

Oxidizing Agents

Potassium permanganate: It acts as a powerful **oxidizing** agent, and oxidizes toxins and bacteria to make them inert. It is used as a **disinfectant** and **deodorant,** but as soon as the oxygen is liberated it loses its germicidal activity. It is also used to disinfect ponds and wells. To disinfect bed pans and septic discharges, it is used in a strength of 1:100 to 1:500. Solutions of 1:4,000 to 1:1,000 are used as gargle or mouthwash in **stomatitis,** and to wash **infected ulcers** as well as for irrigating serous cavities. It is used as gastric lavage in the treatment of poisoning after ingestion of compounds like **opium** and **strychnine. Pure crystals** are applied locally promptly in cases of snake bite.

Hydrogen peroxide: As a 3 percent solution, this agent has been extensively used for cleaning wounds. The compound is unstable and nascent oxygen is released, particularly on contact with organic matter. The evolution of oxygen mechanically loosens pus and tissue debris, and also kills the bacteria. **The action is weak, short-lived, and the agent has poor penetrating power.** It is widely used for cleansing wounds and discharging ulcers. A dilute solution (5%) can be used as a **mouthwash** and **deodorant** in aphthous stomatitis, tonsillitis, and diphtheria. It should never be used in a closed or hollow cavity which has no exit for the liberated oxygen.

Phenolic Compounds

Phenol: Phenol reacts with proteins to form insoluble proteinates, coagulates cell protein, destroys cell membrane, and acts as a protoplasmic poison. It is also effective against fungi and many viruses. **It is ineffective against spores or acid-fast organisms.**

Dettol is a liquid germicide containing 4.8 percent chloroxylenol (chlorinated phenol). A 5 percent solution is used for cleansing wounds, and a 5 percent solution in 70 percent alcohol is used for disinfection of surgical instruments.

Cresol: This compound (cresol) is about 10 times more active than phenol, with about the same toxicity. It is not too soluble in water and is used as a soapy emulsion referred to as Lysol.

Hexachlorophene: Hexachlorophene (G_{11}) is a halogenated phenol. **Staphylococcus aureus** is sensitive to it even in high dilutions. It is incorporated in a variety of **soaps** meant for scrubbing. It is also useful for the treatment of **acne, impetigo, furuncles, carbuncle,** and **fungal infection.**

Surface-active Agents (Surfactants)

Surface-active agents are also called **detergents** or wetting agents. **Soaps are anionic, and organic quaternary ammonium-compounds are cationic surface-active agents.**

Anionic Surfactants

Soaps: Soaps are active against gram-positive organisms only. The mode of action of soaps is a physical one, and by **emulsification** of the lipoidal secretions of the skin in which bacteria reside, they have a cleansing action.

Cationic Surfactants

These agents are generally more effective than the anionic compounds. They can be used in more dilute solutions (1:5,000 to 1:20,000) and their antimicrobial activity covers a wider range of organisms including some gram-negative bacteria and fungi. In strengths of 0.1 to 1.0 percent they are used for **preoperative skin preparation.** Commonly used agents are **benzalkonium chloride; benzethonium chloride;** and **cetylpyridinium chloride.** These agents are usually employed as 10 percent solution or 0.1 percent tinctures.

Cetrimide (cetavlon): Cetrimide is a **cationic detergent** with bactericidal activity. A 0.5 to 1.0 percent solution is used for disinfecting and cleansing wounds, and for preoperative **preparation of the skin.** It is also useful for disinfecting utensils and to **sterilize surgical instruments.**

Nonionic Surfactants

Nonoxynol-9 is a nonionic detergent used as a **spermicide.** It is incorporated also into antimicrobial hand soap preparations.

Alcohols

Ethyl alcohol (Ethanol): Ethyl alcohol is extensively used for cleaning the skin prior to parenteral injections. **It is ineffective against spores and viruses responsible for serum hepatitis.** Maximum antiseptic effect is possessed by 70 percent ethanol by weight (78% by volume). Ethanol may be rubbed on the skin to prevent **bed sores.**

Halogens

Iodine: It is one of the oldest antiseptics. Solutions containing elemental iodine are antiseptics and are **lethal to bacteria and other spore-bearing organisms.** It also possess high **fungicidal** and **virucidal** activity. The germicidal activity is slowed down in the presence of organic matter.

Many preparations of iodine are available: (i) **Iodine tincture** is a 2.5 percent solution of elemental iodine with 2.5 percent potassium iodide in water, and 44 to 50 percent ethyl alcohol; (ii) **Iodine solution** contains approximately 2.5 percent iodine and 2.5 percent potassium iodide in water; (iii) **Strong iodine solution** (Lugol's solution) contains 5 percent iodine, and 10 percent potassium iodide. It is used in the treatment of iodine deficiency, thyroid disease and thyrotoxicosis; and (iv) **Compound paint of iodine** (Mandl's throat paint) contains 1.25 percent iodine; and 2.5 percent potassium iodide in alcohol, and glycerin. This paint is applied over the mucous membrane of the throat and tonsils in pharyngitis and tonsillitis.

Iodine stains the skin and is locally **dermatotoxic.** Hypersensitivity reactions are known as **iodism.**

Iodophores: They are large organic molecules carrying loosely bound iodine which is liberated slowly. They are expensive and are more effective than elemental iodine solutions. A popular preparation is **Povidone-Iodine.** This iodophore is prepared by the interaction of **iodine** and **polyvinylpyrrolidone.**

Chlorinated lime (Bleaching powder) contains not less than 30 percent w/w of available chlorine. When it comes in contact with water and air, chlorine is liberated. The onset of action is quick but short-lasting. It is used as a **disinfectant** and **deodorant,** and is a useful disinfectant for water closets, faeces, urine, drains, ponds, and tanks specially during epidemics of *cholera* and *gastroenteritis.*

Because of difficulties in handling chlorine in the form of gas and instability of chlorine water, chlorine-releasing substances like **chlorinated lime,** surgical **chlorinated soda solution** (Dakin's solution), Strong sodium hypochlorite solution**, calcium hypochlorite solution** (Eusol), **Chloramine T, Halazone** and **chloroazodin** may be used. Free hypochlorous acid is responsible for their bactericidal effect.

Aldehydes

Formaldehyde: Formaldehyde precipitates protein, and hardens skins and other tissues. Therefore it is used for **preserving pathological specimens.** It is an effective germicide in a concentration of 1:200, which kills both spore forming and non-spore forming organisms. Formaldehyde solution can be used as a disinfectant against bacteria, fungi and viruses but acts slowly on spores and acid fast bacteria. As a mouthwash or gargle it is used in a strength 1:500 for hardening the gums. It is extensively used for *disinfecting surgical instruments* and excreta. Formaldehyde also has an **anhidrotic action** when applied to the palms and soles, but not axillae.

Glutaraldehyde: It is rapidly **sporicidal** and possesses **tuberculocidal** activity. A 2 percent aqueous solution buffered with sodium carbonate (0.3%) to a pH of 7.5 to 8.5 may be used to disinfect and sterilize surgical and endoscopic instruments, and plastic and rubber apparatus. Like formaldehyde it has **anhidrotic** action when applied to palms and soles.

Acridine Dyes

Acriflavine Hydrochloride, Profalvine hemisulphate: These acridine dyes are yellow in colour, and act as **bacteriostatic** agents. Gram-negative organisms are much less sensitive, compared to the gram-positive organisms. *Pseudomonas aeruginosa*, *Proteus vulgaris* and acid-fast bacteria are resistant to the acridines. These agents have a very low toxicity, and do not cause local irritation. Used for the treatment of wounds, burns and other infections of the skin and mucous membranes. Acriflavine is usually employed in a strength of 1:1000 in isotonic saline; and proflavine in a strength of 1:100 in isotonic saline.

Triphenylmethane Dyes

Gentian violet: It is also known as crystal violet, and is toxic to gram-positive organisms. It is specially effective against **Staphylococci, C. diphtheriae** and **P. pyocyanus**. Acid-fast bacteria and gram-negative organisms are resistant to this dye. In the form of jelly or lotion (0.5%) it is used as an application for burns. Often it is combined with **brilliant green and proflavine hemisulphate (triple dye)** as a first aid treatment for burns.

Brilliant green: Like gentian violet, this agent is also an antiseptic and disinfectant. It is used as a 0.05 to 0.1 percent solution in water or hypertonic saline in infected wounds, and may be usefully combined with gentian violet and profalvine in the treatment of burns.

Silver Compounds

Silver nitrate: A few drops of a 1 percent solution of silver nitrate are instilled into the conjunctival sac of infants as a prophylaxis against *gonococcal ophthalmia neonatorum.*

Colloidal silver preparations (strong silver protein, mild silver protein, and silver halide) are used in the form of microsuspension (solution). A 1 to 5 percent solution of mild silver protein with ephedrine is used as drops for nasal infection.

Zinc Salts

Zinc salts are mild **antiseptics.** They are also **astringents** and **corrosives.** They are used as antiseptics and astringents on mucous membranes and skin. **Zinc oxide ointment** (10%) can be used in skin diseases like *eczema, impetigo, varicose ulcers* and *psoriasis.* Zinc oxide as calamine is astringent, antiseptic and antipruritic. Solution of **zinc sulphate** (0.1 to 1.0%) is used as antiseptic eye drops. **Zinc chloride** is used in dentistry as an astringent and a local analgesic.

Antibiotics

Bacitracin, polymyxin B, neomycin, framycetin and **tyrothricin** are some antibiotics used for their local effects.

Chlorhexidine (Savlon)

Chlorhexidine salts (acetate, hydrochloride, gluconate) have their primary effect on the bacterial cell membrane. They are used for disinfection of skin pre-operatively, and in obstetrics and wound cleansing. Occasional hypersensitivity reactions may occur.

ECTOPARASITICIDES

Ectoparasiticides are drugs which eradicate or kill the parasites infesting the external surface of the body. This section includes drugs used in the treatment of scabies (caused by **Sarcoptes scabiei,** the itch mite), and pediculosis (infestation with **Pediculus humanus** and **Pediculus capitis,** varieties of lice).

Scabicides are drugs used to eradicate the infestation of the skin caused by the itch mite. The drugs commonly used are *benzyl benzoate application, crotamiton, precipitated sulphur, and gamma benzene hexachloride.* **Pediculicides** are drugs used to eradicate body infestation by lice.

Benzyl benzoate application: Benzyl benzoate is an effective **scabicide.** The patient is first scrubbed with soap in a hot bath to open up the burrows, and immediately after drying benzyl benzoate application is applied over the whole body surface below the neck. A second application is made on the following day. Alternatively three applications may be made at 12-hourly intervals. Clothing and bedding should be changed to prevent reinfestation. Benzyl benzoate can also be used as a **pediculicide,** and an insect repellent. It must not be allowed to come in contact with eyes. Benzyl benzoate 25 percent emulsion (Ascabiol) is also available for use in *scabies* and *pediculosis.*

Cortamiton (Crotorax): Crotamiton is a very effective scabicide, and is applied as a 10 percent cream or lotion over whole of the body surface below the neck. Preliminary bathing of the skin is not essential, but if done the skin should be absolutely dry before applying crotamiton. A second application is made 24 hours later. A third application usually is sufficient for complete cure.

Crotamiton is a potent **antipruritic** agent, and local application gives rapid relief from itching. It is used for the relief of *pruritus ani, vulvae* and *scroti,* and *senile pruritus* or itch associated with various dermatoses.

Precipitated sulphur: This compound may be applied topically as a 6 percent (range 5% to 10%) ointment in petrolatum to treat **scabies.** It is applied by friction on three consecutive nights, followed by soap water bath on the fourth day. The clothings are boiled to avoid reinfestation. Sulphur is an **antiseptic** and a **fungicide** as well.

Sulphur dioxide obtained by burning sulphur is used to disinfect rooms, furniture and books. If taken by mouth, sulphur is a mild purgative.

Dicophane (DDT, Dichlorodiphenyl trichloroethane, Chlorophenothane): It is an effective *insecticide* and *larvicide*, and is used in the prevention and treatment of *arthropod infestation. Mosquitoes* and their larvae, flies, bed bugs, fleas and lice are susceptible to this agent. It is used as a watery suspension, solution or dust. It stimulates the **campaniform organs** (peripheral sensory structures peculiar to arthropods) and results in a convulsive state and ultimately death. It is thus a contact poison.

For **prediculosis,** a single application of 2 percent DDT is highly effective. It may be *combined with benzyl benzoate* for the treatment of scabies.

Gamma-benzene hexachloride (Gammexane, Gamma-BHC, Lindane): This agent is effective in all forms of *scabies* and *pediculosis.* It is irritating to the skin, eyes and mucosa. Allergic contact dermatitis may occur. It is absorbed through intact skin, and systemic toxicity is usually manifested as CNS stimulation and convulsions. Gamma benzene hexachloride is also an effective **insecticide.**

In the treatment of scabies gamma-benzene hexachloride (1%) in vanishing cream base is applied all over the skin below the face, as a thin film. Preliminary bath is not required, and the application is removed after 24 hours, followed by a soap bath.

Antifungal Agents

Antifungal agents are drugs used to kill or inhibit the growth of common mycotic infestations. From the therapeutic standpoint, fungal infections may be divided into two categories: superficial and deep **(Chap. 9.13)**.

Autacoids

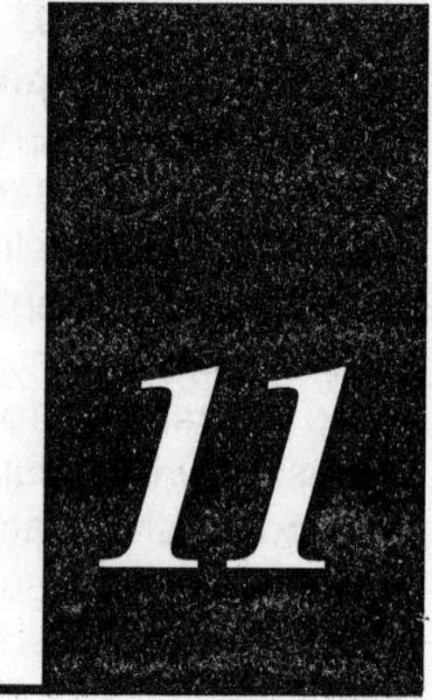

11.1 HISTAMINE AND ANTIHISTAMINES

A number of substances, designated as **autacoids** are formed in various tissues of the body, and are believed to function as **local hormones.** The important autacoids include **histamine, 5-hydroxytryptamine (serotonin), prostaglandins,** and the **kinins.**

HISTAMINE

Histamine is a biogenic amine, and as the name implies (*Hist* = tissue) it occurs in many tissues in almost all forms of life. Histamine plays a role in the *regulation of gastric secretion*, in the *body's protective mechanism* at the site of injury (triple response, acute inflammation), and as a *mediator* in allergic and anaphylactic conditions.

Synthesis, Storage and Metabolism

Histamine is synthesized from the amino acid **histidine** by the action of **histidine decarboxylase.** It is present in high concentrations in **lung, skin** and **intestine.** In the brain histamine occurs in high concentration in the **hypothalamus.**

The activity of histamine is terminated within 5 to 15 minutes by monoamine oxidase (MAO). Another histaminase (diamine oxidase) also deaminates histamine.

Mode of Action

Histamine acts on *two* separate and distinct receptors termed H_1- and H_2-receptors. Contraction of the smooth muscle of the **bronchi** and the **intestine,** and most of the **depressor effect on blood pressure** (BP) are mediated by H_1-receptors, and antagonized by classical antihistamines like **mepyramine** and **diphenhydramine.** In contrast, the H_2-receptors mediate the actions of histamine on the **gastric secretion, cardiac acceleration,** and **inhibition of the rat uterus**. These actions are antagonized by **cimetidine** and **ranitidine.** Both, the classical and the new type of antihistamines act as **selective competitive antagonists.**

Pharmacological Actions

Cardiovascular System

Histamine sharply lowers BP. Histamine produces dilatation of the cerebral vessels and produces severe **throbbing headache.** Histamine may induce **postural hypotension** due to venous pooling of blood. With large doses, venous pooling leads to **shock.** The permeability of the capillaries and small venules is increased, leading to **tissue oedema, haemoconcentration**, and **elevation of the haematocrit.** Such a tissue oedema is the cause for urticarial lesions.

Smooth Muscle

Histamine is a powerful direct stimulant of the

nonvascular smooth muscles. **Bronchiolar constriction** and **intestinal hypermotility** are the important manifestations of the generalized smooth muscle stimulation.

Gastric Secretion

Histamine causes maximal secretion of **acid** and **pepsin** by the stomach. It is present in high concentration in the gastric mucosa. Histamine exerts its effect on the **parietal cells of the oxyntic gland area** of the stomach.

Anaphylactic Shock

The similarity between anaphylactic shock and the actions of histamine suggest that histamine may be a **mediator of anaphylactic shock.** In addition, other autacoids like **bradykinin, prostaglandins, 5-hydroxytryptamine** (serotonin), and an unsaturated fatty acid called **slow reacting substance of anaphylaxis** (SRS-A) are liberated in varying amounts.

Clinical Uses

1. Gastric analysis

Histamine is useful for the differential diagnosis of pernicious anaemia from other stomach diseases on the basis of achlorhydria.

2. Diagnosis of pheochromocytoma

Histamine (3 mcg/kg IV) may be employed for the diagnosis of pheochromocytoma.

ANTIHISTAMINES

All the antihistamines are **competitive antagonists** at the histamine receptors, and can be divided into two groups: **H_1-receptor antagonists,** which comprise the large group of older classic agents; and the **H_2-receptor antagonists** namely cimetidine and ranitidine.

Allergic Disorders

The term 'allergy' refers to an exaggerated susceptibility to some underlying **antigen/antibody reaction.** Allergic reactions are often categorized as being either **immediate** or **delayed.**

Mode of Action

Both H_1- and H_2-receptor antagonists do not influence the formation or release of histamine, but **selectively** and **competitively** antagonize its action presumably at specific receptor sites. The antihistamines effectively block the actions of **exogenously** administered histamine in man.

H_1-RECEPTOR ANTAGONISTS (ANTIHISTAMINES)

Classification

1. *Alkylamines:* Chlorpheniramine, triprolidine, pheniramine, dimethindine, dexchlorpheniramine, brompheniramine.
2. *Phenothiazines:* Promethazine, trimeprazine, methdilazine.
3. *Piperazines:* Cyclizine, chlorcyclizine, meclozine, buclizine, cinnarizine.
4. *Ethylenediamines:* Tripelennamine, mepyramine, pyrilamine, methapyrilene, antazoline.
5. *Ethanolamines:* Diphenhydramine, dimenhydrinate, clemastine, carbinoxamine, embramine.
6. *Miscellaneous:* Cyproheptadine, azatidine, terfenadine, astemizole, fexofenadine, loratadine, mizolastine, cetirizine.

The older agents (***classical or first-generation antihistamines***) cause appreciable sedation– **dimenhydrinate, promethazine,** and **trimeprazine** are more sedating, whereas **chlorpheniramine, cyclizine** and **mequitazine** are less sedating. The non-sedating agents (**Second-generation antihistamines**) like **acrivastine, cetirizine, fexofenadine, loratadine,** and **mizolastine** cause least sedation and psychomotor impairment.

Pharmacological Actions

Central Nervous System

In therapeutic doses the antihistamines produce **depression** and **sedation** of the central nervous system.

Peripheral Nervous System

The antihistamines have **anticholinergic, local anaesthetic** and **antiserotonin** actions in different measures. The compound **cyproheptadine** has significant antiserotonin activity in addition to its antihistamine action.

Absorption, Metabolism and Excretion

The antihistamines are readily absorbed on oral or parenteral administration. The actions are manifested within 30 minutes but their potency, duration of action, and sedative effect varies with different agents. They are metabolized in the liver.

Therapeutic Uses

Hypersensitivity states: Antihistamines are effective in the management of *hay fever, vasomotor rhinitis, acute and chronic urticaria. Atopic* and *contact dermatitis* and for treating the *pruritus, erythema* and *oedema of insect bites.*

The antihistamines play only a **secondary role** in the therapy of *anaphylactic shock, angioneurotic oedema, serum sickness* and *bronchial asthma.* For an acute anaphylactic reaction *adrenaline* 0.3 to 0.6 mg (1:1000 solution) is injected IM or IV. The glucocorticosteroids may also be used.

Antihistamines like diphenhydramine have been used in the treatment of **parkinsonism,** and drug-induced extrapyramidal reactions. The piperazines (cyclizine and others), promethazine and diphenhydramine are useful in the prevention of **motion sickness,** and nausea and vomitting following radiation exposure. **They may be used to manage mild blood transfusion reactions.** Promethazine and diphenhydramine have been used for their sedative effect, and for **preoperative medication.** There is little evidence that the antihistamines influence the course of common cold. **Cyproheptadine accelerates weight gain, and stimulates linear growth in children.**

Adverse Reactions

Usually depression of the CNS, **dizziness, tinnitus, incoordination, diplopia** and **fatigue** develop. Sedation is the most common adverse effect. Hence the patient using antihistamines should be **warned not to drive a vehicle or operate machinery** as accidents may occur.

Some antihistamines (diphenhydramine, promethazine) possess appreciable anticholinergic activity and produce **xerostomia, dysuria, blurring of vision, impotence and constipation.** Depression of bone marrow, **leucopenia** and **agranulocytosis** occur rarely.

Drugs Interactions

Alcohol and certain CNS depressants can potentiate the sedative effect of antihistamines, and the patients should be warned about concomitant use of alcoholic beverages.

H_2-RECEPTOR ANTAGONISTS

In 1975 **cimetidine,** an H_2-receptor antagonist was introduced. In contrast to the H_1-antagonists, the H_2-receptor antagonists are less lipid-soluble compounds, and do not cross the blood-brain barrier, and as such do not cause sedation. The newer H_2-receptor antagonists—**ranitidine, nizatidine** and **famotidine** are detailed in **Chapter 12.**

Cromolyn Sodium

Cromolyn sodium (disodium cromoglycate) was introduced as an adjunct for the management of **severe perennial bronchial asthma.** It is administered in the form of a dry powder by means of an oral inhaler.

Cromolyn sodium appears to 'stabilize' the membrane of the sensitized mast cells, **preventing the release of histamine, serotonin, bradykinin, SRS-A, acetylcholine** and **other mediators of hypersensitivity reactions.**

Cromolyn sodium is **poorly absorbed on oral administration,** and has to be **inhaled** by means of a device known as 'spinhaler'.

Cromolyn sodium is most useful in the control or prevention of **exercise-induced asthma,** and 'extrinsic' asthma. It is used in a dose of 20 mg (micronized forms) every 4 to 6 hours by inhalation.

Adverse effects are not common. Inhalations may occasionally cause **transient broncho-constriction** and irritation in the throat.

Nedocromil Sodium

Nedocromil sodium has actions similar to cromolyn sodium. It is used for the *prophylaxis of asthma* in doses of 4 mg (2 puffs) four times daily by aerosol inhalation. **Side effects** include irritation in the throat, headache, nausea, dyspepsia, abdominal pain, and bitter taste.

Ketotifen is an agent which resembles cromylyn sodium. It is used in the *prophylaxis of asthma.*

11.2 SEROTONIN AND SEROTONIN ANTAGONISTS

Serotonin (5-hydroxytryptamine, 5-HT) is not a therapeutic agent itself, but it is important with respect to the action of certain other drugs and diseases.

Occurrence, Biosynthesis and Metabolism

Serotonin is widely distributed throughout the body being concentrated in the **enterochromaffin cells** of the gut (90%), and in the brain and **platelets.** Some fruits like bananas contain high concentrations of 5-HT, but there is no threat of poisoning as it is not well absorbed from the gut, and is rapidly metabolized.

The amino acid **tryptophan** is hydroxylated to 5-hydroxytryptophan by tryptophan hydroxylase which is then decarboxylated to 5-HT by aromatic L-amino acid decarboxylase. 5-HT is stored in association with ATP within the **intestinal chromaffin cells, platelets** and the **specific 5-HT containing (serotonergic) neurones** of the brain. The amount of 5-HT in the CNS is highest in the **hypothalamus** and **mesencephalon.**

Tumours of the enterochromaffin cells, known as **carcinoid tumours,** produce excess of 5-HT.

Pharmacological Actions

Cardiovascular system: It acts directly to constrict the arteries, and increases the peripheral vascular resistance.

Gastrointestinal tract and nervous system: 5-HT stimulates *intestinal, bronchial* and *uterine* muscles, the *adrenal medulla* and *ganglia* of the ANS. It is a stimulant of the sensory nerve endings and induces pain when applied to an exposed blister base.

Role in Physiology and Pathophysiology

The localization of 5-HT in platelets and its vasoconstrictor action are suggestive of its role in blood clotting. The role of 5-HT in mood and behaviour disorders is supported by various evidences. The strongest evidence being that LSD exerts a powerful psychotomimetic effect, i.e., it produces hallucinations. 5-HT also possibly plays a role in intestinal motility. 5-HT appears to be involved in the causation of **migraine** and **vascular headaches.**

SEROTONIN ANTAGONISTS (ANTISEROTONINS)

1. **Cyproheptadine:** Cyproheptadine has equal potency at both H_1-histamine receptors, and 5-HT receptors as an **antagonist.** It **increases the appetite** and **promotes weight gain** and linear growth in children. In addition, it may be used for the symptomatic treatment of **carcinoid syndrome,** and for **prophylaxis of migraine**.
2. **Lysergic acid diethylamide (LSD):** LSD has potent antiserotonin activity by which it causes a *toxic psychosis* (model psychosis). LSD because of its high dependence liability is not a useful therapeutic agent.
3. **Phenothiazines (Chlorpromazine)** and the **sympatholytics** (phenoxybenzamine and phentolamine) in addition to their alpha-adrenoceptor blocking activity also block responses to 5-HT.
4. **Ondansetron:** It is a 5-HT_3 antagonist and approved for use in the prevention of nausea and vomiting associated with *cancer chemotherapy*. It is also being evaluated for its *anxiolytic* and *antipsychotic* activity.

11.3 PROSTAGLANDINS AND OTHER EICOSANOIDS (THROMBOXANES, LEUKOTRIENES AND RELATED COMPOUNDS)

The *prostaglandins* are a group of 20-carbon essential fatty acids. In addition, the other structurally related lipids include the **thromboxanes (TXs),** the **hydroperoxy-eicosatetraenoic acids (HPETEs),** the **hydroxyeicosatetraenoic acids (HETEs),** the **leukotrienes (LTs),** the **lipoxins (LXs),** and **epoxyeicosatetraenoic acids (EETEs).** These agents are potent naturally occurring autacoids.

Occurrence, Biosynthesis and Metabolism

The basic 20-carbon skeleton of prostaglandins is named as *prostanoic acid.* They are synthesized from **arachidonic acid** by the action of prostaglandin synthetase (cyclooxygenase), an enzyme which is almost universally distributed in the body. This step forms the cyclic endoperoxides (PGG_2, PGH_2) and can be blocked by non-steroidal anti-inflammatory agents like **aspirin and indomethacin** by inhibiting the enzyme prostaglandin synthetase. The endoperoxides have a short half-life and further synthesis may follow three different paths forming several **prostaglandins, thromboxanes and prostacyclin.**

On the basis of their chemical structure the prostaglandins have been divided into six groups: A, B, C, D, E and F. The prostaglandins are virtually synthesized by every tissue.

Pharmacological Actions

Smooth muscle: The human **arteriolar smooth muscle** is relaxed by PGE_2 and PGI_2. In contrast, TXA_2 and PGF_2 alpha act as vasoconstrictors, specially on veins. The effect on the **gastrointestinal smooth muscle** is complex. The **respiratory smooth muscle** is relaxed by PGE_1, PGE_2 and PGI_2 while it is contracted by TXA_2 and PGF_2 alpha. The **genitourinary smooth muscle** (specially the gravid uterus at term) is contracted by PGE_2 and PGF_2 alpha.

Platelets: PGE_1 and PGI_2 effectively inhibit platelet aggregation, while TXA_2 markedly facilitates aggregation.

Reproductive Organs

PGE_2 and PGF_2 alpha have marked **oxytoxic action,** and when administered intravenously they produce abortion in about 80 percent of cases. There is about 20 times more PGE than PGF in fertile semen, though the ratio varies among individuals. Men with low seminal concentration of PGs are relatively infertile.

Nervous system: PGE_1 and PGE_2 increase body temperature more so when administered intracerebroventricularly. Pyrogens release interleukin-1, which promotes the synthesis and release of PGE_2. This synthesis is blocked by aspirin and aspirin-like antipyretics.

Mode of Action

PGs have marked effects on the function of cyclic mononucleotides (c-AMP, c-GMP) in cells, and these may function as mediators of PG action. The PGs lead to stimulation of c-AMP production and calcium utilization by various cells. *It has been suggested that c-AMP and c-GMP are opposing limbs of a bidirectional intracellular control mechanism. Thus the PGs act directly on smooth muscle, and not through neural mechanisms.*

Therapeutic Uses and their Basis

1. **Therapeutic abortion:** They are usually employed for **first** and **second trimester abortion,** and for ripening the cervix before abortion.

   Dinoprost tromethamine (Prostin F_2 alpha) is given as a single 40 mg intra-amniotic injection. The abortion is usually completed within 20 hours.

   Carboprost tromethamine (15 methyl-PGF_2 alpha, prostin/15M) 250 mcg IM initially repeat at 1½ to 3½ hour interval; may increase to 500 mcg IM per dose, if necessary (maximum dose 12 mg) for abortion.

Dinoprostone (Prostin E_2), a synthetic PGE_1 analogue may be administered as 20 mg vaginal suppositories. One suppository is inserted high into the vagina; repeat at 3-5 hour intervals until abortion occurs.

Abortion pill: Recently the antiprogestin, **mifepristone** (RU-486) in combination with PGE_2 has been found to produce effective early abortion.

2. **Induction of labour:** The two drugs PGE_2 and PGF_2 alpha, effectively initiate and stimulate labour.
3. **Dysmenorrhoea:** NSAIDS (aspirin, indomethacin) effectively inhibit the formation of these PGs and offer relief in 75-85 percent of cases.
4. **Hypertension and vasospastic disease:** PGE and PGA compounds have been used in *hypertensive* patients.
5. **Thrombosis:** Prostacyclin (PGI_2) inhibits platelet aggregation, and high doses of aspirin may nullify the beneficial effect by inhibiting PGI_2 production from the vascular endothelium. *Thus low dose aspirin therapy is recommended.*
6. **Patent ductus arteriosus:** Patency of the fetal ductus arteriosus is dependent on PGE_2 and PGI_2 synthesis. For palliative therapy of neonates with congenital heart disease the patency of the ductus arteriosus has to be maintained till surgery.
7. **Respiration:** PGE_2 is a strong bronchodilator, but promotes coughing which is its major limitation.
8. **Gastrointestinal system:** PGs also inhibit gastric acid secretion. **Misoprostol** (a synthetic analogue of PGE_1) is used as an *antiulcer* agent. It is also approved for treatment of NSAID-induced gastric ulcers.
9. **Immune system:** Monocyte-macrophages are the main cells of the immune system which can synthesize all the eicosanoids. The eicosanoids in turn modulate the effects of the immune system.

Acute organ transplant rejection is a cell mediated immune response. PGI_2 given to renal transplant patients reverses the rejection reaction in some cases.

Aspirin and related anti-inflammatory agents inhibit cyclooxygenase activity, and this is its mechanism of action in relief of arthritis. The NSAIDs in addition offer benefit in rheumatoid arthritis by **reducing free radical formation.**

11.4 THE KININS

The kinins are **vasodilator polypeptides.** Among them *bradykinin* and *kallidin* are of importance.

Occurrence, Biosynthesis and Metabolism

The kinins have effects somewhat similar to those of histamine on vascular smooth muscle, capillary permeability, bronchial and intestinal smooth muscle.

The important kinins are **bradykinin** (a non-apeptide), **kallidin** (lysyl bradykinin, a decapeptide), and related vasodilator peptides. Both *bradykinin* and *kallidin* are formed from the same circulating *$alpha_2$ globulins* (kininogens) by the action of specific proteolytic enzymes (kallikreins). Glandular tissues such as salivary glands and pancreas, and also urine are among the rich sources of kallikrien.

The kinins are rapidly destroyed in blood (t½ less than 1 minute) by kininases, yielding inactive peptides.

Role in Physiology and Pathophysiology

Kinins have been implicated in many physiological functions including **reactive hyperaemia, regulation of tissue blood flow, blood pressure control,** and **neonatal circulatory changes.** Kininogen has a role to play in **blood clotting.** Kinins may be involved in many pathological states like shock, allergy, inflammation, pancreatitis, and bronchoconstriction.

Pharmacological Actions

An interesting relationship seems to exist between **bradykinin** and **angiotensin.** Both are polypeptides split from plasma proteins. *Angiotensin is a potent vasoconstrictor while bradykinin is a vasodilator*. The converting enzyme in the angiotensin system is a strong inactivator of bradykinin.

On the cardiovascular system bradykinin has a potent **relaxant effect on the vascular smooth muscle,** causing a fall in blood pressure and increase in capillary permeability.

Aprotinin, a peptide obtained from bovine lung, inhibits kallikrein, plasmin and other proteases. Aprotinin is used in patients at high risk of blood loss during and after *open heart surgery*.

Aprotinin is administered by slow IV injection, with a loading dose of 2000,000 units, and maintenance dose of 500,000 units until the end of the operation.

Drugs Acting on the Gastrointestinal System

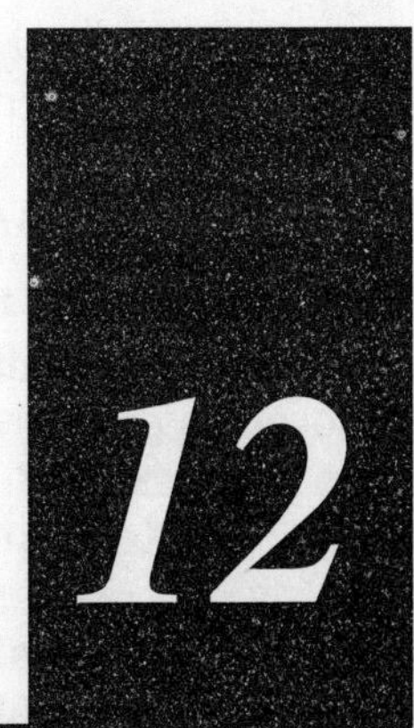

APPETITE STIMULANTS (APPETIZERS, BITTERS)

Bitters are used to stimulate the appetite when it has been impaired by illness. Bitters are divided into **simple** and **aromatic bitters.** The former are simple solutions, containing bitter alkaloids, e.g., **quinine, gentian** and **tincture nux vomica.** Aromatic bitters are preparations containing volatile oils like **tinctures of orange** and **lemon.** Alcoholic drinks and spices also function as appetizers. **Cyproheptadine,** an antihistamine-antiserotonin compound, also has been employed to stimulate appetite and promote growth. It is used in some cases of **anorexia nervosa.** The usual dose is 2-4 mg 3 or 4 times a day.

APPETITE SUPPRESSANTS (ANOREXIANTS)

Anorexiants are used as adjuncts in the management of **obesity** due to excessive food intake. The **amphetamines** stimulate the 'satiety centre' in the hypothalamus and block the impulses reaching the 'eating centre'. The commonly used anorexiants include the amphetamines, and other sympathomimetics like **diethylpropion hydrochloride, phenmetrazine hydrochloride** and **fenfluramine hydrochloride.**

CARMINATIVES

Carminatives are volatile oils which mildly irritate the gastric mucosa and relieve the feeling of discomfort and distension after meals. This they do by causing eructation and movement of gas from the stomach. Carminatives used clinically include **compound tincture of cardamom,** and **tincture of ginger.** Other agents like **camphor, peppermint, spearmint, aniseed, coriander, cloves, fennel** and **nutmeg** may also be used.

ANTIFLATULENTS

Antiflatulents reduce the symptoms of excess gas production in the gastrointestinal tract.

Simethicone is a silicone derivative possessing defoaming action which helps relieve flatulence by dispersing gas pockets trapped in the GI tract. The gas is then expelled by belching or by flatus. The pain of dyspepsia, spastic colon, diverticulitis, and postoperative atony is relieved. Usual dosage is 40-125 mg qid. It is available in combination with antacids.

Charcoal is an inert **adsorbent** and can adsorb toxins and gas onto the surface of its particles, reducing the volume of intestinal gas and provides relief from cramping and flatulence.

DEMULCENTS

Demulcents form aqueous solutions with the ability of soothing the irritated mucous membranes or abraded surfaces. This they cause by coating and protecting the underlying cells from irritant stimuli. The demulcents may be applied to the gastrointestinal tract in the form of **demulcent drinks,** or enemas, and to the throat in the form of *gargles* or *lozenges*. Some known demulcents are acacia, tragacanth, glycyrrhiza, carboxymethylcellulose sodium, diluted glycerine, and propylene glycol.

PROTECTIVES AND ADSORBENTS

Insoluble salts like **bismuth subnitrate** and **subcarbonate** and **magnesium trisilicate** are employed as protectives in the management of ulcers of the stomach and intestines. They may be employed in cases of diarrhoea as non-specific remedies. The main gastrointestinal adsorbents are **pectin, kaolin, aluminium hydroxide** and **magnesium trisilicate.**

ASTRINGENTS

Astringents are locally acting agents that precipitate the protein. Metallic ions like **zinc** and **aluminium** have an astringent quality. Of the vegetable astringents **tannic acid** may be employed orally for the symptomatic treatment of diarrhoea.

DIGESTANTS

The digestants promote the process of digestion in the gastrointestinal tract. The agents employed are **hydrochloric acid, pepsin, pancreatic enzymes** and **bite salts.**

EMETICS AND ANTIEMETICS

Nausea and vomiting may be symptoms of serious organic disturbances involving any of the viscera of the chest or abdomen, or produced by drugs, radiation, movement, infections, metabolic and emotional disturbances, neoplasms or painful stimuli.

Mechanisms of Vomiting

Emesis (vomiting) is a **complex reflex** that is coordinated by the vomiting centre in the medulla. Wang and Borison over 40 years ago proposed that vomiting involves the 'vomiting centre' located in the *lateral reticular formation.* Emetic stimuli directly related to the vomiting centre include tactile *pharyngeal stimulation, distention of viscera, rotation or unequal stimulation of the labyrinths, increased intracranial pressure, pain and psychologic factors like sight, memory* and *smell.* On the contrary blood borne emetic substances first act upon the **chemoreceptor trigger zone** (CTZ) in the ventral surface of the fourth ventricle. The CTZ alone cannot induce vomiting, but does so indirectly through the vomiting centre (**Fig.12.1**). There is evidence that in part this mechanism is **dopaminergic,** the main mechanism being **cholinergic.**

Emetics

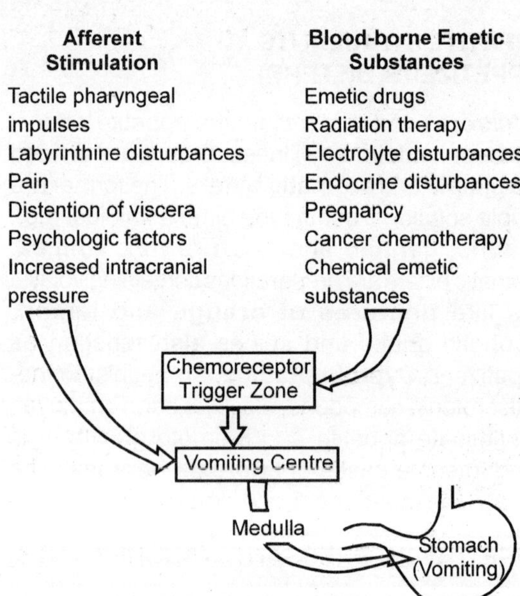

Fig. 12.1: *Mechanisms of vomiting.*

Apomorphine Hydrochloride

Apomorphine acts directly on the CTZ and induces vomiting within 10 minutes of intramuscular or subcutaneous injection. Its action is more efficient if 200 to 300 ml of water is given by mouth before the injection. Apomorphine usually produces some degree of **depression of the CNS,** and the patient becomes drowsy afterwards. Like all emetics, apomorphine is **contraindicated** in the unconscious patient, advanced age, or when caustic substances have been ingested.

Apomorphine hydrochloride is available as 6 mg soluble tablets which must be mixed with water just prior to administration. The usual dose is 6 mg in adults, or 0.06 mg/kg in children IM or SC injection.

Ipecac Syrup

Ipecac is sometimes preferred in young patients because it produced less of CNS depression. Ipecac syrup acts both **reflexly** on the gastric mucosa as an **irritant,** and after absorption **stimulates the CTZ** centrally and induces vomiting within 20 to 30 minutes. The emetic action is increased if 200 to 300 ml of water is taken immediately after the ingestion of the syrup. In adults, ipecac syrup 20 ml orally, followed by 200 to 300 ml of water is given.

Antiemetics

The main groups of agents used as antiemetics are: (i) the ***anticholinergics;*** (ii) the ***antihistamines;*** (iii) the ***phenothiazines;*** and (iv) ***miscellaneous drugs.***

ANTICHOLINERGICS

Scopolamine (Hyoscine)

Scopolamine is a natural alkaloid related to atropine. Its anticholinergic action possibly *blocks afferent impulses to the vomiting centre.* It reduces conduction at the labyrinthine receptors which accounts for its use in **motion sickness. Scopolamine hydrobromide** may be used in a dose of 0.6 to 1.0 mg SC. **Transdermal scopolamine** in the form of circular flat discs is also available. It adheres to the skin behind the ear.

Antihistamines

The antiemetic activity amongst the antihistamines is almost restricted to the **ethanolamines** (diphenhydramine, dimenhydrinate) and the **piperazines** (cyclizine, meclozine, buclizine).

Their antiemetic action is the result of depression of neural functioning at the labyrinthine receptors which makes them specially effective in **motion sickness,** *Meniere's disease,* and vestibular disturbances. *Side effects* include drowsiness and xerostomia. In higher doses excitement, convulsions, dilated pupils, flushed face and fever may occur.

Phenothiazines

Certain phenothiazines are of proven value in controlling the nausea and vomiting due to **drug toxicity, radiation sickness, carcinomatosis, gastrointestinal disturbances,** and **operative procedures.** Their antiemetic action is exerted at the CTZ. They essentially have an **antidopaminergic action.**

The most common side effect of phenothiazines at therapeutic doses is sedation. The incidence of **hypotension** is greater with the aliphatic phenothiazines, while **extrapyramidal reactions** occur more often with the piperazines.

Metoclopramide

Metoclopramide is a **dopamine receptor antagonist** with a dual action, i.e., it sedates the CTZ and inhibits vomiting induced by copper sulphate (peripheral action). It is a smooth muscle stimulant largely acting on the upper GI tract to increase gastric contractions and facilitate peristalsis in the duodenum and jejunum.

Therapeutic uses include: (i) treatment of **gastroesophageal reflux** not responding to conventional therapy; (ii) prevention of **nausea and vomiting of cancer chemotherapy;** (iii) treatment of acute or **chronic gastroparesis** (gastric stasis); and (iv) for facilitation of **small bowel intubation.**

Dosage: Metoclopramide is available as tablets (5, 10 mg), syrup (5 mg/5 ml), and injection (5 mg/ml). The usual dosage is 10-15 mg orally upto qid, 30 minutes before meals and at bedtime. For **cytotoxic chemotherapy-induced vomiting,** initially 1-2 mg/kg by slow IV infusion is given 30 minutes before starting chemotherapy. **Side effects** noted at high parenteral doses are drowsiness, fatigue, restlessness and diarrhoea.

Cisapride

Cisapride is a potent stimulant of gastric emptying. It acts by **facilitating the release of acetylcholine** from the myenteric plexus. It has no antiadrenergic, antidopaminergic or cholinergic side effects. Patients of **gastroparesis** who have failed to respond to metoclopramide frequently respond to cisapride. It also improves the motility of the small intestines and colon in cases of **chronic constipation.**

Domperidone

Domperidone is another drug used to accelerate gastric emptying. It is primarily a **peripheral dopamine antagonist.**

Therapeutic uses: It is used for nausea and vomiting following cytotoxic therapy or radiotherapy in a dose of 200-400 mcg/kg every 4-8 hours. **Side effects** include galactorrhoea and gynaecomastia Dystonic reactions may occur rarely.

Cannabinoids

Dronabinol

Nabilone

Dronabinol is delta -9-tetrahydrocannabinol (THC), the main psychoactive substance found in *Cannabis sativa* or marijuana. **Nabilone** is a synthetic cannabinoid. They are effective antiemetics, specially in **controlling vomiting due to cancer chemotherapy.** Their use should be reserved for patients not responding to conventional therapy.

Dronabinol is given in a dose of 5-7.5 mg/m^2 orally 1-3 hours before, and every 2-4 hours after chemotherapy. **Nabilone** is given in a dose of 1-2 mg 1-3 hours before, and every 8-12 hours after chemotherapy.

Adverse reactions to cannabinoids include drowsiness, elation, dizziness, impaired thinking ability, altered perception, irritability, euphoria, memory impairment, nightmares and ataxia.

Cinnarizine

Cinnarizine is used for vestibular disorders like vertigo, tinnitus, nausea and vomiting in **Meniere's disease** and motion sickness. **Dose:** 15-30 mg orally bid or tid.

Betahistine

Betahistine is a vasodilator like histamine. It improves microcirculation. It is used to relieve vertigo, tinnitus, nausea and vomiting and hearing loss in **Meniere's disease. Dose:** Initially 16 mg tid with food; maintenance 24-48 mg daily.

Ondansetron, a 5-HT$_3$ inhibitor, has been approved for use in the *prevention of chemotherapy induced nausea and vomiting.* The benzodiazepines may be used to control anticipatory nausea and vomiting.

PROKINETIC AGENTS

Agents which specifically ***promote gastrointestinal peristalsis*** and ***accelerate gastric emptying*** are termed as *prokinetic agents.*

Metoclopramide and **cisapride** (see above) are promoted as selective GI motility stimulants or *prokinetic agents.* Both these drugs release ACh from cholinergic neurones in the myenteric plexus, and also sensitize intestinal smooth muscle to the action of ACh. These agents hasten oesophageal clearance, accelerate gastric emptying, and shorten the small intestine transit time. Both these agents exert an antiemetic effect. **Domperidone** (see above) also accelerates gastric emptying and has a prokinetic effect of the gut.

GASTRIC ANTACIDS

Antacids are weak bases that react with gastric hydrochloric acid to from salt and water. They are employed in the treatment of **hyperchlorhydria** and **peptic ulcer,** collectively known as **acid-peptic disease.**

Administration of antacids remains the basis of management of acid-peptic disease. Newer approaches to the medical management include the use of *anticholinergic drugs, H_2-receptor antagonists, carbenoxolone sodium, tricyclic anti-*

depressants, the substituted prostaglandins (PGE_2 compounds) *proton pump inhibitors,* and *eradication of Helicobacter pylori infection.*

Mechanism and Control of Acid Production

Gastric acid secretion is divided into two periods : (i) **interprandial** (basal secretion); and (ii) **post-prandial** (stimulated secretion during and after meals). Three phases of acid output are recognized in the postprandial secretion, namely **cephalic, gastric** and **intestinal.**

The final *common pathway* for both vagal effects and effects of gastrin, involve the release of **histamine** which acts on H_2 receptors and the parietal cells are stimulated to release acid. **Prostaglandins** (E series) appear to modulate the release of histamine. Histamine, vagal stimulation, and gastrin promote pepsin secretion.

Mode of Action

The antacids diminish the quantity of free hydrochloric acid in the stomach by *three* mechanisms: (i) **direct neutralization** of preformed acid;(ii) **buffering of preformed acid;** and (iii) **adsorption of hydrogen ion plus adsorption and inactivation of pepsin.**

Classification

Antacids are divided into *two* classes: (i) **systemic** antacids of which sodium bicarbonate is the only example; and (ii) **non-systemic** *buffer* antacids e.g., calcium carbonate, magnesium hydroxide, magnesium trisilicate, and aluminium hydroxide.

Systemic Antacid

Sodium bicarbonate has a rapid onset and short duration of action and offers rapid relief of pain.

$$NaHCO_3 + HCl \rightarrow NaCl + H_2O + CO_2$$

It is not recommended for long-term use because it produces *systemic alkalosis.* If large quantities of milk or a calcium-containing antacid are taken simultaneously, *hypercalcaemia* and *renal calcinosis* may occur (milk-alkali syndrome). It makes the pH almost neutral or alkaline and thus *interferes with the peptic digestion of food.* Sodium bicarbonate is not much used now. *Dose* 1 to 5 g.

Non-systemic Buffer Antacids

Calcium carbonate produces a more prolonged reduction in gastric acidity.

$$CaCO_3 + 2HCl \rightarrow CaCl_2 + H_2O + CO_2$$

As calcium carbonate acts slowly rebound acid secretion is minimal. Frequent use causes constipation. *Dose* 1 to 5 g.

Magnesium Hydroxide

In the stomach it reacts with HCl:

$$Mg(OH)_2 + 2HCl \rightarrow MgCl_2 + 2H_2O$$

Magnesium chloride is soluble, but the magnesium ion is poorly absorbed from the gut. It acts as an osmotic purgative. The duration of action is prolonged. It is used as an antacid-laxative mixture. The dose for milk of magnesia is 5 to 10 ml as an antacid, and 25 to 50 ml as a laxative.

Magnesium Trisilicate

It acts both as an antacid and adsorbent:

$$2MgO_3\,SiO_2 \times H_2O + 4HCl \rightarrow MgCl_2 + 3SiO_2 + (x + 2)\,H_2O$$

This reaction is slow and prolonged. Magnesium chloride and hydrated silicic acid are formed. Silicic acid is gelatinous in consistency and has good adsorbent property. The magnesium chloride formed reacts with the bicarbonate in the intestine as under:

$$MgCl_2 + 2NaHCO_3 \rightarrow MgCO_3 + 2NaCl + H_2O + CO_2$$

The magnesium carbonate formed is eliminated in the faeces. It has a *laxative* effect and *hypermagnesaemia* may occur. *Dose* 0.5 to 2 g depending on the patient's need.

Aluminium Hydroxide

In the gel form it is a **nonabsorbable buffer antacid** with slow onset of action, and a low neutralizing capacity:

$$Al(OH)_3 + 3HCl \rightarrow AlCl_3 + 3H_2O$$

In the intestine aluminium chloride is converted to the hydroxide. The gastric contents are not completely neutralized, and the pH is maintained between 3.5 to 4.0.

The *advantages* are its relative palatability, and its lack of serious toxic effects. The most common side effect is **constipation,** which can be countered by combining with a magnesium-based antacid. Aluminium hydroxide gel is used in a dose of 7.5 to 15 ml, depending on the patient's need. *Dose* range 5 to 30 ml.

Dihydroxyaluminium sodium carbonate: It is converted to *aluminium hydroxide* in the presence of gastric hydrochloric acid, releasing carbon dioxide. It gives a rapid but transient neutralizing effect. *Chewable tablets* (334 mg) are available, and the dose is 1-2 tablets tid to six times a day.

Hydroxymagnesium aluminate: It is a synthetic combination of *aluminium* and *magnesium hydroxides* and sulphuric acid. It does not produce acid rebound and has a low incidence of diarrhoea and constipation. It is available in the form of a suspension 540 mg/5ml; tablets 480 mg; chewable tablets 480 mg. The usual dose is 480-1080 mg tid to six times daily between meals and at bedtime.

Other Agents

Milk

Milk is a weak antacid and also possesses some protective action and a 'milk drip' containing *aluminium hydroxide gel* administered through a Ryle's tube into the stomach may promote healing of the ulcer.

Anticholinergic Drugs

Anticholinergic drugs like **propantheline** reduce the inter and postprandial secretion of gastric juice, since these phases are partly under cholinergic control. In peptic ulcer patients, where gastric hypermotility and muscle spasms are marked, anticholinergics may be useful. They successfully prevent night pain in duodenal ulcer if taken immediately before retiring. **Adverse reactions** to anticholinergic drugs include xerostomia, constipation, blurred vision, retention of urine and precipitation of glaucoma.

Sedatives and **tranquilizers** have also been employed in the treatment of duodenal ulcers. They reduce emotional tension but have little effect on acid secretion.

DRUGS PROMOTING ULCER HEALING

H_2-RECEPTOR ANTAGONISTS

Cimetidine

Cimetidine was the first *histamine H_2-receptor antagonist* available for clinical use. It reduces fasting and stimulated acid and pepsin secretion by competitively antagonizing the action of histamine on H_2 receptors. It is effective in promoting healing of gastric and peptic ulcers.

Cimetidine given in tablet form (200 mg three times daily, and 400 mg each evening) for 4 weeks heals duodenal ulcers in about 60 percent of patients, and after 8 weeks therapy the healing occurs in more than 80 percent of patients. When healing has occurred therapy is continued for upto one year in a reduced dose (400 mg twice daily). *Duodenal ulcers usually recur in most patients.* Cimetidine is also effective in treating **oesophagitis.** Intravenous administration of cimetidine is found to be helpful in the treatment of **haemorrhagic gastritis** or **stress ulceration.**

Side effects include drowsiness, itchy skin rashes, gynaecomastia, interstitial nephritis, acute pancreatitis, cardiac arrhythmias and impotence.

Ranitidine

Like cimetidine, it has a low incidence of toxicity. **Side effects** include confusion, anicteric hepatitis, and cardiac arrhythmias on IV dosing. **Dose:** Ranitidine hydrochloride is available as tablets (150, 300 mg), and as an injectable. The oral dose is 150 mg bid or 300 mg before bedtime. The IV dose is 50 mg every 8 hours.

Famotidine

On oral administration the onset of effect is within 1 hour. The **usual oral dose** is 20 mg bid or 40 mg at bedtime. The IV dose is 20 mg every 12 hours.

Nizatidine: Side effects are as with other H_2-receptor antagonists. Gynaecomastia may occur rarely. The **usual dose** for gastric and duodenal ulceration is 300 mg at night, or 150 mg bid for 4-8 weeks, maintenance, 150 mg bid for 4-8 weeks, 150 mg at night upto 1 year.

Roxatidine

It is 4 times more potent than cimetidine. The usual **dose** is 150 mg twice daily, or 300 mg at bedtime, maintenance 150 mg at bedtime.

OTHER AGENTS

Carbenoxolone Sodium

It **accelerates the healing of gastric ulcers,** but the mode of action is controversial. An *increased production of gastric mucus,* and prolongation of the life span of gastric epithelial cells is the possible mechanism involved in the healing. It has a **local anti-inflammatory action.** Carbenoxolone is given in a dose of 100 mg two or three times daily for 4-8 weeks. **Side effects** like oedema and mild hypertension can be controlled by thiazides diuretics.

Pirenzepine: It is a ***antimuscarinic agent*** with relative selectivity for gastric M_1 muscarinic receptors. It inhibits gastric acid and pepsin secretion with fewer peripheral side effects. It does not cross the blood-brain barrier, and is as effective as H_2-receptor antagonists in healing gastric and duodenal ulcers. Pirenzepine is also used in conjunction with H_2-receptor antagonists in resistant cases. **Dose:** 50 mg bid increased if necessary to a maximum of 150 mg/day in 3 divided doses before meals for 4-6 weeks.

Prostaglandins

Prostaglandins of the A, E and I type inhibit gastric acid secretion. They have a **cytoprotective action** and stimulate mucus and bicarbonate secretion by the gastric mucosa.

Misoprostol: It is a synthetic analogue of PGE_1 (alprostadil), and inhibits gastric acid secretion, promoting gastric and duodenal ulcer healing. It can protect against **NSAID-induced gastric ulcers.** It is also used for the treatment of peptic ulcer disease. The recommended dosage is 800 mcg daily in 2-4 divided doses, with main meals and at bedtime, for 4-8 weeks. **Side effects** include diarrhoea, abdominal pain, flatulence and menstrual irregularities (menorrhagia, and postmenopausal bleeding).

Proton Pump Inhibitors

Omeprazole: It inhibits gastric acid secretion by blocking the H^+-K^+-adenosine triphosphatase (ATPase) enzyme system (the 'proton pump') of the *gastric parietal cells.* It is used to treat **gastric and duodenal ulcers and erosive oesophagitis.**

Dosage: For gastric and duodenal ulcers, reflux oesophagitis, and ulcers complicating NSAID therapy 20 mg daily for 4 weeks. For Zollinger-Ellison syndrome, initially 60 mg once daily; usual dose range 20-120 mg daily. *Side effects* include diarrhoea, headache, flatulence, skin reactions, and photosensitivity.

Lansoprazole

It is a proton pump inhibitor. Both *basal* and *stimulated* acid secretion, and even the stimulus-independent acid secretion is inhibited. It is used for short-term treatment of *gastric and duodenal ulcer, reflux oesophagitis, stricturing and erosive oesophagitis. Dose:* 30 mg OD in the morning for 4-8 weeks. In refractory cases the dose may be increased to 60 mg OD for 8-12 weeks. *Adverse reactions* include diarrhoea, nausea, abdominal pain, headache, dizziness, rhinitis and rash.

Pantoprazole is another proton pump inhibitor with similar actions and uses. *Dose:* 40 mg OD in the morning for 2 weeks, followed by further 2 weeks if the ulcer is not fully healed.

Sucralfate

It is an aluminium hydroxide sulphated sucrose complex which is only minimally absorbed from the GI tract. *It probably acts by selectively binding to necrotic ulcer tissue, where it acts as a barrier to acid, pepsin and bile.* Sucralfate is used for gastric and duodenal ulceration, and chronic gastritis. The *usual dose* is 2 g twice daily on rising and at bedtime, or 1 g 4 times daily 1 hours before meals and at bedtime, for 6-12 weeks. **Side effects** include constipation, diarrhoea, indigestion, dry mouth, pruritus, insomnia, vertigo and dizziness.

Colloidal Bismuth

Colloidal bismuth promotes *healing of duodenal ulcers.* The **antipepsin activity** may be partly responsible, but in addition bismuth may react with necrotic tissue in the ulcer crater, denaturing the protein and creating a physical barrier protecting the viable tissue.

HELICOBACTER PYLORI ERADICATION REGIMENS

Nearly all duodenal ulcers and most gastric ulcers are caused by *Helicobacter pylori.* Acid inhibition with antibiotic treatment is highly effective in the eradication of *H pylori* leading to long-term ulcer remission. Reinfection is rare.

Triple therapy (a proton pump inhibitor + a macrolide + either amoxycillin or metronidazole) given for 1 week is recommended, and provides high eradication rates.

PURGATIVES

Purgatives are drugs used to promote the evacuation of faeces from the bowel.

As a group the purgatives are used in the treatment of **constipation** which is a functional disturbance of the gastrointestinal tract, and a symptom of many underlying diseases. They are one of the much abused drugs by the laity. Sometimes regular diet habit and high residue diet, and adequate intake of water is all that is needed to treat constipation.

Classification

1. **Bulk purgatives:**
   - i. **Osmotic purgatives:** *Magnesium sulphate, magnesium hydroxide, sodium sulphate* and *sodium potassium tartrate.*
   - ii. **Hydrophilic colloids:** *Methylcellulose, agar, and psyllium.*
   - iii. **Vegetable fibres:** *Ispaghula husk* and *bran.*
2. **Irritant purgatives:**
   - i. **Anthraquinone (emodin) purgatives:** Rhubarb, Senna, Cascara sagrada and aloes
   - ii. Castor oil
   - iii. Phenolphthalein
   - iv. Bisacodyl
   - v. Sodium picosulphate.
3. **Lubricant purgatives:**
   - i. Liquid paraffin
   - ii. Dioctyl sodium sulphosuccinate
   - iii. Glycerine suppositories and soap water enema.

Osmotic Purgatives (Saline Purgatives)

Magnesium Sulphate (Epsom Salt)

It is a potent osmotic purgative as both *magnesium* and *sulphate* ions are minimally absorbed by the small intestine. It has a bitter taste and rapid action, and may cause considerable loss of water from the body. *Dose:* 5 to 20 g.

Magnesium hydroxide (Milk of magnesia): It acts like magnesium sulphate, but is *less potent.* In addition it is an *antacid. Dose*: 10 ml of magnesium hydroxide mixture.

Sodium sulphate and sodium potassium tartrate may also be used as saline purgatives in a dose of 15 g and 10 g orally respectively. The Seidlitz powder contains sodium potassium tartrate 7.5 g with sodium bicarbonate 2.5 g (in blue paper), and tartaric acid 2.5 g (in white paper). The contents of the blue paper are dissolved in water, and the contents of the white paper are added. This results in an effervescing drink.

Hydrophilic Colloids

Methylcellulose: It absorbs water and swells to form a gel so that faecal bulk is increased. It produces a bulky, moist, well formed stool, and should be taken with a substantial volume of water. Rarely intestinal obstruction may occur. *Dose*: 1 to 3 g.

Agar is derived from seaweeds, and has a similar action as a methylcellulose. *Dose:* 4 to 12 g.

Psyllium seeds: They are dried ripe seeds of *Plantago psyllium*. They contain a lot of muscilage which swells in the bowel to form a soft, bulky muscilagenous mass. It imbibes water. It increases peristalsis and a soft formed stool is passed. *Dose*: 5 to 15 g.

Vegetable Fibre

Ispagula husk (Isogel): Ispagula husk obtained from *Indian plantago seeds* has similar properties to those of psyllium, and is used as a bulk purgative. *Dose*: 3 to 5 g.

Bran

Bran is the residue of *husks after the milling of wheat.* It acts as *roughage* and promotes intestinal motility. The usual way of taking bran is in the form of a *breakfast cereal.*

Irritant Purgatives

Anthraquinone (emodin) purgatives: Anthraquinone purgatives includes **senna, cascara, rhubarb** and **aloes**. The active principles (emodin and chrysophanic acid) are liberated by hydrolysis of parent glycosides in the small intestine. These are absorbed and re-excreted into the colon, where *they stimulate the myenteric plexus* and induce colonic contractions. They are administered late in the evening, and exert their action next morning. Repeated use of anthraquinones may cause *degeneration of the myenteric plexus.* Senna pod 600 mg per tablet, administered as 2 tablets at bedtime.

Castor Oil

Castor oil is a fixed oil obtained from the castor bean *Ricinus communis*. It is hydrolysed in the small intestine liberating **ricinoleic acid**. This mildly irritates the intestine and peristalsis is increased. Sometimes it causes severe griping, and it has an unpleasant taste and smell. *Dose* : 15 to 60 ml orally.

Phenolphthalein: Phenolphthalein is a synthetic purgative. It irritates the mucosa of the small intestine and colon. Some of it is absorbed in the small intestine, and is then exerted in the bile. Purgative effect is produced in 6 to 12 hours. *Dose*: 60-180 mg.

Bisacodyl: It resembles phenolphthalein in its action, but is not absorbed from the intestine. It stimulates reflex peristalsis by mucosal irritation. Formed faeces are passed 1 hour after inserting a suppository, or 8 to 12 hours after oral administration. The dose is 15 mg orally and 10 mg by suppository.

Sodium Picosulphate

It exerts laxative action within 10-14 hours, and is devoid of serious toxic effects. It irritates the colon and stimulates propulsive activity. It also promotes accumulation of water in the colon. This laxative action is restricted to the colon resulting in a soft, formed stool without excessive loss of water and electrolytes. *Indications :* Constipation in patients with cardiovascular disease, hernia, anorectal disorders, the elderly, and postoperatively. It is also used for *bowel evacuation prior to abdominal radiological procedures, endoscopy and surgery. Dose:* 5-15 mg orally as a single dose at bedtime.

Lubricant Purgatives

Liquid paraffin: Liquid paraffin is a mineral oil, which is minimally absorbed by the alimentary tract. It mixes with and coats the intestinal contents, leading to the formation of soft oily faeces. It has no other action. The oil may trickle down to the anal sphincter, and leakage occurs which is messy and embarrassing to the patient.

Dioctyl sodium sulphosuccinate: It is an anionic surface active emulsifying and wetting agent, and softens the stool by lowering surface tension. It increases the water content of the stool. It is safe, effective and useful in the treatment of painful anal lesions like fissures or following *haemorrhoidectomy. Dose*: 50 to 360 mg daily. It is available in tablet and syrup form.

Glycerine: It can be introduced into the rectum as a *suppository,* and defaecation usually occurs within 30 minutes.

Enemas: Enemas evacuate faeces from the bowel by providing the *distention stimulus,* and by simple lavage. Water alone may be used, but traditionally slightly soapy water is used. The fluid (200-250 ml) is instilled into the rectum, and evacuation generally occurs within a few minutes.

Therapeutic Uses

The purgatives are used in the following conditions: (i) the treatment of **helminthic infestations** of the bowel; (ii) in bowel disease accompanied by chronic constipation, e.g., **megacolon** without aganglionosis; (iii) **before surgery on the large bowel** and the rectum; (iv) **before proctoscopy** or **sigmoidoscopy** or **radiology** of the bowel; (v) **in haemorrhoids** or **anal fissure;** (vi) in cases of **poisoning;** (vii) treatment of **hepatic precoma** and **coma;** (viii) to relieve constipation produced by drugs; (ix) during **convalescence from myocardial infarction, pulmonary embolism and cerebral haemorrhage;** and (x) to relieve **cerebral oedema** hypertonic magnesium sulphate is used.

Contracindications

Purgatives should not be used in cases of **undiagnosed abdominal pain.** Purgatives are contraindicated in cases of **intestinal obstruction,** or **faecal impaction.** Purgation should be *avoided* during the later stages of pregnancy.

Adverse Effects

Occasional use of purgatives is relatively safe, but on continued use they induce **habituation,** which is not easy to break. Withdrawal may lead to anorexia, irritability, myalgia, occipital headache, malaise, and insomnia. Other effects are colicky abdominal pain, diarrhoea leading to dehydration and electrolyte imbalance. The anthraquinone purgatives on prolonged use are **likely to damage the myenteric plexus** of the colon.

ANTIDIARRHOEAL DRUGS

Diarrhoea is a symptom marked by a frequent passage of semisolid or liquid faeces. Prolonged diarrhoea, whatever the cause, leads to **electrolyte loss**. The use of antidiarrhoeal drugs only offers a **symptomatic relief**.

The Opiates: They have been used for many years for the symptomatic control of diarrhoea. **Paregoric** (camphorated tincture of opium) 4ml; **laudanum** (tincture of opium) 0.3 to 0.6ml; and **codeine sulphate** 16 to 32 mg reduce the propulsive movements of the colonic muscle, permitting the faeces to remain longer in the lumen and water is reabsorbed.

Diphenoxylate hydrochloride: Diphenoxylate is related to pethidine and acts like the opiates. It may be combined with atropine. The usual dose is 5 mg three times daily. A newer agent is **loperamide** which is related to diphenoxylate. The usual dose is 4 mg followed by 3 mg after each stool is passed to a maximum of 16 mg/ day.

Antispasmodic Agent

Anticholinergic agents like **propatheline bromide,** and **dicyclomine hydrochloride** may be used to diminish intestinal motility, and the associated abdominal cramps also subside.

Hydrophilic agents: Agents like **methylcellulose, isogel** and **psyllium seeds** may be used as they absorb water forming a gelatinous mass. Such an action reduces the free water content of the stool. These agents have already been described under purgatives, but they are of value both in constipation and diarrhoea because of their hydrophilic nature.

Demulcents: *Bismuth subcarbonate* 2 g orally; calcium carbonate. 2 g orally; and magnesium oxide, 1 g orally may be used as demulcents to provide a soothing effect to the irritated intestinal mucosa.

Adsorbents

They supposedly adsorb irritants, bind water and reduce mucus secretion. **Activated charcoal** 1 to 6 g orally; **Kaolin** 3 g orally; and **Kaopectate** (mixture of kaolin and pectin) 15 ml orally; may be used. Kaopectate has both demulcent and adsorbent property.

Oral Rehydration Therapy (ORT)

Oral rehydration therapy (ORT) is today recognized as the **first line** treatment in most cases of acute diarrhoea. Antibacterial agents are required only in infectious diarrhoea where pathogens have been identified. The oral rehydration salts (ORS) solution recommended by the WHO contains glucose (20.0 g) and three salts–sodium chloride (3.5 g), trisodium citrate dihydrate (2.9 g), or sodium bicarbonate (2.5 g), and potassium chloride (1.5 g) to be mixed in 1 litre of water. The composition of this ORS formulation is optimum for the rehydration of patients of all ages—infants, children and adults—with dehydration due to acute diarrhoea of any aetiology. Its efficacy rests in the fact that **glucose linked sodium reabsorption mechanism** in the small intestine remains largely intact during acute diarrhoeal states, and serves to promote sodium entry into the body. The ORT has been described as 'potentially the most important medical advance of this century'.

OTHER THERAPEUTIC AGENTS

Lactulose

Taken orally, it passes unchanged to the lower alimentary tract, where it is hydrolysed by **carbohydrate fermenting bacteria** and thus provides nutrition to them. The growth of these organisms lowers the faecal pH, and thereby lactulose exerts a **mild laxative effect.** Lactulose is of value in the treatment of **hepatic encephalopathy.** It is available as a 50 percent w/w solution and 50 ml is given orally twice or thrice daily. It may be used in the treatment of **chronic constipation** in a dose of 10 to 20 g after breakfast, but it may take 2 to 3 days to exert a purgative effect.

Cholestyramine

Cholestyramine is an ion exchange resin which absorbs bile salts. Taken orally it prevents the reabsorption of bile salts by the distal ileum thereby facilitating the depletion of the bile salt pool. It is of value in **cholestatic syndromes,** and the itching associated with high serum concentrations of bile salts is relieved.

DRUG TREATMENT OF TRAVELLER'S DIARRHOEA

Upto 50 percent of travellers or tourists to the tropics develop diarrhoeal illness. It is characterized by **abdominal cramps, watery diarrhoea, flatulence** and **fatigue.**

The first measure in the treatment is **oral rehydration** of the patient. Effective early treatment regimen include: (i) **doxycycline** 100 mg qid for 48 hours; or (ii) **trimethoprim-sulphamethoxazole,** one regular strength tablet bid for 5 days; or (iii) **bismuth subsalicylate** 30 to 60 ml every half hour for eight doses.

Drugs Acting on the Respiratory System

Chronic obstructive pulmonary diseases (COPD) include **bronchial asthma, chronic bronchitis** and **emphysema**. The bronchodilator drugs are the mainstay in the drug management.

BRONCHODILATOR DRUGS

The *tone* of the bronchial muscle is controlled by *humoral factors*, and by the *autonomic nervous system*. The *parasympathetic* system causes bronchoconstriction mediated by acetylcholine. The *sympathetic* stimulation mediated by nor-adrenaline causes increased pulmonary blood flow, **bronchodilation**, and vasodilatation of the pulmonary circulation.

Classification

1. **Anticholinergic agents**
   Ipratropium
   Tiotropium
2. **Sympathomimetic amines**
   a. *Drugs stimulating alpha- and beta-receptors* Ephedrine
   b. *Drugs stimulating beta$_1$- and beta$_2$-receptors* Orciprenaline
   c. *Drug stimulating beta$_2$-receptors*
      Salbutamol
      Terbutaline
      Isoetharine
      Rimiterol
      Formoterol
3. **Theophylline derivatives (Methylxanthines)**
   Aminophylline
   Choline theophyllinate
   Diprophylline

Mode of Action

Beta-adrenoceptor activity is mediated by c-AMP. The beta-adrenergic drugs increase adenylcylase activity which promotes the conversion of ATP to active c-AMP, and this in turn relaxes the bronchial muscle (**Fig. 13.1**). Cyclic-AMP is broken down by the enzyme phosphodiesterase. The Methyl-xanthines inhibit this enzyme, thereby conserving c-AMP in the bronchial muscle cell. **Thus, the adrenergic agonists cause bronchodilation by promoting the formation of c-AMP, and the methylaxanthines act by inhibiting the destruction of c-AMP.**

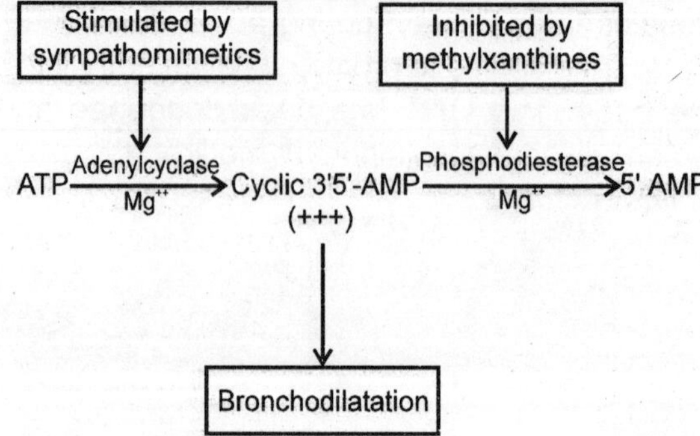

Fig.13.1 : *Mode of action of sympathomimetics and methylxanthines as bronchodilators*

Anticholinergics

Ipratropium

Ipratropium is a new synthetic anticholinergic agent. It is claimed that ipratropium has some **bronchoselectivity,** producing bronchodilation without unwanted anticholinergic side effects. Ipratropium is available in a **metered dose inhaler** delivering 0.02 mg per inhalation. The usual dosage is one or two puffs three or four times daily. **Tiotropium** is a newer agent used as maintenance treatment of COPD. **Dose:** 1 capsule (18 mcg) to be inhaled once daily.

Sympathomimetics

Ephedrine

Ephedrine stimulates both alpha- and beta-receptors. It is readily and completely absorbed after oral or parenteral administration. **Side effects** include CNS stimulation, vomiting, sweating, tremors, nervousness, insomnia and cardiac irregularities.

Ephedrine is used for mild or moderately severe bronchial asthma. The adult dose is 30 to 60 mg orally three or four times daily.

Orciprenaline

Orciprenaline is a long-acting derivative of isoprenaline. It stimulates both beta$_1$- and beta$_2$- receptors, although it is claimed that it has little effect on the heart muscle. Orciprenaline given orally reduces the frequency and severity of asthmatic attacks. Inhaled as an **aerosol,** it acts promptly and the action lasts for 3 to 6 hours. Orally it is given in a dose of 20 mg every 6 hours. The metered aerosol produces 0.75 mg per dose, and adults may take upto 12 doses in 24 hours.

Beta$_2$ Agonists

Salbutamol

Salbutamol is the most widely used **beta$_2$-receptors stimulant.** It is effective by **oral, intravenous** and **aerosol** inhalation routes of administration, and has a much longer duration of action than isoprenaline. It is virtually devoid of cardiovascular effects in usual doses. The **oral** dose in the treatment of bronchial asthma is 2 to 4 mg three times daily. For **inhalation** 100 to 200 mcg may be repeated 4 hourly with a maximum of 8 inhalations in 24 hours.

Terbutaline

Terbutaline is closely related to orciprenaline but is **more beta$_2$ selective.** Its pharmacological actions and therapeutic uses resemble salbutamol. **Orally** it is given in a dose of 2.5 to 5 mg two or three times daily. It may be administered **subcutaneously** (250 to 500 mcg) or by **inhalation** (200 or 250 mcg metered dose).

Isoetharine

Isoetharine is a **selective beta$_2$-receptor stimulant** and is effective by mouth, but its duration of action is short. Orally it may be given in a dose of 10 mg **delayed release tablets,** with an effective duration of action of 4 to 6 hours. *Aerosol* preparation (350 mcg metered dose) is also available.

Rimiterol

Rimiterol is a **short-acting beta$_2$-receptor stimulant.** Its activity is similar to that of *salbutamol* and *terbutaline*. The **dose** is 0.2 to 0.6 mg (one to three inhalations from a metered aerosol) with not more than 8 inhalations in 24 hours.

Formoterol

Formoterol is a **long-acting beta-2 receptor stimulant**, used in the *prevention of asthma attacks.* It is ineffective in acute asthma. *Usual dose* is 12 mcg (one capsule) every 12 hours by *inhalation.*

Other beta$_2$ stimulants used as bronchodilators are **fenoterol, salmeterol, reproterol and tulobuterol.**

Methylxanthines

The methylxanthines act by inhibiting the enzyme phosphodiesterase and hence have actions which resemble the sympathomimetics. They cause **bronchodilation, myocardial stimulation** and CNS stimulation.

Aminophylline

Aminophylline is a combination of theophylline and ethylenediamine, and is useful in **bronchial asthma** and **pulmonary oedema.** It is often used by slow intravenous injection (250 to 500 mg) as a first line treatment in patients with severe asthmatic attacks. When a large intravenous dose of aminophylline is given rapidly, **convulsions, arrhythmias** or **cardiac arrest** may occur. *Aminophylline suppositories* of 50,100,150 and 360 mg may be used to avoid gastric irritation caused by oral aminophylline.

Choline Theophyllinate

Choline theophyllinate is used for the relief and prophylaxis of mild to moderate bronchospasm. The **adult oral dose** is 400 to 1600 mg daily in divided doses.

Diprophylline

Diprophylline is a theophylline derivative which is used like aminophylline. It causes less of nausea and gastric irritation. The usual dose is upto 15 mg /kg every 6 hourly.

DISODIUM CROMOGLYCATE

Disodium cromoglycate (DSCG, Cromolyn sodium) is *not a bronchodilator.* Its main action is **prophylactic,** reducing the incidence and severity of allergic asthmatic attacks. DSCG administration permits the **reduction in the dosage of corticosteroids** and **bronchodilators** in asthmatic patients.

DSCG *inhibits the release of histamine* and *SRS-A* from the sensitized mast cells, by **stabilizing the mast cell membrane,** and preventing exocytosis. It also prevents exercise-induced bronchoconstriction in normal and asthmatic patients, by inhibiting the local release of prostaglandins.

DSCG has to be administered by **inhalation** from a special dispenser, the **spinhaler**. The initial dose is 20 mg four times daily. DSCG has also been tried in **hay fever, allergic rhinitis, food allergy, allergic conjunctivitis** and **ulcerative colitis.** *Nedocromil* is a newer cromolyn-like compound.

KETOTIFEN

Ketotifen has actions similar to cromolyn sodium, and acts primarily by inhibition of mediator release. It also has anti-histamine properties. It is used in the proplylaxis of bronchial asthma. *Dose*: 2 mg bid orally.

Corticosteroids in Bronchial Asthma

Glucocorticoids are **life-saving** in an acute attack or status asthmatics. Probably they function as **non-specific anti-inflammatory agents** to provide relief from congestion and exudation.

Beclomethasone dipropionate is a chlorinated analogue of betamethasone. It acts **locally** on the respiratory mucosa, and the metered dose inhaler delivers 42 or 50 mcg/puff. Baclomethasone inhalation allows 'topical' treatment without major adverse effects like the suppression of the pituitary adrenal axis. It is highly effective locally but **poorly absorbed.** However, topical corticosteroids may lead to **local atrophy** of the pharyngeal mucosa, and **superinfection** with Candida.

Antihistamines in Bronchial Asthma

The antihistamines are almost ineffective in the treatment of bronchial asthma. This is probably because histamine is released from the sensitized mast cells in very high concentrations near the target cells, and the competitive blockade produced by antihistamines is *ineffective.*

ANTITUSSIVE DRUGS

Coughing is a protective reflex. The **cough receptors** lie in the mucosa of the bronchial tree. The impulses from these receptors are transmitted through the **vagus** and the **glossopharyngeal**

nerve to the cough centre in the medulla. It is often not advisable to completely suppress cough in cases of **chronic bronchitis** or **bronchiectasis,** as it may result in the retention of secretions in the tracheobronchial tree.

Classification

I. **Centrally-acting antitussives**
   i. *Narcotic antitussives*
      Codeine, ethylmorphine, oxycodone
   ii. *Non-narcotic antitussives*
      Dextromethorpan, noscapine, propoxyphene, caramiphen.
II. **Peripherally-acting antitussives**
   i. *Mucosal anaesthetics*
      Benzonatate, chlophedianol
   ii. *Bronchodilators*
      Ephedrine
   iii. *Hydrating agents*
      Steam, aerosols, fluids
   iv. *Miscellaneous*
      Bromhexine, candy, syrup.

Narcotic Antitussives

Codeine

Codeine is an opium alkaloid, available both as sulphate and phosphate in tablet, elixir or syrup form. It is a very effective antitussive agent and **depresses the cough centre** in the medulla, resulting in an elevation of the cough threshold. When large doses are used **respiratory depression** may occur. Codeine has a potential for the development of dependence like the opioids. The **usual adult dose** is 10 to 15 mg orally every 4 to 6 hours. The **side effects** include nausea and vomiting, constipation, drowsiness, pruritus and respiratory depression.

Ethylmorphine and **oxycodone** have codeine-like antitussive action.

Non-narcotic Antitussives

Dextromethorphan

Dextromethrophan is a synthetic morphine derivative, and a very useful antitussive agent. It has a very **low addiction liability.** The usual adult dose is 10 to 30 mg every 4 to 6 hours.

Noscapine

Noscapine (Narcotine) is an opium alkaloid. It has a **potent antitussive action,** almost equaling that of codeine. It is well absorbed from the gut. The **usual dose** is 15 to 30 mg three or four times daily. It has a wide margin of safety.

Propoxyphene Napsylate

Propoxyphene is separable into its l-form and d-form. *The laevoform has antitussive properties, while the dextroform has analgesic action.* The antitussive action of l-propoxyphene (50 mg) was found to be equivalent to 15 mg of codeine. It does not depress the CNS and respiration. The usual **dose** is 50 to 100 mg every 4 hours. The **side effects** include nausea, epigastric discomfort, skin rashes, urticaria, drowsiness and dizziness.

Caramiphen Ethanedisulfonate (Taoryl)

Caramiphen raises the threshold of the cough reflex, and is less active than an equal dose of codeine. It has an **atropine-like action,** and exerts antisecretory and mydriatic effects. The oral dose is 10 to 20 mg three or four times daily.

The *peripherally-acting antitussives* are mucosal anaesthetics, bronchodilators, hydrating agents or demulcents. They provide a soothing effect by correcting the irritation to the cough receptors.

EXPECTORANTS AND MUCOLYTIC AGENTS (MUCOKINETIC AGENTS)

Expectorants and mucolytic agents alter the viscosity of the sputum, and promote the removal of secretions from the bronchial tree. In **infections** such as bacterial bronchitis, pneumonia, chronic bronchitis, or bronchiectasis the secretion is usually *thick, tenacious* and *frequently mucopurulent. It is in these situations that expectorants and mucolytic agents (collectively named as mucokinetic agents) play an important role.* They are classified as under:

I. Inhalational agents (also effective orally)
   i. **Water**
   ii. **Saline solutions:** hypotonic, isotonic, hypertonic
   iii. **Hygroscopic agents:** Glycerol guaiacolate, propylene glycol
   iv. **True mucolytic agents:** Acetylcysteine, trypsin, chymotrypsin.
   v. **Volatile agents:** Balsams and other volatile oils

II. Oral Agents
   i. **Vagal stimulants:** Creosote derivatives, terpenes, guaifenesin.
   ii. **Direct mucokinetics:** Potassium iodide, ammonium chloride, bromhexine, ambroxol.

Glycerol guaiacolate is the most commonly used expectorant. It is used singly or in combination with *dextromethorphan*. The usual *dose* is 100 to 200 mg three or four times daily. *Side effects* are rare.

Propylene glycol is a hygroscopic agent with a sweet taste and demulcent properties. A 2 percent solution in water is isosmotic with serum, and is therefore non-irritating to the airways.

Acetylcysteine is a mucolytic agent, both effective *in vivo* and *in vitro*. It acts by lowering the viscosity. Acetylcysteine can be given by means of a **nebulizer** or **instilled** directly into the trachea. The **usual dose** is 3 to 5 ml of 20 percent solution with a bronchodilator and saline when nebulized.

Creosote derivatives: Hard woods such as beech are used as a source of creosote, which is a mixture of phenols having a characteristic odour. The most important components are **creosol** and **guaiacol.** Creosote is an antiseptic with an expectorant quality.

Guaifenesin is a guaiacol derivative which has replaced creosote as a mucokinetic agent. It is less irritating to the bowel, and is absorbed more reliably. The usual dose is 100 to 200 mg every 3 to 4 hours.

Terpenes are volatile oils related to turpentine, and are used in many cough remedies for their expectorant action. Such drugs include *anise oil, eucalyptus oil, lemon oil, pine oil, terpin hydrate* and *thymol*.

Terpin hydrate is the most popular agent. It is usually employed in combination with other agents in a dose of 125 to 300 mg every 6 hours.

Potassium iodide increases bronchial secretion by reflex stimulation of the gastric mucosa. It also increases the volume and decreases the viscosity of salivary, nasal and lacrimal secretions. The use of potassium iodide may lead to unpleasant hypersecretion, parotid swelling, thyroid enlargement and brassy taste may be troublesome. The usual dosage is 0.3 g as plain or enteric coated tablets 3 to 4 times daily.

Bromhexine is an oral mucokinetic agent. It is obtained from the plant *Adhatoda vasica*. It acts by **depolymerization of the mucopolysaccharides** in the mucus, thereby lowering the viscosity. The usual dose is 8 to 16 mg orally three times day.

Ambroxol: Ambroxol is a metabolite of bromhexine with similar action and uses. *Dose*: 30 to 120 mg orally in 2 or 3 divided doses. It may be given by inhalation or rectally.

The use of expectorants in the treatment of chronic bronchitis and emphysema is beneficial. *Adequate hydration*, *postural drainage* and *chest physiotherapy* are effective in acute and chronic conditions to mobilize bronchial secretions.

OXYGEN THERAPY

Supplemental oxygen is widely used in patients with **acute respiratory distress.** There are many situations in which simultaneous mechanical assistance and oxygen is required, e.g., **central respiratory depression due to narcotic drugs, severe shock, acute and chronic pulmonary disease.** The pre-requisites for oxygen administration are, a patent and adequate airway, maintained if necessary by *tracheal intubation* or *tracheostomy,* and a *positive pressure device* and *masks*.

Technique of Oxygen Administration

Oxygen from the cylinder should preferably be bubbled through water to humidify if before it is delivered to the patient's airway.

i. **Oxygen tent:** Concentration of 25-50 percent oxygen can be reached.
ii. **Head tents or hoods:** Concentrations from 50-80 percent can be reached as they are smaller than tents.
iii. **Nasal catheter or cannula (Prongs):** Concentrations from 40-60 percent can be reached, and this technique is adequate for most purposes.
iv. **Endotracheal tube or facial masks:** 80 to 100 percent concentrations can be delivered by these methods.
v. **Hyperbaric oxygen:** Oxygen can be administered under pressures greater than 1 atmosphere, and as high as 3 atmospheres in special pressurized chambers.

Mode of Action

Atmospheric air contains 20.9 percent oxygen, which exerts a partial pressure (PO_2) of 159 mm Hg in the inspired air. **Under usual conditions haemoglobin is almost completely (96%) saturated with oxygen (except in anoxic anoxia).**

Therapeutic Uses

Oxygen administration is indicated in cases of anoxia: (i) **anoxic anoxia** due to inadequate ventilation; (ii) **anaemic anoxia,** when the blood haemoglobin content is low, or in cases of shock; (iii) **stagnant anoxia** as in cases of shock; and (iv) **histotoxic anoxia** as occurs in cases of **cyanide poisoning** which exerts its lethal effect due to inactivation of cytochrome oxidase.

The chief clinical indications for oxygen therapy are: *Acute respiratory failure or arrest; arterial hypoxia due to acute or chronic respiratory disease; congestive heart failure* or *vascular insufficiency; severe anemia* or *haemolysis* and certain poisons like *cyanide* and *carbon monoxide.*

Oxygen Toxicity

Adverse reactions induced by oxygen administration are: (i) **respiratory tract irritation;** (ii) **respiratory depression** due to carbon dioxide wash out; and (iii) **retrolental fibroplasia** in premature infants.

Preparations

Medical oxygen is available in cylinders which are painted white at the valve and down to the shoulder, and the remainder is painted black (white shoulder, black body) according to *British convention.* The chemical symbol O_2 is clearly stamped on the cylinder valve. According to *American convention* oxygen cylinders are painted green. Commercial oxygen or welding oxygen is equally pure and may be used if necessary.

Hyperbaric oxygen: (Oxygen administration between 2 and 3 atmospheres, but never more than 4 atmospheres) administered in pressure chambers is effective in the treatment of **carbon monoxide poisoning** and **gas gangrene.** At 3 atmospheres pressure and 100 percent oxygen, enough oxygen is dissolved in the blood (6ml/100ml) to meet the tissue needs, without haemoglobin desaturation. *Oxygen toxicity is increased at higher pressures.* The value of hyperbaric oxygen in clinical practice is due to *three* biologic effects: the **relief of hypoxia** and **anoxia**; the **potentiation of ionizing radiation effect (radiosensitization);** and the **inhibition of bacterial growth** and **toxin production**.

RESPIRATORY STIMULANTS

The use of drugs to act as respiratory stimulants has been *disappointing* as drugs which have a specific stimulant effect on the respiratory drive are not available.

Essentially analeptics are CNS stimulants and some of them stimulate the respiratory centre in the medulla. They do not have a specific action on this area, and stimulate the cerebrospinal axis at all levels causing general arousal and in larger doses produce convulsions. The commonly employed analeptics are *caffeine sodium benzoate* and *doxapram* **(Chap. 2.9).**

Heavy Metals and Chelating Agents

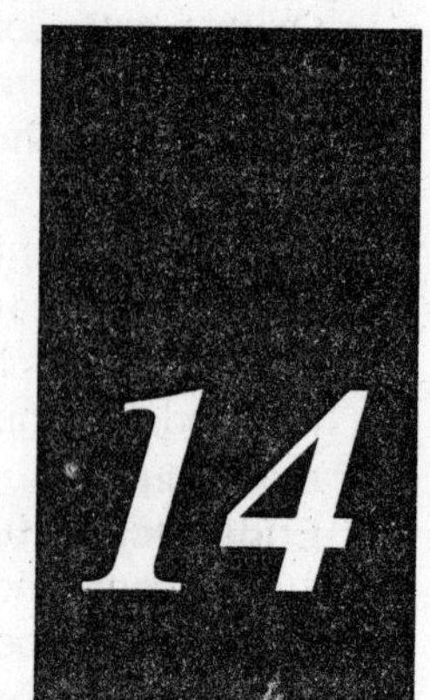

The heavy metals are employed in industrial processes and a large number of workers are at risk of poisoning.

HEAVY METALS

The heavy metals have a special affinity for **sulphydryl groups,** which are essential for the activity of many enzyme systems.

Arsenic

Arsenic is a transition element or **metalloid.** Certain arsenicals used as pesticides, fungicides and rodenticides, or used in glass, electroplating, dyestuff, paint and cosmetic industries can cause poisoning. Arsenicals are absorbed through mucous membranes. Arsenic poisoning is treated with **dimercaprol.**

Antimony

Antimonials such as *antimony potassium tartrate* are used in the treatment of **schistosomiasis.** The The toxicity is similar to that of arsenic and the treatment is the same.

Mercury

Mercury is used in the manufacture of herbicides, and fungicides. Treatment is by chelation with **dimercaprol.**

Bismuth

Insoluble bismuth salts are used in the treatment of *peptic ulcer*. The toxic effects are similar to those of mercury, treatment is by chelation with **dimercaprol.**

Gold

Gold compounds are used in the treatment of **rheumatoid arthritis.** Treatment of poisoning is with **dimercaprol.**

Lead

Lead has many industrial uses and poisoning can occur during the manufacture of paints, batteries, rubber and glazed pottery. Inhalation of lead is a hazard in industry. Lead from water pipes can contaminate water and food.

Treatment is by chelation of lead with **calcium disodium edetate** and **dimercaprol.**

Silver

Silver compounds are used only for their local action. **Silver nitrate** sticks are used for their caustic (corrosive) action to prevent the formation of granulation tissue. Topical **silver sulphadiazine** is used to prevent the infection of burns. Chronic silver poisoning can lead to slate-grey pigmentation of the skin, eyes and mucous membranes (argyria). **Sodium thiosulphate solution** injected into the affected areas may reduce the discolouration. Chelating agents are ineffective in the treatment.

CHELATING AGENTS

Chelating agents are metal binding **antidotal chemicals** which bind the ions of heavy metals by incorporating them into an **inner ring structure** in the molecule, and rendering them biologically inactive. This is brought about by chemical groups called **ligands.** The chemical complex thus formed is called a **chelate**, is stable and nontoxic and is excreted by the kidneys. This process of complex formation is known as **chelation**, and the term is derived from the Greek word '*chele*' which means '*claw*'. The chelating agents are also designated as **heavy metal antagonists.**

Dimercaprol (BAL, British Anti-leuisite)

Dimercaprol was developed during World War II in Great Britain. It was synthesized during a systematic study of possible antidotes against arsenic containing vesicant war gases like **Leuisite** (hence the name BAL). It forms very stable 1:1 chelates with **arsenic, mercury** and **lead**. The chelates formed with **gold, bismuth, antimony** and **nickel** are less stable.

After intramuscular injection dimercaprol plasma levels peak in 30 minutes, and the drug has a very short half-life. **The chelate is excreted in urine.** Liver damage increases the half-life of the drug.

Toxicity

Dimercaprol is a toxic drug. Side effects include pain at the site of injection, hypertension, tachycardia, nausea, vomiting, chest tightness, sweating, abdominal pain, burning and tingling sensations, lacrimation, salivation and rhinorrhoea.

Dose: Dimercaprol (BAL) is available in peanut oil (100 mg/ml) for injection. Dosage ranges from 3 to 5 mg/kg body weight by deep intramuscular injection, and repeated 1 to 4 times daily.

Penicillamine

Penicillamine (Dimethylcysteine) is an inactive degradation product of penicillin. It combines with **copper, iron, mercury, lead** and **arsenic** to form soluble complexes that are excreted by the kidney.

Penicillamine is well absorbed from the gut and is partly oxidized to its disulphide derivative and excreted by the kidney.

Therapeutic Uses

Penicillamine is used for the removal of copper in **hepatolenticular degeneration (Wilson's disease).** Penicillamine has also been tried in cases of **rheumatoid arthritis.**

Toxicity

Side effects include nausea, anorexia, vomiting, rashes, fever, thrombocytopenia, and rarely agranulocytosis and nephrotic syndrome.

Dose: Penicillamine (Cuprimine) is available in 250 mg capsules. The dose for adults is 250 mg four times daily, with gradual increase not to exceed 5 g every day.

EDTA (Ethylene Diamine Tetra-acetic Acid)

EDTA is a powerful chelating agent. Its affinity for metallic ions increases in the written order: Ca, Mn, Fe, Co, Zn, Cu, Ni, Cd and Pb. It has been estimated that its affinity for lead (Pb) is 10^7 times that for calcium (Ca.) It is insoluble in water and is not used therapeutically.

Disodium Edetate is dangerous when injected intravenously, since it chelates calcium and may lead to hypocalcaemic tetany, coagulation abnormalities, or even fatal hypocalcaemia. Its main use is for the topical treatment of lime burns in the eye.

Calcium disodium edetate (Calcium disodium versenate) is used primarily to treat lead poisoning (Plumbism). The chelates formed are stable, water soluble, and readily excreted by the kidneys.

Side effects include thrombophlebitis, hypotension, lacrimation, muscle pain, sneezing and chills. Renal damage and transient bone marrow depression may occur.

Dose: Calcium disodium edetate is available as a solution (200 mg/ml) in 5 ml containers, to be diluted for intravenous infusion. The daily dose should not exceed 50 mg/kg/day in adults, or 30 mg/kg/day in children.

Desferrioxamine Mesylate

Desferrioxamine (Deferoxamine) obtained from *Streptomyces pilosus*, is a chelating agent used in the treatment of **iron poisoning.** It forms stable 1:1 complexes with inorganic iron and can remove iron from *ferritin*, and *transferrin* but not from haemoglobin or cytochromes. It is used in the management of **secondary haemochromatosis** and **thalassemia** to promote iron excretion.

Toxicity

If desferrioxamine is administered intravenously rapidly, it may cause hypotension, urticaria and tachycardia. Long-term treatment may cause blurred vision, diarrhoea, leg cramps and cataracts.

Dose: Desferrioxamine may be infused intravenously at a rate of not more than 15mg/kg body weight per hour to a maximal dose of 80 mg/kg in 24 hours, or it may be administered in a dose of 2 g IM.

Deferiprone

Deferiprone is an orally effective iron-chelating agent developed with an aim to overcome this problem. The drug is available as 250 and 500 mg capsules.

Trientine

Trientine is a ***copper chelating agent*** used in the treatment of Wilson's disease (hepatolentricular degeneration). It is claimed to be less toxic than penicllamine. The adult dose is 1.2-2.4 g/day orally in 2 or 4 divided doses on an empty stomach (1 hour before, or 2 hours after meals).

To summarize, the principal uses of the chelating agents are: **dimercaprol** for arsenic, mercury and gold; **calcium disodium edetate** for lead; **penicllamine** for copper and lead; and **desferrioxamine** for iron poisoning. **Trientine** is a newer copper chelating agent.

Vaccines and Antisera

15

Edward Jenner (1749-1823) the discoverer of vaccine against *smallpox* got the idea from a dairy maid who asserted that she would never get smallpox as she had already had cowpox. Jenner's observation that an attack of cowpox conferred immunity against smallpox was the beginning of therapy with *vaccines* and *sera*.

IMMUNITY

Immunity is a state of relative resistance to disease, which develops after exposure to the specific agent responsible for infection. Immunity may be of two kinds: (i) ***Active immunity***; and (ii) ***Passive immunity.***

Active Immunity

Active immunity may be acquired by administering: (i) **living organisms;** (ii) **attenuated or treated organisms,** e.g. smallpox and rabies; (iii) **dead or killed organisms,** e.g., enteric fever and whooping cough; (iv) **separated exotoxins,** e.g., scarlet fever; and (v) **the toxoid or modified toxin,** e.g., diphtheria and tetanus.

The term **vaccination** interpreted today includes all the above measures for active immunization. The most significant achievement of active immunization is the eradication of smallpox from the world.

Passive Immunity

Passive immunity is conferred by administering immune sera containing **preformed antibodies** or **antitoxins** (prepared from animals or humans who have been actively immunized) to individuals who have either not been previously exposed to the pathogen, or are not immunized adequately. Passive immunization is therefore indicated in cases of **actual infection** with a specific organism. Passive immunization is inferior to active immunization, and the effect is short lived. But it is of immediate value as the borrowed antibodies/antitoxins attack the invaders or neutralize the toxins.

PRODUCTS FOR ACTIVE IMMUNITY

Some of the available varieties are listed below:

1. **Inactivated killed vaccines**
   i. **Bacterial inactivated vaccines**
   Pertussis (whooping cough)
   Plague, Cholera, Typhoid
   ii. **Rickettsial inactivated vaccines**
   Epidemic typhus, Rocky mountain
   Spotted fever, Q fever, Scrub typhus
   iii. **Viral inactivated vaccines**
   Influenza, Measles, Mumps
   Poliomyelitis, Rabies.
2. **Live attenuated vaccines**
   i. **Bacterial live vaccines**
   Plague, Tuberculosis
   ii. **Viral live vaccines**
   Smallpox, Poliomyelitis, Measles
   German measles, Mumps, Yellow fever,
   Rabies.

3. **Toxoids**
   Diphtheria and tetanus, often used together (DT) and sometimes combined with pertussis (DTP) vaccine.

PRODUCTS FOR PASSIVE IMMUNITY

These immune sera (antisera) may contain **antitoxins, antivenins, antibacterial** or **antiviral antibodies.** Hypersensitivity reactions are very likely if the antibodies are derived from animal sera.

Some of the available products are listed below:

1. **Human gamma globulin**
   Immune serum globulin is derived from pools of human plasma. It can be injected IM or SC, but not intravenously. It has been employed clinically for the management of *hypogammaglobulinaemia, viral hepatitis, measles* and *German measles.*
2. **Specific hyperimmune human gamma globulins**
   Tetanus, Rabies, Vaccinia, Chickenpox, Rh sensitization, Pertussis.
3. **Antitoxins and antisera from animals**
   Diphtheria antitoxin, Botulism antitoxin, Tetanus antitoxin, Antivenins, Gas gangrene antitoxin, Rabies antiserum.

Detail of immunization schedules is beyond the scope of this text.

Triple Antigen (DPT)

Diphtheria toxoid is the type of preparation preferred for long-term prophylaxis against diphtheria. It is available alone, or in combination with *tetanus toxoids* (DT) , or with *tetanus toxoids* and *pertussis vaccine* (DTP). The 'triple antigen' is used for active immunization against diphtheria, tetanus, and whooping cough.

It is suitable for immunization of young children. Three doses of 0.5 ml IM at intervals of 4-8 weeks are administered. A fourth booster dose of 0.5 ml IM is given about 1 year later, and another booster dose may be given at the school entry age of 5 years.

Antivenins

Antivenins are concentrated *globulin fractions* of sera of animals (horse) immunized with the venoms of poisonous snakes (Rattlesnakes, vipers, cobras and others), spiders and scorpions.

Haffkine Bio-pharmaceuticals, Mumbai manufacture **antivenin-lyophilized polyvalent anti-snake venom serum** injection for use in the emergency treatment of poisonous snakebite. Kasauli in Himachal Pradesh manufactures antisera against cobra and Ressell's viper (venom of Ressell's viper has strong coagulant activity). Vials of 10 ml are standardized to neutralize 2 mg of cobra venom and 4 mg of viper venom per ml. For dosage and route of administration the manufacturer's directions must be followed, and *testing for hypersensitivity* must be done prior to administration.

The steps in the *management of poisonous snakebite* are:

i. Slow down the spread of venom by applying a **tourniquet,** and **cold compacts.** Immobilize the part, in addition.
ii. Remove as much venom as possible from the site of the bite by **incision** and **suction.**
iii. Neutralize the venom with **antivenin** administered systematically, and also by regional limb perfusion.
iv. **General supportive therapy:** Administer corticosteroids, blood, antibiotics, fluid and electrolytes, tetanus and gas gangrene prophylaxis, and cardiorespiratory support should be instituted, if necessary.

NATIONAL IMMUNIZATION SCHEDULE

The National Immunization Schedule recommended by the government of India to protect women from **tetanus,** and children from six disabling diseases, namely, **tuberculosis, diphtheria, whooping cough, tetanus, poliomyelitis** and **measles** is as under:

For the pregnant woman		
Early in pregnancy	-	T.T. -1 or T.T. Booster (injection)
One month after T.T.-1	-	T.T.-2 (injection)
For the infant		
After 1½ months	-	B.C.G. (injection)
	-	D.P.T.-1 (injection) and
	-	O.P.V.-1 (dose)
After 2½ months	-	D.P.T.-2 (injection) and
	-	O.P.V. -2 (dose)
After 3½ months	-	D.P.T.-3 (injection) and
	-	O.P.V. -3 (dose)
At 9 months	-	Measles (Injection)
At 16 to 24 months	-	D.P.T. Booster (Injection) and O.P.V. Booster dose

If the infant has been delivered in a hospital or clinic, the *BCG injection* and *OPV dose* should be given at birth. Adherence to the above schedule significantly reduces the risk of the mentioned diseases.

Some Special Vaccines

Rabies Vaccine

Active immunization against rabies is primarily an emergency measure used together with ***hyper-immune globulin*** to protect individuals bitten by rabid animals. Sometimes immunization has to be routinely carried out in persons with high risk. Both in post and pre-exposure treatment, the vaccine of choice is the *human diploid cell rabies vaccine* which is more potent and significantly less reactogenic than older vaccines.

Human Diploid Cell Rabies Vaccine (HDCV): It is supplied as 1ml single dose vials of lyophilized vaccine with accompanying diluent. The HDCV has almost entirely replaced the nerve tissue and duck embryo vaccines because: (i) it requires a **lower number of doses;** (ii) it elicits **a more rapid and higher antibody response;** (iii) it does **not** cause serious adverse reactions; and (iv) it has proved **clinically effective** in controlled studies.

For **post-exposure immunization** the complete series consist of six 1 ml IM injections, given on days 0-3-7-14-30-90 (WHO recommendation, 1977). **Specific antirabies hyperimmune globulin (RIG)** is given only once at the beginning of treatment with the first dose of the vaccine, or upto 7-8 days after, if it was not immediately possible. From the 8th day on, passive antibody administration is needless because an active antibody response to HDCV starts by this time. For **pre-exposure immunization** the primary series consists of *three 1 ml doses* of HDCV given IM on day 0-7-28. A booster is then given every 2 years.

Mild local reactions like *pain, erythema* and *swelling* may occur at the site of HDCV injection.

HDCV today is the ideal antirabies vaccine. If it is not available the purified chick-embryo cell (PCEC) rabies vaccine may be used.

Measles Virus Vaccine

Active immunization against measles is **recommended for all children.**

Measles vaccine is a freeze-dried preparation containing live attenuated measles virus. For vaccine production the virus is grown on a **chick embryo cell culture.** Measles vaccine is available as a monovalent (*measles only*). Bivalent (*measles rubella*) and trivalent (*measles-mumps-rubella*) preparation. The dried vaccine is reconstituted before use with diluent, and is given by the subcutaneous or IM route. It *can be given concurrently* with the DPT (Diphtheria and tetanus toxoid and pertussis vaccine) and/or OPV (Oral polio vaccine) administration. Measles vaccine is recommended for use between 9 to 15 months.

Oral Polio Vaccine

For active immunization against poliomyelitis the trivalent **oral polio vaccine** (OPV) is the vaccine of choice for infants, children and adolescents (upto 18 years). Poliovirus has three serological types–called type 1, type 2 and type 3—which possess specific antigens and do not induce reciprocal immunity. Thus, the *trivalent vaccine* is used. Each dose of trivalent vaccine contains about 1,400,000 $TCID_{50}$ (1,000,000 type 1; 100,000 type 2; 300,000 type 3). These doses are usually contained in a volume of 0.1 ml (2 or 3 drops). Ordinary OPV must be stored frozen at -20°C or less, since thawed non-stabilized vaccine maintains its potency for about 3 months at 0–4°C, and for only a few hours at room temperature.

Primary immunization (commenced at 2 or 3 months of age) with trivalent OPV consist of 3 doses, two administered 6-8 weeks apart, and the third 8-12 months after the second dose. A f*ourth reinforcing dose* is then administered before entering school (3 years). Breast feeding does not interfere with the immunizing power of OPV, but some experts recommend water instead of the breast feeds before and after the administration of the vaccine to infants. OPV does not produce any significant untoward effects.

Hypersensitivity Reactions

To safeguard against anaphylactic reactions the following steps must be observed:

1. **Intradermal test:** Diluted (1:10) test material is injected intradermally in an amount of 0.1 ml, which raises a bleb. The site is observed for 15 minutes. The appearance of **erythema** and **oedema** with **wheal** formation within 15 minutes is suggestive of specific hypersensitivity.
2. **Conjunctival test:** May be done as an alternative to the intradermal test. One drop 1:10 dilution of the test material is instilled into a normal conjunctival sac. *Itching lacrimation* and *redness* within 5 minutes is indicative of hypersensitivity. One drop of sterile physiologic sterile is instilled into the other eye to serve as control.
3. Past history of any food or drug allergy must be obtained.
4. A syringe containing 1 ml **adrenaline** (1:1000) must be readily available. Other drugs like **corticosteroids,** and an antihistamine like **diphenhydramine** for injection, and **oxygen** for inhalation must also be at hand in case an anaphylactic reaction occurs. A **tourniquet** and an **intratracheal tube** should be readily available, in case needed.

Appendix - I

WEIGHTS, MEASURES AND EQUIVALENTS

Metrology is the science of weights and measures. The term weight signifies the force with which a body is attracted towards the earth by gravity. There are *two* systems of weighing and measuring drugs; (i) the **Metric system;** and (ii) **Apothecaries' System.**

The Metric System

The **metric** or **decimal** system of weights and measures has been accepted all over the world for mainly *two* merits: (i) its tables are simple, because they are based upon the decimal system of notation; and (ii) its tables of **weights, volume** and **length** are correlated, and the *metre* is the fundamental unit of this system.

The metric system is based on the decimal system using multiples or fractions of 10. The primary units in this system are **metre** (m) for length, **litre** (l) for volume, and **gram** (g) for weight. The unit of weight, the gram is defined as the weight of 1 ml of distilled water at 4°C in vacuo, i.e., at standard temperature and pressure (STP). Under these conditions 1 g of water, and 1ml of water are equal (1g H_2O = 1 ml H_2O at STP).

Table I.1: *Metric system*

Weight		
1 kilogram (kg)	=	1000 grams
1 gram (g, gm)	=	1000 milligrams
1 milligram (mg)	=	1000 micrograms
1 microgram (μg, mcg)	=	1000 millimicrograms
	=	1000 nanograms (ng)
1 millimicrogram (mμg)	=	1000 micromicrograms (μμg)
	=	1000 picograms (pg)
Volume		
1 litre (l, L)	=	1000 millilitres (ml)
	=	1000 cubic centimetres (cc)

Table I.2: *Equivalents (approximate)*

Liquid			*Weight*		
Metric		*Apothecaries*	65 mg	=	1 grain (gr)
30 ml	=	1 fluid ounce	28.35 gm	=	1 ounce (oz)
250 ml	=	8 + fluid ounces	1 kg	=	2.2 pounds (lb)
500 ml	=	1 + pint	**Linear**		
1000 ml	=	1 + quart	1 millimetre (mm)	=	0.04 inch (in)
			1 centimetre (cm)	=	0.4 inch
			2.5 centimetres	=	1 inch
			1 metre	=	39.37 inches

Table I.3: *Household measures (approximate)*

Measure		*Metric equivalent*
1 drop	=	0.1 ml
1 teaspoonful (tsp)	=	5.0 ml
1 dessertspoonful (dsp)	=	8.0 ml
1 tablespoonful (tbsp)	=	15.0 ml
1 tea cup	=	120.0 ml
1 water glass	=	250.0 ml

Conversion Formulae

Temperature

To convert *Fahrenheit to Centigrade*, subtract 32 from °F, multiply by 5/9.
To convert *Centigrade to Fahrenheit*, multiply °C by 9/5 and add 32.

Weight

1 kg	=	2.2 lb	1 lb	=	0.45 kg
1 Gm	=	15.43 grains	1 grain	=	0.065 grams

mg% to mEq/L

In case of solids

$$\frac{\text{mg\%} \times \text{valance} \times 10}{\text{atomic wt.}} = \text{m Eq/L}$$

In case of gases

$$\frac{\text{vol\%} \times 10}{22.4} = \text{mM/L}$$

(For CO_2 use 22.26 instead of 22.4)

Appendix - II

PRESCRIPTION WRITING

A *prescription* is a written order of a registered physician to the pharmacist with directions for the preparation of the prescribed drugs, and their use by the patient. A valid prescription should invariably be written and signed by the prescriber.

Parts of Prescription

Traditionally a prescription order follows a definite pattern. It consists of the following parts:

1. **Name and address of the physician,** and his or her telephone number. This part is usually printed on a prepared pad of blanks.
2. **Patient's name and address,** his or her age and the **date.**
3. **Superscription:** This consists of the symbol Rx, the abbreviation for 'recipe' which means 'take thou'.
4. **Inscription:** This part forms the **body of the prescription** order. It contains the name and the amount of each ingredient. The *metric system* of weights and measures must be used. The inscription consist of four subdivisions: (i) **Basis:** This is the main drug which is responsible for the chief action of the prescription; (ii) **Adjuvant:** It is the helping drug which promotes the action of the main drug; (iii) **Corrective:** It modifies or eliminates the undesirable effects of the basis and adjuvant; and (iv) **Vehicle:** This is the agent used as a solvent or carrier of the drugs into the human system.
5. **Subscription:** Right under the body of the prescription are written the directions to the pharmacist regarding the compounding and dispensing of the prescription. These directions form the subscription.
6. **Signature or signatura:** This includes the directions for the patient. Some physicians prefer the term label, as these directions are written by the pharmacist on the label of the container in which the preparation is dispensed.
7. **Prescriber's signature and Registration number:** It is required by law that the physician's signature and registration number must appear on every prescription order.

Table II.1: *Some commonly used Latin abbreviations*

Abbreviation	*Latin derivation*	*English meaning*
a.c.	ante cibum	before meals
ad lib.	ad libitum	at pleasure (as desired)
b.i.d.	bis in die	twice a day
Caps.	capsula	capsule
h.s.	hora somni	at bedtime
inj.	injectio	injection
p.c.	post cibum	after meals
p.r.n.	pro re nata	as needed
pulv.	pulvis	powder
q.i.d.	quater in die	four times a day
q.s.	quantum sufficit	a sufficient amount
s.o.s.	si opus sit	if needed
sol.	solutio	solution
stat.	statim	at once
tab.	tabella	tablet
t.i.d.	ter in die	three times a day
t.d.s.	ter die sumendum	three times a day

Categories of Drugs

The Drugs and Cosmetics Act, 1940 (and later Amendments) have categorized drugs into various schedules to regulate **storage, sale, compounding** and **dispensing of drugs.** The drugs in schedule H and L should be dispensed only on the prescription of a registered medical practitioner. Drugs other than those included in Schedule H and L may be dispensed without prescription.

Modern Prescription Writing

Prescriptions today are commonly for proprietary remedies. A prescription for a **proprietary remedy** must have the **name of the manufacturer** mentioned.

Compliance

Compliance is the extent to which the patient follows the prescribed treatment. A good doctor-patient relationship greatly improves compliance. There are mainly *four* types of *noncompliance*: (i) the patient fails to *obtain* the medication; (ii) the patient fails to *take* the medication (iii) the patient prematurely *stops* medication; and (iv) the patient takes medication *inappropriately*.

Compliance is reported to be about 75% for short-term therapy, and only 50% for long-term therapy. Patient compliance can be *improved* by simplification of the drug regimen and patient education. Higher the expense on the treatment, lower is the patient compliance.

Appendix - III

Drug Management of Medical Emergencies

In dental practice the dentist must be prepared to promptly manage medical emergencies and their systemic complications, if they occur even after proper assessment and preparation of the patient. Complications are usually mild, but may be serious especially in the young and old individuals. Immediate management measures must ensure delivery of oxygenated blood to vital organs in the body. For this the dentist must be competent in providing basic cardiopulmonary resuscitation (CPR).

Haas (2006) has detailed drugs that must be readily available with the dentist to manage an emergency. They may be considered under two heads: Essential Emergency Drugs, and Supplementary Emergency Drugs.

Essential Emergency Drugs

1. **Oxygen:** It is indicated in almost all emergent situations, except *hyperventilation.* It is administered via a *full-face-mask* in a breathing patient, and via a *bag-valve-mask* in a patient with apnoea. Initially 100% inhalation is advisable. A suggested flow rate is 10 to 15 litres/minute.
2. **Adrenaline:** It is the drug of choice for emergency treatment of *asthma* not responding to salbutamol. Adrenaline is also used to manage cases of *cardiac arrest.* For *asthma* the usual dose is 0.1 mg IV or 0.3 to 0.5 mg IM, available as a 1:1000 (1 mg/ml) solution. For *cardiac arrest* the dose is 1.0 mg IV. Adequate oxygenation and defibrillation are essential measures to treat cardiac arrest or *ventricular fibrillation*.
3. **Nitroglycerin:** This drug is indicated for *acute angina pectoris,* and *acute myocardial infarction* (AMI). The usual dose is 0.3-0.4 mg tablets administered sublingually. If needed the dose may be repeated twice in 5-minute intervals. A precaution is that the systolic blood pressure should not be below 90 mmHg.
4. **Antihistamines:** Injectable antihistamines like *diphenhydramine* (25-50 mg IV or IM), or *chlorpheniramine* (10-20 mg IV or IM) are recommended. Mild allergic reactions can be managed by oral administration.
5. **Salbutamol:** It Is the most widely used *selective beta-2 agonist* used in the management of bronchospasm. When administered as an inhalation it provides selective bronchodilation with minimnal systemic effects. Adult dose is 2 sprays by inhalation, repeated as necessary.

Table 1: *Drug Dosage Schedule for Essential Emergency Drugs*

Drug	Indication	Dosage
1. Oxygen	Almost all emergencies	100% inhalation initially
2. Adrenaline	Anaphylaxis	0.1 mg IV or 0.3 to 0.5 mg IM
	Refractory asthma	0.1 mg IV or 0.3 to o.5 mg IM
	Cardiac arrest	1.0 mg IV
3. Nitroglycerin	Pain of angina	0.3 to 0.4 mg sublingually
4. Antihistamines		
Chlorpheniramine	Allergic reaction	10 to 20 mg IV or IM
Or		
Diphenhydramine	Allergic reaction	25 to 50 mg IV or IM
5. Salbutamol	Asthmatic bronchospasm	2 sprays by inhalation
6. Aspirin	Myocardial infarction	160 to 325 mg

6. **Aspirin:** It is a newly recognized life-saving drug to reduce mortality from *acute myocardial infarction* (AMI). By *antiplatelet aggregation activity* it prevents the progression of myocardial ischaemia to myocardial infarction. It is effective in low doses (160 to 300 mg), given to the patient with pain suggestive of AMI.

Suplementary Emergency Drugs

1. **Glucagon:** This drug allows parenteral management of *hypoglycaemia* in an unconscious patient. For severe hypoglycaemia ideally intravenous administration of 50% dextrose is indicated. As an alternative glucagon 1 mg IM (adults), or 0.5 mg IM (for subjects below 20 kg body weight) may be administered.

2. **Atropine:** This anticholinergic drug is used to manage *hypotension* due to bradycardia. The usual dose is 0.5 mg IV or IM initially, followed by increments, up to a maximum of 3.0 mg, if necessary

3. **Ephedrine:** This is an adrenergic *vasopressor* agent used to manage *hypotension.* It has adrenaline-like cardiovascular actions, but is less potent with a long duration of action lasting for 60 to 90 minutes. The usual dose is 5.0 mg IV or 10-25 mg IM.

Table 2: *Drug Dosage Schedule for Supplementary Emergency Drugs.*

Drug	Indication	Dosage
1. Glucagon	Hypoglycaemia in an unconscious patient	1.0 mg IM
2. Atropine	Significant bradycardia	0.5 mg IV or IM
3. Ephedrine	Significant hypotension	5.0 mg IV or 10-25 mg IM
4. Hydrocortisone	Recurrent anaphylaxis	100 mg IV or IM
	Adrenal insufficiency	100 mg IV or IM
5. Morphine	Angina unresponsive to nitroglycerin	2.0 mg IV or 5.0 mg IM
6. Nitrous oxide/ Oxygen	Unresponsive angina	35% inhalation

Cont.

Cont.

7. Naloxone	Reversal of opioid overdose	0.1 mg IV
8. Lorazepam	Status epilepticus	4.0 mg IM or IV
Or		
Midazolam	Status epilepticus	5.0 mg IM or IV
9. Flumazenil	Benzodiazepine overdose	0.1 mg IV

4. **Adrenocorticosteroid:** Hydrocortisone is used for the prevention of *recurrent anaphylaxis* in a dose of 100 mg IV or IM. It may also be used to treat *adrenal crisis.* But a drawback is its slow onset of action (about 1 hour).

5. **Morphine:** It is indicated in *severe angina pain,* unresponsive to nitroglycerin, and in cases of *myocardial infarction.* The usual dose is 2.0 mg IV or 5.0 mg IM.

6. **Naloxone:** This opioid antagonist is included in the emergency kit to reverse opioid overdose, if it occurs. The usual dose is 0.1 mg IV up to 3 doses.

7. **Nitrous oxide/Oxygen:** It is a second choice to morphine for the management of *myocardial infarction pain.* It is administered in a concentration of 35% with oxygen as an inhalation.

8. **Injectable Benzodiazepines:** Dental procedures in vulnerable Individuals may precipitate recurrent seizures (status epilepticus). *Lorazepam* is the drug of choice in a dose of 4 mg IM or IV. An alternative is *Midazolam* in a dose of 5.0 mg IM or IV.

9. **Flumazenil:** It is *benzodiazepine antagonist*, and may be needed to manage benzodiazepine overdose, in a dose of 0.1 mg IV.

In conclusion, for managing medical emergencies in dental office practice, the above mentioned drugs (*Essential* and *Supplementary*) must be available in the *Emergency Kit.* **The dentist must be competent in performing Cardiopulmonary Resuscitation (CPR) procedures till specialist help becomes available.**

References:

Haas, DA: Management of Medical Emergencies in the Dental Ofice: Conditions in Each Country, the Extent of Treatment by the Dentist. Anesth Prog. 53(1): 20-24, 2006.

Appendix - IV

Short Notes on Commonly Used Medications in Dentistry

A number of different drugs are used by the dentist to provide safe and effective dental care to the patient. *Local anaesthetics* are the most commonly used agents. In addition, *analgesics* and *anxiolytics relieve* pain and anxiety associated with acute dental problems. *Antibiotics, antifungal,* and *antiviral agents* are necessary to combat microbial infection. They are grouped as under:

1. **Local anaesthetics**
2. **Analgesics**
3. **Antibiotics**
4. **Antifungal agents**
5. **Antiviral agents**
6. **Anxiolytics**

1. LOCAL ANAESTHETICS

Lidocaine (Lignocaine): An amide local anaesthetic. Produces local anaesthesia (topical or by injection). Lidocaine (2%) with adrenaline (1:80,000) is the *'gold standard'* local anaesthetic for dental procedures. Onset of anaesthesia is less than 5 minutes. *Dose:* Maximum dose is 4.4 mg/kg, with an absolute sealing of 300 mg.

Bupivacaine: An amide local anaesthetic. It is more potent than lidocaine, and is effective in 0.5% concentration. Onset of anaesthesia is in about 10 minutes, used in combination with adrenaline (1:200,000) concentration. *Dose:* Maximum dose is 1.3 mg/kg with an absolute ceiling of 90 mg.

Mepivacaine: An amide local anaesthetic. Mepivacaine (3%) does not cause vasodilatation like lidocaine and bupivacaine. It has actions like lidocaine, but a slightly longer duration of action. Not an 'ideal' choice for longer procedures. *Dose:* Maximum dose is 4.4 mg/kg with an absolute ceiling of 300 mg.

Prilocaine: An amide local anaesthetic. Prilocaine (4%) is often combined with adrenaline to improve efficacy, and extend its duration of action. It is best utilized for shorter procedures. *Dose:* Maximum dose is 6.0 mg/kg, with an absolute ceiling of 400 mg.

2. ANALGESICS

Paracetamol (Acetaminophen): It is an analgesic-antipyretic used for the treatment of mild-to-moderate pain, and can also be administered with narcotics like hydrocodone or oxycodone. It acts by decreasing the synthesis of prostaglandins (PGs), the chemical mediators of inflammation and pain. *Dose:* 0.5-1.0 g every 4-6 hours.

Non-steroidal Anti-inflammatory Drugs (NSAIDs)

Ibuprofen: It is a peripherally-acting NSAID, and relieves pain with a significant inflammatory component, e.g., pain following surgical procedures. It inhibits the enzyme cyclooxygenase, which converts arachidonic acid to prostaglandin H2, from which other prostaglandins are formed. *Dose:* 1.0-1.2 g daily in divided doses.

Naproxen: It is also a peripherally-acting NSAID, prescribed for mild-to-moderate pain following dental procedures or pain of odontogenic origin. *Dose:* 250 mg twice daily, with meals if gastric discomfort is experienced.

Opioid Analgesics

Codeine: It is a prototype opioid analgesic, and can be used in combination with *paracetamoil, aspirin* or *ibuprofen.* Used for mild-to-moderate pain of odontogenic or post-procedural origin. *Dose:* 30-60 mg every 4-hours.

Oxycodone: It is used for the treatment of mild-to-moderate pain, and can be combined with *paracetamol, aspirin* or *ibuprofen.* It is 1.5 to 2 times as potent as morphine in oral form. *Dose:* Initially 5 mg 4-6-hourly, increased to a maximum of 400 mg according to the severity of pain.

3. ANTIBIOTICS

Antibiotics are essential drugs for effective and safe practice of dentistry. Bacteria within the periodontal pockets can cause progressive infection in the surrounding soft tissue. Moreover bacterial contamination of the dental pulp can extend into the alveolar bone.

Penicillins

Penicillin and its derivatives share the same chemical structure including the beta-lactam ring. This structure forms the core skeleton of *cephalosporins* and *monobactam* antibiotics. Penicillins remain choice agents for treating orofacial infections caused by aerobic, gram-positive streptococci, and anaerobes. Penicillins weaken the bacterial cell wall and cause ultimate rupture of bacteria through *osmotic lysis*. This is responsible for their *bactericidal activity.*

Amoxycillin: A broad spectrum beta-lactam antibiotic, used to treat infections like a dental abscess, and other periodontal pockets of infection. *Dose:* 250-500 mg orally thrice daily, or 500-1000 mg IV for serious infections.

Amoxycillin & Clavulanic acid: In resistant infections many bacteria produce *beta-lactamase,* and treatment with penicillin alone becomes ineffective. This combination can effectively control such infections. *Dose:* Amoxycillin 250 mg and clavulanic acid 125 mg (Augmentin tabs 375 mg), prescribed as one tablet thrice daily. Higher dose tablets/preparations for oral/IV administration are also available.

Cephalosporins

Cephalexin: It is a first-generation cephalosporin, used as an alternative to treat dental infections in patients allergic to penicillin. *Dose:* 250 mg four times daily.

Cefuroxime: It is a second-generation cephalosporin, and used for prophylaxis against infection in oral and maxillofacial surgery. *Dose:* 1.3 g 8-hourly IM/IV.

Macrolides

Clindyamycin: It is a derivative of lincomycin, and acts by inhibition of bacterial protein synthesis by binding to the 50S ribosomal RNA (rRNA) subunit of susceptible bacteria. It is used to treat dental infections that have progressed to the bone, and do not respond to beta-lactam antibiotics. *Dose:* 150-300 mg orally QID, or 0.6-2.7 mg/kg IV/IM daily, over 2 to 4 doses.

Azithromycin: It is derived from erythromycin, and is *bacteriostatic* in nature. It can interfere with the efficacy of oral contraceptives. It is an alternative antibiotic for orofacial infections. *Dose:* 500 mg once daily for 3-5 days.

Tetracyclines

Doxycycline: It is used to treat orofacial infections and periodontal disease. *Dose:* 200 mg on the first day, then 100 mg daily for 5 days. Staining of teeth is a notable unwanted effect. Thus, it should not be prescribed to pregnant and nursing mothers, and children under 8 years of age.

Minocycline: A tetracycline used to treat bacterial infection. It can produce *oral candidiasis* as a side effect. *Dose:* 100 mg twice daily.

4. ANTIFUNGAL AGENTS

Antifungal agents are prescribed less frequently compared to antibiotics and analgesics. They are mainly used to treat candidiasis caused by *Candida albicans.* In addition, patients taking oral antibiotics and cytotoxic drugs can develop *oral candidiasis.*

Nystatin: It is a polyene antifungal drug , commonly prescribed as an oral suspension (400,000-600,000 units) four times daily; or as dissolvable troches (200,000-400,000 units) four times a day. It is also available as an ointment for topical application.

Azole antifungals

Fluconazole: It is a triazole antifungal agent, used to treat *oropharyngeal candidiasis* not responding to nystatin *Dose:* 15-100 mg daily for 15 days.

Ketoconazole: Used for systemic and oropharyngeal candidiasis, and severe resistant *mucocutaneous candidiasis. Dose:* 200 mg once daily for 14 days.

Clotrimazole: It is available as a topical cream or troches. *Dose:* Troches (10 mg) are to be dissolved in the mouth, 4-5 troches/day, for 14 days. It is also available as a topical cream.

5. ANTIVIRAL AGENTS

Acyclovir: It is an antiviral agent used to treat *recurrent herpes labialis* infection, caused by reactivation of *herpes simplex virus-1* (HSV-1) from its dormant state. *Dose:* 200 mg QID for 5 days. Other antiviral agents include *ganciclovir, penciclovir,* and *famciclovir.*

6. ANXIOLYTIC AGENTS

Many people consciously or subconsciously fear dental procedures, and approach a dentist only in an emergency. Some patients develop *anxiety* or even *panic* disorders. In such patients *anxiolytics* are used to calm down the patients, and the choice agents are the *benzodiazepines*..

Diazepam: It has *anxiolytic* and *anticonvulsant* properties. Used for sedation and preoperative preparation of the patient. Dose: 2-10 mg three times a day for anxiolysis; and 5-10 mg as premedication prior to a dental procedure.

Triazolam: It has a rapid onset of action, and a short half-life (2-5 hours), and does not cause extended sedation. It is administered the night before the dental procedure. *Dose:* 0.25 mg orally.

Lorazepam: It is used for short-term treatment of anxiety, and as a preoperative sedative. *Dose:* 1-4 mg daily in divided doses.

Nitrous Oxide/Oxygen Inhalation

Conventional dental use of this gas/oxygen mixture (30% nitrous oxide and 70% oxygen) in dentistry is to minimize discomfort of tooth extraction.

In conclusion, judicious use of these medications can make dentistry a safe procedure assuring well-being of the patient. *For detailed pharmacology of the above described agents consult respective Chapter(s) in the main text.*

References:

1. Becker DE, Reed KL. Essentials of local anesthetic pharmacology. *Anesth. Prog.* 53(3): 98-109, 2006.
2. Haas DA. An update on local anesthetics in dentistry. *J. Can. Dent. Assoc.* 68(9): 546-551, 2002.
3. Malamed SF. The chronicles of anesthesia: part 1. *Dimensions of Dental Hygiene.* 4(1): 22-24, 2006.
4. Meechan JG, Seymour RA. *Drug dictionary for dentistry.* First Edition, Oxford University Press, Oxford, 2002.
5. Silverman M, Hexem J. Nitrous oxide/Oxygen sedation and the single-dose sedative. *Inside Dentistry.* 7(8): 42-54, 2011.

Index

D

P

Q

R